Contemporary Issues Series

Wanted: A National Health Care Program

A Critical Analysis of the Federal Government's Role in Providing Access to Health Care in the United States

Scott Deatherage

National Textbook Company
a division of *NTC Publishing Group* • Lincolnwood, Illinois USA

Published by National Textbook Company, a division of NTC Publishing Group.

Manufactured in the United States of America.

3 4 5 6 7 8 9 VP 9 8 7 6 5 4 3 2 1

Contents

Introduction

Thirty-seven million Americans have no health insurance; fifty million more are underinsured. Important medical needs are commonly excluded from coverage: AIDS, alcohol and drug dependency, mental health, prenatal care, preventive medicine, to name a few. Sizable groups have unmet needs: the elderly, urban poor, rural Americans. Despite these gaps in coverage, health care costs are rising at an astronomical rate. In 1991 we spent $540 billion on medical care, nearly twelve percent of gross national product.

This crisis in American health care has in recent years brought demands for major systemic reform from nearly every quarter. Where the notion of national health insurance once invoked the horrible specter of socialized medicine, today its advocates can be found in academe, business, government, law, and even medicine. The problem for policymakers is that no one can agree on a direction for health care reform. Should reform aim primarily at reducing health care costs, leaving millions still uninsured? Alternatively, ought reform accept underinsurance for the presently insured as the cost of providing basic services to all? These are but two of the questions that illustrate the dichotomies facing health care decision makers in the 1990s. After all, the health care crisis contributed substantially to the downfall of the Bush presidency, and newly elected President Bill Clinton has staked his political credibility on his ability to improve the system. Health care reform won't be easy; whatever plan is adopted, there will be powerful and vocal critics to remind us of what has been left out.

All of this will make for interesting debate. This volume introduces some of the central issues that high school debaters are called on to consider in the coming year. The issues covered herein are not exhaustive; literally dozens could be covered in a volume like this. The ones selected do, however, strike at the heart of the central issues in the national health insurance debate. As an introduction, they should prepare readers for the most important issues that will be debated in the coming year and provide a foundation for expanding the scope of the topic.

The introductory article by David Mechanic of the Institute for Health,

Health Care Policy and Aging Research at Rutgers is an excellent overview of the issues facing the health care industry in the '90s. Mechanic assesses American health care from the ground up, tackling issues like access for disadvantaged groups, the role of preventive care, the need for long-term care, and the relationship between medicine and public health. Mechanic discusses the common major solutions found in the literature, including the Canadian system, cost controls, competition, and cost containment measures. This essay is particularly instructive for those interested in debating about national health insurance because the critique is systemic; that is, Mechanic's argument explicates the substantial interrelationships between the various problems addressed. For instance, he argues that a substantial commitment to long-term care is essential in order to relieve pressure on crisis care, thereby enhancing care access for everyone. In short, Mechanic's overview is one of the best introductions to the topic available.

The Office of Technology Assessment's September 1992 report "Does Health Insurance Make a Difference?" is an essential work for any debater starting on the health care topic. The OTA study, the most extensive available on the relationship between insurance and health, concludes that the uninsured go without care until emergencies arise, thus increasing their morbidity and mortality. Also striking among their conclusions is the argument that publicly insured persons (those on Medicaid or Medicare) receive substantially worse care than those who have private insurance.

Fred Barnes contests strongly the findings of the OTA. His argument, published in the May 1993 issue of the *American Spectator*, is that "[t]here is no health crisis." His conclusion, critical of President Clinton's proposed health care reforms, is that America's medical care is second to none and available to all. Together, the OTA report and the Barnes article provide an interesting contrast in perspectives that describes the extremes in the health care access debate.

In the May 1993 issue of the *Journal of Health Politics, Policy and Law*, Jeffrey Buck and Mark Kamlet assess the potential for closing the coverage gap through the Medicaid system. They argue that there are severe limitations to the Medicaid system in terms of benefits, cost sharing, managed care, cost containment and provider payment that would make expansion of the system untenable. As structured, they conclude that Medicaid cannot be the vehicle by which a national system of health care is implemented.

President Clinton's proposed health care system reforms revolve around the notion of "managed competition." Essentially, the concept encourages large groups of health consumers to promote price competition among health care suppliers. The concept is the brainchild of Dr. Alain Enthoven of Stanford. Enthoven's proposals, now twenty years old, have been the subject of substantial recent controversy, and his explanation and defense of managed competition is featured in a special 1993 supplemental edition of *Health Affairs*. Enthoven argues that managed competition is compatible with Americans' desire for both individual choice and universal coverage. He warns that much of the criticism directed at the managed competition concept is in fact grounded in misunderstandings and inadequate study of the concept.

Paul Starr and Walter Zelman are key players in developing Clinton's plan for managed competition. In the same supplement of *Health Affairs*, Starr and Zelman argue that managed competition can work in unison with cost containment concepts like global budgeting to provide quality affordable care. Starr and Zelman conclude that a scheme of managed competition would successfully join competing free market and regulatory perspectives to provide the best possible health care for all Americans.

A different perspective on managed competition comes from Rick Carlson in the May/June 1993 issue of *Healthcare Forum Journal*. Carlson argues that managed competition may slightly reduce health care costs, but he claims that it will ultimate fail to change fundamentally the demand culture inside the health care industry. Carlson offers several alternatives for systemic change that he claims are necessary if the health care crisis is to be truly addressed.

Whatever the plan for addressing the tremendous insurance gaps that exist, adequate financing must be attained. Indeed, the financing structure of the American health care industry today is complex and confusing and itself contributes to the high cost of medical care. An interesting approach to cost containment and access is offered by Walter Jones and Robert Broyles of the Medical University of South Carolina and their associate Bernard Reilly of Widener University. These authors argue that the various public financing schemes employed in recent years fail because they don't address the methods used to finance the use of services. Essentially, present approaches throw good money after bad without addressing the fundamental issue of how payment is structured. The authors argue that health care professionals must lead the way through private, market-based user fees. They conclude that only a unified method of financing service use, that is, major insurance reform, will adequately contain costs and guarantee that all Americans have access to quality medical care.

An alternative perspective on the financing issue is offered by Thomas Bodenheimer and Kevin Grumbach of the University of California at San Francisco. Bodenheimer and Grumbach argue for a public approach to the financing problem. Consistent with their notion that health care is a fundamental right, these authors argue that a social insurance approach is necessary. They explain that such an approach can combine tax-based financing methods with premium payment features so as to spread the total cost of universal health insurance.

Steven Smith of Duke and Michael Lipsky of MIT attack the problems of private health care from a different angle. Their argument is that the relatively common practice of contracting government health services to private providers is inefficient, costly and fraught with politics. Their contention is that the contracting decision process must be reformed if privatization is to be the vehicle by which government health insurance is provided. In principle they offer no objection to privitization, but instead they claim that it will continue to be a failure without their proposed changes.

Some advocates have argued for health care rationing, a concept that has received substantial negative publicity because of the negative histories associated with rationing. Essentially, detractors object to the notion of limiting or allocating health care because the concept is contradictory to the American notion of choice in health care. Daniel Callahan thoroughly reviews the arguments against rationing and concludes that it is an essential first step toward national health insurance. He claims that any scheme for universal coverage will fail unless we recognize that health care is finite and that basic care is a fundamental right.

Rationing has received a cool reception inside the medical community. Still, Dr. Ron Anderson, president and CEO of the Parkland Memorial Hospital in Dallas, argues that as long as medical resources are allocated on the basis of ability to pay rather than on the basis of need, substantial gaps in care will continue to exist. He concludes that despite the distaste for rationing among his colleagues in the medical profession, the reality of unmet need makes rationing essential.

All of these proposals are informed by relatively substantial experience in other industrialized countries. Canada, Germany, Japan, Sweden and the United Kingdom, among others, have undergone major overhauls in their health care systems in recent years. These changes have been the subject of much debate in the United States. Many proposals for coverage contain elements of reform that are based on the experiences of one or more of these nations. The Canadian system has, in fact, been suggested as a baseline model for American health care reform by numerous authors. In a very interesting cross-national study, William Hsiao of Harvard compares the experiences of several nations grappling with the problems of health care coverage. His data demonstrates that in the United States we spend more money per capita and have the shortest life expectancy and highest infant mortality rate of all of the other countries included in the study. Hsiao seeks to draw from the experiences of these other Western industrialized countries to make recommendations for reform of the American health care system.

A contrasting view on the experiences of other nations comes from John Iglehart, editor of *Health Affairs*. In a 1992 article in *Health Management Quarterly*, Iglehart argues that "[t]hough we can learn valuable lessons from other nations, Americans still must make painful decisions for themselves [regarding health care]." He warns against relying too heavily on cross-cultural comparisons, arguing that the profit motive in the American health care economy affects significantly the dynamic of health care reform.

One significant issue that has slowed progress towards universal health insurance is the impact that such coverage would have on small businesses in the United States. Most of the 190 million Americans who do have health insurance coverage have it through cost sharing arrangements tied to their jobs. But millions still are employed with small-sized firms, businesses that do not offer health benefits as a matter of employment. Any plan that relies on the current system of employee-based insurance to achieve the goal of universal health coverage must account for this problem. Opponents of national health insurance have argued that a universal scheme would cripple small businesses. Those same opponents argue against government-provided care. In the March/April edition of *Society*, Robert Smith, a Senior Program Evaluator of Managed Medical Care with Aetna Health Plans, proposes a comprehensive approach that would localize health care and accumulate groups of small businesses for insurers. Smith concludes that "[n]ear-universal coverage can be created if the government structures conditions for the small business market."

One final issue addressed in this volume concerns prescription drug prices. Drug companies have been the target of substantial criticism. Critics charge that the companies put profits ahead of lives and that the profit margins of most major pharmaceutical manufacturers are excessive. In fact, President Clinton has pointed the finger at drug makers, charging that their practices are a major cause of the cost crisis in American medicine. Viveca Novak, writing in the Winter 1993 issue of *Business and Society Review*, details the criticisms launched at the pharmaceutical industry and discusses the relationship between comprehensive national health insurance and the need for controlling drug prices. One specific case that has brought substantial criticism in the direction of the drug companies is their handling of the AIDS drug AZT. The ethical and legal issues surrounding AZT are complex. Law professor Mary Griffin outlines the history of the AZT controversy, particularly in regard to industry pricing of the drug, and suggests some legal standards for conduct aimed at preventing similar instances or price gouging.

The national health insurance debate is an interesting and timely one. Virtually every commentator agrees that we should strive for universal coverage, high-quality care, and reasonable cost. Most consider it unconscionable that so many Americans have no health insurance. Regardless of perspective, every authority is concerned about maintaining the highest possible quality in health care. And all agree that universal coverage is not possible without cost containment; cost and coverage are opposite sides of the same coin. There is much disagreement, however, about how these goals ought to be achieved. Working from both market and regulatory paradigms, authorities in the field have presented thousands of potential plans to reform our health care system. The debate will be fierce when President Clinton presents his health reform package to Congress this summer. And it will continue into the '90s and beyond. Of this, at least, we can be certain: Americans will continue to demand access to individually provided high-quality care. Any program that sacrifices either is doomed to failure, universal coverage or otherwise.

America's Health Care System and Its Future: The View of a Despairing Optimist

David Mechanic

FIFTY YEARS OF LOOKING AHEAD

The history of *Medical Care Review* is intimately tied to the School of Public Health at the University of Michigan. Odin Anderson (1991) recalls his early years at Michigan working for Dr. Nathan Sinai, who developed the Bureau of Public Health Economics within the new school.

> The Bureau of Public Health Economics subscribed to many journals, which I was supposed to peruse for relevant articles and trends. As an almost incidental spinoff of this activity, I started composing a monthly abstract . . . some participants saw these abstracts and suggested that they should have general circulation. The result was a periodic abstract of articles and events, which interested parties subscribed to. It was called *Public Health Economics.* (Long after my departure from the bureau, this project became *Medical Care Review,* with the addition of original articles . . .) (p. 103)

It is fitting, thus, that a presentation given to celebrate the fiftieth anniversary of the School of Public Health at Michigan in September 1991 should be adapted to celebrate another major event, the fiftieth anniversary of the *Medical Care Review.* The institutions have grown, side by side, and each has been intimately

---

This is a revised version of a presentation prepared for the 50th Anniversary Symposium, September 21, 1991, School of Public Health, the University of Michigan, Ann Arbor.

Address correspondence and requests for reprints to David Mechanic, Ph.D., René Dubos Professor of Behavioral Sciences and Director, Institute for Health, Health Care Policy, and Aging Research, Rutgers University, New Brunswick, NJ 08903.

involved through the decades in discussions of health care reform, an old issue now rising with new vigor on the nation's agenda.

My purpose here is to examine some future possible structures for health care. To do this responsibly requires us to consider ways in which the health care system can increase its role in maintaining and enhancing health and function. We cannot simply focus on treating disease. In recognizing the health-producing potential of the health care system, we must nevertheless keep in mind that macro forces set limits on the contributions of health services. Medical care cannot compensate for economic deprivation, social disorganization, personal alienation, and low levels of education and social integration, although it can offer assistance and support for those affected by such forces. These situations of deprivation impoverish human lives, incite conflict and violence, contribute to deleterious personal and group behavior, and explain many of the observable disparities in health status. Achieving more equal health outcomes requires a more equitable society in which all groups have a stake.

The theme of this article lies in the presumption that despite American medicine's extraordinary experience with decades of change in technology, economic growth, organizational arrangements, and government involvement, its core culture has remained relatively stable and resilient. Through all of the changes, the system has maintained an individual perspective in contrast to a community view, with an emphasis on aggressive intervention, and a focus on cures and on more narrow biomedical concerns such as changes in physical parameters. Despite many intrusions from government and other third parties, medicine and (particularly) its technical subspecialties have retained their dominance. Countervailing influences have not had as substantial a modifying effect on the power base and direction of medical work as we might have expected (Mechanic 1991b).

The directional thrust of medical work is not an inevitability (Rosenberg 1987; Stevens 1989); there are alternative ways to approach a society's health care needs and problems. These are only dimly perceived, however, largely because of medicine's intellectual and ideological dominance over public conceptions of health and disease. Medicine has a remarkable capacity to absorb competing perspectives and approaches—in a manner that assures them a low priority. Despite much rhetoric about prevention and caring, and the broad public acceptance of the two concepts, the medical care system is focused on increasingly sophisticated diagnostic and curative interventions, and not on broader social objectives.

Following Deep Throat's advice to "track the money," we can see that the technologic imperative is as strong as ever. One need look no further than the example of childbirth, an area where dissatisfaction and pressures from women have substantially altered the ambience of obstetrical practice. But a deeper look reveals more aggressive interventions, more cesarean deliveries, standard use of electronic fetal monitoring, and continuing medicalization of a natural process.

The presence of maternity care centers and nurse-midwives may support the illusion that care has fundamentally changed, but these alternatives are simply a diversion from the main road that obstetrical practice follows.

In this article I argue for an alternative view of medicine, one organized around a framework of equitable access related to need, greater sensitivity to the plight of the disadvantaged, strong attention to a process of care that seeks to promote and support function among the chronically ill and disabled, and greater focus on prevention and community health. This does not imply denigration of the extraordinary developments made possible by advances in science and technology. It does require, however, that these developments be applied within a broader framework of values and priorities. None of these caring goals is foreign to medicine, and each is pursued now somewhere in our large and heterogeneous system of care. The challenge is to elevate the priority of elements that are now tangential to the main course of health care activity.

As we look to the future, it is also clear that much that concerns medicine will inevitably change—patterns of disease, the scope of our knowledge, the range of technologies, directions of economic organization, expectations of patients, and much more. Unexpected problems and new disease will emerge, for as René Dubos (1959) reminded us, "fitness requires never-ending efforts of adaptation to the total environment, which is ever changing." The emergence of other new diseases such as AIDS, with their devastating consequences for individuals and societies, will pose unexpected challenges. The future is unpredictable, and I am deeply skeptical of efforts to foresee it. The future of population health depends not only on changes in the natural environment and on emerging strains of viruses and bacteria, but also on the emergence of new social and environmental problems and their related morbidities. It also depends on the evolution of our economy and politics, and on our ways of managing new developments in science and technology.

Thus, the plan of this article is to examine how health care can be organized to promote the nation's health effectively. Effectiveness depends both on the content of the work of health professionals and on the financial and organizational frameworks within which their work is embedded. Although I present a view of what health care needs, I see myself as a "despairing optimist," a designation René Dubos adopted some years ago. On the other hand, only a fool fails to recognize those interests with a stake in current perspectives and priorities, and their determination to resist fundamental change, as a cause for despair. On the other hand, our rich professional and material resources, and the large numbers of dedicated, creative, and energetic health professionals committed to change, offers hope for a more constructive future.

The article begins with a discussion of the culture of American medical care and the extent of its goals for a system of care with greater capacity to promote health, including increased attention to disadvantaged populations. I then turn to a discussion of the evolution of our health care system and of our present inefficiencies and disarray. The core of this essay addresses the current debate about the organizational and financial framework of the nation's health care, the structural directions I believe most desirable, and those more likely to occur.

THE CULTURE OF AMERICAN MEDICAL CARE: TECHNOLOGY AND INTERVENTIONISM

Americans have great admiration for the possibilities of technology, and have continued to support research investments aimed at increasing technological capacities in health care. The extraordinary advances in transplantation, dialysis, noninvasive imaging technologies, state-of-the-art cardiovascular interventions such as angioplasty, and many other technologies capture the imagination of the public and suggest magnificent future potential.

Some years ago, Victor Fuchs (1968) described the bias among physicians toward the technological imperative—the tendency to try everything possible, on behalf of the patient, that offered any potential however small. In subsequent years there has been much discussion on managing care and on related concepts such as cost effectiveness, balancing, and rationing. Capitated systems such as HMOs have had clear incentives to moderate the use of expensive modalities, in contrast to fee-for-service medicine where providers are more encouraged to be technically aggressive in marginal situations (Luft 1987). The introduction of new technologies continues unabated, however, encouraged by aggressive marketing by industries that manufacture and sell medical and hospital equipment and drugs (Waitzkin 1983), by economic incentives, and by public and professional support.

The aggressiveness of American medicine in the uses of technology transcends skillful marketing or even the economic incentives that make its adoption highly profitable. American culture is individualistic and oriented to intervention, and we act as if technology offers a potential solution to almost any of our problems (Payer 1988). New technology diffuses rapidly, often well before any systematic evidence of its value is available, and almost always before its cost effectiveness is assessed. The rapid diffusion and wide acceptance, for example, of specialized intensive care units and fetal electronic monitoring remains impervious to evidence from controlled clinical trials in which their superiority, and even their equivalency, to more traditional and mundane forms of medical management, comes into question (Mechanic 1989b).

Culture is difficult to change, of course, particularly when it is reinforced by occasional spectacular successes, aggressive marketing, and profitable opportunities. After World War II and in recent decades, American hospitals grew enormously, capitalizing on the opportunities offered by federal funding, first through the Hill-Burton program and then through favorable incentives for writing off depreciation under the Medicare program. In the latter case, instead of paying for depreciation in terms of original cost, depreciation was defined in terms of current replacement costs, giving hospitals considerable incentive for further expansion. In addition, 2 percent of reimbursable costs was added under Medicare for what was viewed as necessary capital enhancement, and for-profit hospitals were additionally guaranteed a substantial return on equity capital as an allowable cost (Stevens 1989, 296–97). These opportunities stimulated enormous capital expansion by allowing hospitals to pass the costs on to government and other third party payers.

Stimulated by a competitive, entrepreneurial ethos, the hospital sector grew in a way that offered state-of-the-art technology almost everywhere, often duplicating expensive technologies and introducing specialized units that were frequently underutilized. Many of these little used facilities could not provide care of quality comparable to that of the facilities carrying out a higher volume of specialized procedures. Further, the incentive structure that affected adoption and use of new technology was encouraging utilization where little benefit was expected. This was true both for the often administered basic diagnostic tests and for the "big ticket" items such as imaging studies and expensive surgical interventions.

Much of the success of American medicine has derived from its openness to new cutting-edge technologies, and its aggressive pursuit of innovative medical, surgical, and drug treatments through increasingly complex—and expensive—research and development. The causes of most major diseases remain unknown, and many of our interventions are what Lewis Thomas has called "half-way" technologies (Thomas 1977). Many have faith that our increased basic scientific knowledge will lead to technological approaches that are more specific and targeted, and as a result, most cost-effective—that fully curative technologies will one day substitute for less efficient half-way approaches. Moreover, with increased technological capacities, it seems reasonable to anticipate that many commonly used technologies will become less expensive over time.

Warner (1987) has suggested that an appropriate set of economic incentives can lead to the substantial development of cost-saving approaches and to increased motivation among health professionals to seek less costly alternatives. There is not much indication of a strong tendency in this direction, although the Health Care Financing Administration (HCFA) is intent on considering the cost effectiveness of new technologies in its reimbursement decisions. In theory, technical advances such as the continued development of computers, which have made access to sophisticated information bases relatively inexpensive, should bring about efficiency and cost savings. But translating an increased capacity for efficiency into cost savings is a managerial and organizational process, and the introduction of computerization in business has not resulted in the anticipated reductions in secretarial and clerical personnel. Achieving efficiency requires a change in those attitudes that form a major barrier to changing behavior. Economic incentives can help change the behavior of physicians (Eisenberg 1991), but not as much or as quickly as many people assume.

Looking to the future, I doubt that new technologies will solve our most pressing dilemmas. I have no doubt that there will be new cures and major advances in noninvasive diagnostics, in the development of synthetic body parts, in miniaturization, in computerization, and in the collection and processing of medical information. I anticipate new vaccines, drugs, prostheses, and materials. Computerization at the bedside will make note-writing and medical records obsolete, and information retrieval will be rapid and efficient. I am confident that these changes will contribute to improved care if they are used wisely, but I anticipate that aggregate costs will increase as well. I am sure that we will have fundamental breakthroughs in some areas, and that some new technologies will save costs. Overall, however, I anticipate many more expensive halfway measures that add small increments to health at large cost. Many chronic conditions such as cardiovascular disease develop over a lifetime, and it is naive to expect some future "quick fix."

The danger is that the excitement engendered by new technologies will divert us from the more simple organizational measures that promote prevention; reach out to underserved people; and provide ready access to basic health monitoring, health education, primary medical care, and appropriate referral. We have much new to learn but we also have to learn to implement better what we already know.

GOALS FOR A HEALTH CARE SYSTEM

Much of the progress in medicine during this century came from pursuing a relatively narrow paradigm—the concept of specific etiology—which was a powerful model for identifying causes of controllable infectious disease (Mechanic 1978c). As the disease picture changes, and as the population ages, the major causes of disease and disability are long-term chronic conditions resulting from many causes and not susceptible, this time, to a "magic bullet." We need a health care system that is responsive to the need for prevention and continuing care for the chronically ill—one that maintains and enhances the ability to function.

The Changing Societal Structures

Medical care plays a broad role in modern societies, in part a result of the erosion of the influence of religion, the family, and other major institutions. At present rates, two-fifths of U.S. children will experience family breakups before age 18 (Cherlin, Furstenberg, Chase-Lansdale, et al. 1991), and more adults than ever before live in single-person households with few social supports. Religion is a less powerful influence on people's lives, and problems that in the past were appropriate for the family or the church to deal with have been redirected to human services interventions, including medical care. The boundaries of medicine have expanded enormously in recent decades, dealing increasingly with wide ranging social and psychosocial problems traditionally handled in other ways. Physicians deal with many patients whose visits are motivated by feelings of depression, anxiety, worry, and social isolation. Depression and other adverse psychological states increase perceived ill health, actual disability, and utilization of health care services. Recent findings from the Medical Outcomes Study, a large multisite investigation of more than 11,000 outpatients, indicate that depression is more disabling than many of the most serious chronic medical conditions that physicians typically deal with (Wells, Stewart, Hays, et al. 1989); it thus requires attention in the primary health care sector. In addition, growing evidence of the extent to which personal behavior and lifestyle relate to risks of morbidity and death (Assistant Secretary for Health 1979, 1990) suggests that physicians must take broader responsibility for patients' education and efforts to modify behavior.

The Role of Prevention

Despite much lip service to prevention, we have done relatively little either to educate physicians in the appropriate use of behavior modification for the reduction of noxious behaviors, or to enable them in their practices to devote the time necessary for serious health maintenance. Much of prevention, of course, requires a broad educational effort at the community level and the encouragement of everyday family, work, and recreational activities in a manner actively disposed toward positive health outcomes. Successful prevention is a product of culture and the social arrangements of everyday activities (Mechanic 1990). But the influence of physicians should not be overlooked. They commonly encounter patients when the latter are feeling anxious and uncertain-when they are particularly amenable to influence (Frank and Frank 1991). The physician still remains a respected and credible authority figure who can have an important influence on specific behaviors such as smoking, eating habits and diet, and substance abuse. The quality of doctor-patient interaction is also important in general in achieving satisfactory understanding and adherence to medical advice. Studies suggest that successful behavior modification requires appropriate knowledge, coping skills to overcome barriers to achieving the desired behavior, and reinforcement of the emergent behavior changes (Mechanic 1991c; Mechanic and Aiken 1991; Leventhal, Prohaska, and Hirschman 1985). A variety of techniques are available to assist physicians in fostering successful adherence to prescribed medical regimens (Svarstad 1986).

Sufficient time to communicate clearly, to elicit questions, and to provide appropriate feedback is a key element in many of the educational and preventive approaches. But in medicine, time is money—and educational efforts are not remunerative. Although ultimate conversion to a resource-based relative value system may eventually give higher value to cognitive and educational services, the prospects are not promising for making such services competitive with technical interventions. Nor is capitated care a particularly likely solution, since physicians in HMOs work under strict time constraints, and with ever-increasing cost-containment efforts these pressures, too, are likely to increase. Preventive educational efforts even within these time constraints may be cost-effective, but physicians facing workload pressures may not see the issue in this light.

Preventive education is one area where a clinical perspective, in contrast to an epidemiological viewpoint, is deceptively discouraging. A very brief counseling session with a physician can decrease the rate of patient smoking. Of a sample of patients given counseling for one or two minutes during a routine consultation, reinforced by a four-page pamphlet on how to give up smoking, 5 percent stopped smoking within one month following the intervention and were abstinent over a one-year period (Russell et al. 1979). This rate of success can probably be increased further by linking patients to smoking clinics and prescribing nicotine chewing gum (Russell, Stapleton, Jackson, et al. 1987). Even modest change is important because of the noxious effects of long-term cigarette use. Assuming that a physician counseled 100 patients, three would terminate smoking as a matter of course, and five might quit as a result of physician intervention. Although a 5 percent termination rate relative to the modest aggregate time expended is perhaps one of the most cost effective things a physician can do, physician perception is unduly influenced by the vast majority of patients who do not change their behavior. On the basis of these experienced failures physicians commonly develop a negative attitude toward health counseling. This, of course, is an excellent reason to ensure that young physicians become familiar with the principles of clinical epidemiology.

In future years preventive and educational efforts will require both the increased use of nonphysicians and more creative use of communication technology. Nurse-practitioners do well in primary care partly because they take more time with patients, providing a climate in which patients can ask questions and receive appropriate answers comfortably. These are important conditions for the successful use of behavioral interventions, and physician extenders can compensate for more physicians who fail to take the necessary time. Moreover, there is substantial room for creativity in using video and other communication technologies to prepare patients for medical procedures and to inform them about health issues, their particular illness problems, and ways of living with and managing chronic symptoms. Follow-up to elicit feedback and answer questions is essential for individualized treatment, but good software can reduce the educational demands considerably. Much of the unproductive time patients spend waiting in hospitals and clinics could be used constructively for both specific instruction and general health education.

The Need for Long-Term Care

Chronic disease is concentrated in later life, and much of medical care focuses on treatment of the elderly, where the challenge is typically less that of effecting a cure (or cures) and more one of enhancing function. Since the end of the Second World War American medical care has turned its major attention to chronic disease (Fox 1986), but care continues to focus more on acute episodes and exacerbations of disease then on the longitudinal issues necessary to maximize function. Between 1960 and 1980, the number of persons in the age group over 85 increased 174 percent, and a 110 percent increase is expected between 1980 and the end of the century (Rice and Feldman 1983). By the year 2000, more than one-quarter of the expected elderly population of 36 million will be older than age 80. As we look further into the future when the baby boom birth cohorts begin to approach old age (beginning in about 20 years), the elderly population is expected to constitute 17 percent of the population (Office of Technology Assessment 1985). As the numbers of old elderly patients increase, strategies that allow individuals to retain their independence become even more important.

The changing demographics of the population highlight a significant need for a national long-term care policy. In the absence of such a policy Medicaid has been the de facto federal long-term care program with 14 percent of elderly Medicaid beneficiaries accounting for 36 percent of Medicaid payments, two-thirds of which go for nursing home care (Ball and Bethell 1989). Many elderly persons who enter nursing homes rapidly deplete their resources and become eligible for Medicaid, drawing resources away from other important Medicaid populations. The share of nursing home care financed by the federal government actually decreased from 53.4 percent in 1981 to 48.6 percent in 1988 (Office of National Cost Estimates 1990). Most nursing home care continues to be financed privately, typically from personal and family resources rather than insurance. The magnitude of expenditures for services provided by nonfacility-based home care agencies has increased rapidly from $1.3 billion in 1980 to $4.4 billion in 1988 (Office of National Cost Estimates 1990). These estimates, however, do not include expanded services such as adult day care, respite care, and supportive social services. Rivlin and Wiener (1988) have estimated annual spending, under an expanded definition of home care services, as $8.7 billion. Needs for such services, and related financing, are likely to grow dramatically in coming decades.

Some development of private long-term care insurance has occurred in recent years, but such insurance is costly, with significant eligibility restrictions; it also has limited coverage, provides inadequate and limited duration of benefits, and involves uncertainties concerning renewability (Ball and Bethell 1989). Although long-term care insurance may contribute toward part of an ultimate solution, it is not a viable strategy by itself (Rivlin and Wiener 1988; Ball and Bethell 1989). On the other hand, budgetary constraints and the uncertainties of predicting cost have made government reluctant to assume responsibility. The Pepper Commission (1990) recommended a long-term care program that would include a requirement for insurance for home- and community-based care and for the first three months of nursing home care, and a floor to protect persons with long nursing home stays against impoverishment. Under this proposal the federal government would subsidize persons with low incomes. The commission estimated that the program would cover 4.4 million people at an increased federal cost of $42.8 billion. Others have suggested developing a long-term care program under Medicare, for example, a "part C" (Somers 1987) or expansion of Medicaid eligibility (Pauly 1988).

Little consensus has been reached on the philosophy of a long-term care policy or on the emphasis to be given to providing front-end care versus protecting private assets through catastrophic insurance. A reasonable federal role is to ensure that persons receive needed care, while the protection of personal assets may more properly be a role for the private sector. Most agree, however, that a financially viable long-term care program would require considerable sharing of government and private responsibility, cost sharing related to capacity to pay, and stringent gatekeeping to ensure the financial viability of the program. Effective gatekeeping is particularly important as the service mix comes to include more home and community care, because it is in these areas that substitution of formal services for informal care is most likely to occur. Effective long-term care policy will require the capacity to target for services those groups that would be at high risk of institutionalization without intervention (Weissert 1991). It is well known that the extension of new community services attracts new clients who are not at highest risk for institutional care, but such services mostly supplement informal services rather than substituting for them (Kemper, Applebaum, and Harrigan 1987). Ball and Bethell (1989) have suggested a framework of goals for long-term care: a universal plan to which most contribute, integrated into the Social Security System; coverage of anyone who becomes chronically ill or disabled; coverage of both home and nursing home care; service to both patients and informal caregivers; emphasis on support for independent functioning; direct payment for necessary services; encouragement of alternative long-term care services; cost sharing; and stringent cost and quality controls. It appears evident that development of a long-term care policy will continue its long gestation.

Significant future efforts in medicine will focus on disabilities and their secondary complications. This is due both to the aging of the population and to the increasing demands of persons with disabilities that their concerns be made more central to medical care processes. Because of the multiple definitions of disabilities, it is difficult to reach a firm estimate of their prevalence. The National Health Interview Survey, based on a sampling of the noninstitutionalized population, reported that in 1988 more than 33 million people (13.7 percent of that population) had an activity limitation resulting from a chronic condition(s) (Institute of Medicine 1991). Almost ten million of these people could not carry out the major activity for someone their age, and more than another 13 million were limited in the amount or kind of major activities they could carry out. Such limitations were found to increase with age, affecting almost two-fifths of the population 70 years or older.

Integration of Medicine and Public Health

Many of the determinants of disability and death are products of social conditions and personal risk factors that are largely preventable through social policy interventions and changes in behavior. Accidents, suicide, and homicide account for increasing proportions of deaths, particularly among young people, and much premature morbidity and mortality is linked to the abuse of alcohol and drugs, smoking, poor nutrition, and the high-risk behavior associated with HIV infection. It is difficult to anticipate how our society will deal in the future with such conflict-laden issues as jobs, income distribution, toxic waste and the environment, abortion, tobacco, gun control, and numerous other factors related to health outcomes. It is more predictable that major efforts will be introduced to modify personal risk factors. Creating a tobacco-free society would by itself have enormous implications for the magnitude of disease, disability, and death, and for the demand for specific types of specialized medical care (Warner 1987). Whatever the political likelihood of banning tobacco (or the lack thereof), progress will continue in changing the culture surrounding smoking and in lowering the prevalence of smoking in the population as well as in modifying the conditions that foster other health-damaging behaviors.

These changes and their influences on patterns of disease occurrence will modify the clinical picture that the average physician sees. At one end of the age spectrum, the challenge will be the "new morbidities" associated with personal and social disruptions and alienation, and with family dissolution. Much illness, however, will be delayed to later life where the crucial challenge will lie in maintaining function in numerous ways, for example, by aiding in control of urinary incontinence, teaching techniques for coping with decrements in memory and orientation, and helping provide social attachments for persons whose personal networks have been depleted. Traditional medical approaches are ill-suited to these and other impending health challenges; such tasks will require major modifications in professional education and in the design of medical practice (Robert Wood Johnson Foundation 1992).

The concerns of public health and medicine need to be integrated more fully in the years ahead. If medicine is to be an effective instrument for maintaining and enhancing health, substantial attention to populations and to the potentials for prevention is required. Relatively few resources in either research or practice go to broad community preventive programs or even to individual preventive interventions, in contrast to the very intensive delivery of remedial medical care. Medicine in essence is an individual treatment endeavor and will remain so. But it is foolish and futile to spend increasingly vast resources to save damaged lives, while paying little attention to the conditions that erode reasonable chances for healthful life and function.

The pessimism many physicians feel about prevention undermines efforts in areas where valuable strategies and technologies are available, as in the smoking counseling example. Further, data from the U.S. immunization survey indicate that approximately two-fifths of American children 1–4 years of age are not immunized against measles, rubella, polio, or mumps.[1] DPT (diphtheria, pertussis, tetanus) nonimmunization reported rates, somewhat lower at 35 percent, are still unacceptable. Among nonwhites, a group of greater risk because of poverty and less adequate nutrition, less than half report being immunized for any of

1. These data, reported in the Household Interview Survey, probably underestimate actual vaccination. Data from 1985, with a subsample that consulted vaccination records, show higher rates, more in the vicinity of 75 percent for most vaccinations, and 87 percent for DPT. Among nonwhites, rates vary from three-fifths to two-thirds, with the exception of DPT where 75 percent report vaccinations (National Center for Health Statistics 1991, Table 42).

these childhood diseases (National Center for Health Statistics 1991). The recent outbreak of measles in a number of major cities, and the continuing occurrence of preventable deaths, attests to our neglect. The incongruity between current efforts to save low-birthweight children and the limited efforts to deliver inexpensive and routine preventive measures to high-risk mothers and children raises grave questions about our priorities and wisdom. Average costs for neonatal intensive care for low-birthweight infants ranged from $11,670 to $39,420 in 1984, and average costs for infants under 1500 grams varied from $26,737 to $60,015 (Office of Technology Assessment 1987). Such low-birthweight infants predominante in high-risk disadvantaged groups. Concentrated efforts to identify high-risk mothers and to provide appropriate prenatal and child care is probably far more effective in the long run than is high-technology care concentrated on one early stage of infant development.

Prevention, of course, is not a simple matter, nor is it always cost effective. In many instances we lack the knowledge and technology to modify disease risk or change behavior with any success. In other areas, the risks are so low, and the target populations so large, that even preventive efforts that are inexpensive per individual administration become extraordinarily costly in the aggregate relative to the gains achieved. They do not give value for the money (Russell 1986). Yet the future of medicine and the value of the enormous resources we expend depend on the success of the strategies we develop to prevent disease, limit disability, enhance function, and support and maintain the chronically ill and disabled, in our efforts to contribute to a better quality of life.

THE CHALLENGE OF DISADVANTAGE

Sophisticated observers from other nations admire the scientific and technological accomplishments of American medicine but are incredulous at our vast outlay of resources while large segments of our population are uninsured and underinsured, and persistent barriers are raised against offering every person access to basic health care. It seems peculiar, indeed, that a nation that spends so much on health care tolerates the massive inequities in care characteristic of the American situation.

In an appalling illustration of the consequences of inequality, McCord and Freeman (1990) examined mortality rates in the central Harlem health district in New York City for the period 1979–1981. This community is 96 percent African American, and two-fifths of the population live below the poverty line. Mortality in central Harlem was more than double that of the American population during the period studied, and survival to age 65 for the African American men was lower than in Bangladesh, a country notorious for its poverty and lack of development. Excess deaths in Harlem relative to the rest of the American population were explained primarily by cardiovascular disease, cirrhosis, homicide, and neoplasms. Deaths due to drug dependency, homicide, alcohol use, and cirrhosis were from 10 to 283 times more likely to occur in Harlem than in the national population. Although the Harlem health district had the highest mortality in New York City, 54 of the 353 health districts in the city had at least double the expected deaths using the American population as a standard. All but one of these health districts were impoverished areas made up largely of African Americans and Hispanic Americans. These findings reaffirm the observations of the task force of the secretary of the Department of Health and Human Services (*Report of the Secretary's Task Force* 1985), which estimated 42.5 percent excess deaths among the African American population in the United States in the period 1979–1981. There is little evidence of improvement since then. While limited access to medical care plays some role in explaining health disadvantage, it is clear that much of the observed morbidity, disability, and mortality is due in large part to the social and economic circumstances of African Americans, other minorities, and the disadvantaged in general (Bunker, Gomby, and Kehrer 1989).

Persons of lower socioeconomic status are, as we know, at higher risk of morbidity, disability, and mortality than more affluent persons (Bunker, Gomby, and Kehrer 1989; Dutton 1986). Not only are the former exposed to more risk factors and more vulnerable when exposed, with fewer resources to counter harmful situations; their level of access to medical care relative to need also falls below that of the more advantaged. Further, they continue to face many barriers to receiving services routinely available to more affluent patients, such as prenatal and child care and preventive services. The poor, and especially poor African American and Hispanic populations in large cities, receive a disproportionate amount of their care from emergency rooms and hospital outpatient clinics, a pattern that interferes with continuity, preventive appraisals and interventions, and health maintenance. Such episodic care typically involves long waiting times, little follow-up, and poor coordination of care. Even though much of the care of disadvantaged patients is hospital based, they are less likely than affluent patients to be referred to specialized care and "cutting edge" treatments for serious physical or mental conditions (Mechanic and Aiken 1989). The dynamics of differential referral processes are not fully clear, but certainly a major influence on differences in treatment is the lack of any insurance or the difficulties inherent in public insurance, such as Medicaid, that pays physicians much less than other insurance programs (Hadley, Steinberg, and Feder 1991).

It has been apparent for decades that the emergency and episodic treatment that characterizes so much of the care of disadvantaged groups is exceptionally wasteful, because continuity in care is so important in dealing with their complex socio-medical problems. Conversely, impressive evidence from studies of community health centers supports the importance of well-organized basic services in contributing to the health of these populations, reducing morbidity, and increasing patient satisfaction (Dutton 1986; Freeman, Kiecolt, and Allen 1982). But we continue to lose ground in organizing primary care services for the disadvantaged. In the 1990s we will have to resurrect the commitment of the 1960s that led to the development of the Office of Economic Opportunity health centers.

A major advantage of the community health approach is its conception of medical problems in their larger social context, thus maintaining a more responsive approach to living conditions that affect the course of a patient's illness, the chances of secondary complications, and the ability of the patient to adhere to medical advice. Such health programs are more likely not only to engage in outreach efforts that identify needs and assist patients in gaining eligibility for other types of required assistance, but to engage also in community development efforts. In poverty areas, the separation for patients between medical care and other types of needed basic assistance—education, sanitation, food supplies—presents major barriers to achieving effective care outcomes. Thus, although the community approach to care is an old model, its relevance for disadvantaged populations is as great as ever (Kark and Steuart 1962; Geiger 1984).

During the 1960s the nation was focusing on issues of access to health care and other welfare entitlements and on meeting the needs of disadvantaged populations. As the emphasis turned to cost containment in the 1970s, attention to these priorities declined, and welfare efforts eroded or failed to keep pace with the growth of the poverty population. The erosion of insurance has placed particular stress on public hospitals and on that segment of nonprofit general hospitals that provides substantial care for indigent persons. Access has again become a salient issue on the national and state agendas of the 1990s, but in a more complex context of budget deficits and cost-containment pressures. In the interim, we have lost sight of the unique potential of community health care centers to wage a multifaceted attack on the devastating conditions that continue to exist in our urban ghettos and some of our rural areas.

THE EVOLUTION OF CURRENT DILEMMAS

American health care as we know it is largely a post-World War II phenomenon. In 1940, the United States spent $4 billion on health, 4 percent of the gross national product. By 1950, as a result of the enormous postwar growth and inflation, expenditures tripled but expenditures as a proportion of GNP rose only modestly to 4.5 percent. In the post-1955 years, with the growth of health insurance, total health expenditures accelerated more rapidly than GNP, beginning an upward trajectory that continues (National Center for Health Statistics 1991, 184). The introduction of Medicare and Medicaid in 1966, greatly expanding the numbers of people covered by insurance under an openended reimbursement system, accelerated the rate of health expenditures so that by 1990, the latest year for which definitive figures are available, expenditures had risen to $666 billion, 12.2 percent of GNP, and $2,566 per capita (Levit, Lazenby, Cowan, and Letsch 1991). Current estimates for 1992 are in excess of $800 billion and are approaching 14 percent of our gross national product.

At various points in American history, strong efforts have been made to develop a national system of health coverage. President Truman asked Congress to pass a national health program, based on models that had been germinating throughout the 1930s. Opponents of a national system supported and encouraged private hospital insurance as an alternative, a pattern that had been developing since the Great Depression. The rapid growth of Blue Cross and Blue Shield in the 1950s and 1960s helped to deflate momentum for a federally sponsored system. The decision by the War Labor Board in 1942 to allow fringe benefits of up to 5 percent of wages, under a wage-controlled situation, encouraged health insurance coverage (Stevens 1989, 259). Nonprofit and commercial health insurance could expand rapidly in the post-World War II years because health coverage became an important part of fringe benefit programs associated with employment, and, because of tax advantages, workers could get through health benefits more than what they could get in increased wages. Individuals outside the employment system were least protected, and the elderly were the most visible and politically important subgroup lacking protection. In the political debates of the early 1960s over health coverage for the elderly, sagacious political maneuvering by Wilbur Mills, with the assistance of Wilbur Cohen, resulted in the enactment of Medicare and Medicaid in 1965 (Marmor 1973).

The notion of national health insurance continued to percolate on the federal agenda throughout the optimistic years of the 1960s and into the 1970s. The issue during these years was less whether a national program was needed or not than its structure and operation. As is often common in the American context, the debate was over whether a new program should build on the existing, *private* health insurance model or adopt a radical new *public* approach involving the organization of a national health service with major planning and regulatory involvement. During these years unionized labor backed Senator Edward Kennedy's Health Security proposal based on a planning model, while the health care industry and physicians supported an expansion of the existing system with federal assistance. By the early 1970s, the Nixon administration was stating a preference for a health insurance plan in contrast to the simple expansion of categorical entitlements, and President Nixon endorsed national health insurance (Starr 1982). Senator Kennedy, seeing little support for his planning concept, joined Wilbur Mills in a proposal that shared many features with the administration's thinking, one that would use private insurers to administer the system. National health insurance seemed imminent. Ironically, organized labor, holding out for the original Kennedy concept, undercut the political momentum and its opposition resulted in a stalemate (Rivlin 1974). Changes in the economic fortunes of the nation, the persistently escalating costs of health care, growing concern about the federal deficit and American competitiveness, and antipathy to new taxes then pushed health insurance off the national agenda.

After a hiatus of more than 15 years, universal health insurance is again an item on the social and political agenda. Although recession, the federal deficit, and concern about American competitiveness in world markets still encourage caution in addressing the issue, the continuing inability to control medical care costs and the large size of the uninsured and underinsured populations together are drawing policy attention to the poor state of present arrangements and the need for reform. One major innovation is the growing tendency of various states to take the policy initiative—to develop approaches for extending insurance, regulating providers, and reallocating health expenditures (Aaron 1991).

The most immediate crisis in health care is the extraordinary segmentation of the health insurance marketplace, which has pushed large numbers of people outside the protective net of insurance. This reflects (1) the historical ties of health care protection to employment; (2) the changing character of the labor market that has developed with the loss of numerous industrial jobs and the addition of poorly paid service jobs offering less in fringe benefits; and (3) the continuing momentum of growth in medical technology and health care costs that adds to increases in the financial burden for employers. Hospitals have served the uninsured by shifting costs to other payers, but government and other payers are increasingly restricting or protesting these transfers. Cost shifting continues to drive premiums up, pushing many small employers and individual enrollees out of the health insurance market. These trends create considerable instability in insurance coverage, affecting many more people than is generally recognized. Twenty-eight percent of the population (more than 60 million people) did not have health insurance coverage during at least one month between February 1985 and August 1987 (Aaron 1991). This combination of influences has resulted in an extraordinarily bizarre health care system that spends more and more money but disenfranchises a significant minority of the population.

In its early years Blue Cross followed a philosophy of encouraging maximum community enrollment through setting rates that pooled risk across large segments of the public (Somers and Somers 1961). This concept of "community rating" encouraged insurance coverage for comparatively unhealthy persons who otherwise might have become indigent patients upon failing ill. It was attractive to the hospital sector and worked exceedingly well when Blue Cross was the dominant insurer. In 1945 Blue Cross controlled 61 percent of the hospital insurance market, but by 1951 private commercial policies covered a majority of enrollees (Law 1974). By the late 1950s, it was clear that Blue Cross was losing the community rating battle, as commercial insurance attracted lower-risk persons at reduced premiums, requiring Blue Cross to increase its premiums to cover its more medically needy enrollees. By the 1970s, some Blue Cross plans were still trying to maintain the community rating ideal, fighting against the tide and not succeeding very well. Data reported by the Health Insurance Association of America (1990, Table 2.2) indicates that Blue Cross and Blue Shield's share of the population of privately insured persons had decreased from 47 percent in 1970 to 41 percent in 1988. In the 1980s, the Employee Retirement Income Security Act (ERISA), by exempting self-insured firms from state mandates for specified health benefits, encouraged self-insurance and further segmentation of risk (Fox and Schaffer 1989).

It is difficult to fault Blue Cross or employers for capitulating to the competitive ethos that destroyed health insurance as a community contract. In the early years, the social ideal served to expand the health insurance market and to support the growth of hospitals. It also weakened the case for national health insurance, and thus received support from conservative interests (Stevens 1989, 192). But it would be unrealistic to expect individual employers in a competitive economy to refrain from seeking to reduce their subsidies to the general population. Moreover, by the late 1970s, the private insurance market had about reached its peak without additional forceful government intervention. Hospitals and various physician groups began to appreciate the notion, following their experiences with Medicare, that national health insurance would probably be in their interest by providing payments for patients who were now the recipients of charity or subsidized care.

Although it is easy to understand the development of the historical connection between employment and health insurance in the United States, that connection increasingly has become a source of gaps in coverage. The largest gaps are found among low-paid workers in the small businesses that fail to provide insurance, or in those businesses that exclude coverage for dependents or offer insurance at rates that many employees find prohibitive (Pepper Commission 1990). Insurance benefits are often nonportable, increasing the discontinuity in coverage that occurs when workers move from one job to another or when they become unemployed. Students beyond their teens, often too old to be covered on parental policies but not yet in stable employment situations, are also at high risk of uninsurance. Moreover, employer-based insurance creates a highly complex system, with widely varying coverage among employees and significant administrative costs.

One possibility for dealing with this situation, of course, is to undertake a significant restructuring of the American health care system. It seems plausible that current spending of roughly $800 billion a year, and a projected $1.6 trillion by the year 2000 (16.4 percent of GNP) (Sonnefeld et al. 1991), should be more than sufficient to ensure all Americans a reasonable level of health care. Much of this article addresses various aspects of this potential challenge. Yet no one familiar with our health care system and American politics can fail to appreciate the obstacles to significant restructuring. Health care, now one of our largest social and economic sectors, is a major source of employment and profit, and it serves many important and powerful interests exceptionally well. Thus, however enthusiastic we may be about planning yearly expenditures of 800 billion, a trillion dollars, or more, little in the history of American social policy, in our political experience, or even in international endeavors suggests its likelihood. This does not mean that we will not have substantial and meaningful change; but we must think very carefully about the structures that set the context for our future.

Politics generally involves a short-term frame of reference, usually bounded by the limited terms of office before public officials come up for re-election. A longer historical perspective suggests the possibility of major transformations in the arrangement of our country's health affairs (Mechanic 1979; Starr 1982). Government support of managed care systems, prospective payment of hospitals, a resource-based relative value scale for the payment of physicians, and many other increasingly accepted practices would have seemed subversive just a few decades ago. But the current concern with the federal budget deficit, and short-term perceptions of fiscal practicability, have encouraged even liberal forces to advocate relatively modest incremental improvements.

Bureaucracy and Administration

American medicine preserves the mirage of a private system at enormous administrative cost. Government directly pays for more than two-fifths of health care expenditures (Levit, Lazenby, Cowan, and Letsch 1991) and indirectly accounts for more through massive tax subsidies to businesses and individuals (Enthoven 1985). We create a large paper bureaucracy to maintain the illusion of free enterprise—and then we regulate health providers more intensively and more intrusively than anywhere else in the world (Mechanic 1981).

Health care has become incredibly bureaucratized. As each new problem arises, and the problems are countless, government responds with additional regulatory requirements. In any given instance a requirement seems focused and responsive to the issues that motivated it, but in its totality the system is weighted down by massive and inconsistent requirements that put enormous drag on daily operations. Woolhandler and Himmelstein (1991) estimated that health care administration cost between $96.8 and $120.4 billion in 1987, 19.3 to 24.1 percent of all expenditures. Between 1970 and 1982, while the total number of health personnel increased by 57 percent, administrative personnel grew by 171 percent (Himmelstein and Woolhandler 1986). Administrative expenditures between 1983 and 1987 in constant dollars increased by 37 percent (Woolhandler and Himmelstein 1991). There is room to quibble about the size of these estimates, but no one who has even modest contact with the health care sector can doubt the size, complexity, or burdens associated with the paper bureaucracy.

Simply dealing with billing and payment consumes enormous resources. Woolhandler and Himmelstein (1991) report that Blue Cross of Massachusetts employs 6,682 workers for an enrollee population of 2.7 million. This is more than the total number of administrators in Canada's health system, which covers 25 million people. Aggregated over the population, the time costs and frustration involved in processing multiple bills for many millions of episodes each year must be incredible, not only for the health system but also for the patients and professionals who must cope with this complexity.

PUBLIC PERCEPTIONS OF OUR HEALTH CARE SYSTEM

Major dissatisfaction with the health care system is evident. A recent Harris survey, for example, found only 10 percent of respondents agreeing that "on the whole the health system works pretty well, and only minor changes are necessary to make it better" (Blendon and Taylor 1989). In contrast, most of the respondents endorsed the need for fundamental change, and three-tenths thought that so much is wrong with the system that we need to "completely rebuild it."

General attitudes, however, are not as informative as they may at first appear. Responses are substantially influenced by the wording and order of questions and the context in which they are asked. When the questions are practical, people are more likely to respond in accord with their personal interests than with overall impressions about social institutions and their contributions to the community. Survey researchers have long recognized major incompatibilities between respondents' reports of general attitudes about health care versus their own experiences (Andersen, Kravits, and Anderson 1971). In surveys that address respondents' personal experiences, considerable satisfaction with one's personal physician and treatment is typically expressed. Even in the Harris survey just noted, a majority of respondents who used services were very satisfied with their physician visits and hospitalization experiences, and only small minorities were dissatisfied—13 percent with physician visits and 15 percent with hospital care (Blendon and Taylor 1989). Other studies show even more profound contradictions, depending on the wording of key items (Jajich-Toth and Roper 1990, 1991).

A variety of hypotheses have been advanced to explain the high measure of personal satisfaction. It may, for example, reflect a psychological need to report satisfaction or the fact that most people are reporting on their experiences when they are relatively healthy, with deficiencies in care forgotten or no longer salient. However, our efforts to survey populations with the greatest needs for care have not substantially increased the levels of reported personal dissatisfaction.

One suspects that the public's image of the deficiencies of our health care system are shaped more by the mass media, and the pronouncements of experts, than by their own experiences. Health care is a highly playable theme for television, newspapers, and the national weekly magazines, and consumers are exposed to much expert criticism on uncontrollable costs, the plight of the uninsured, the inadequacies of long-term care, excessive profit making and other abuses, and the loss of caring practitioners. The media interpret health care to be in perpetual crisis, and all but the most oblivious of adult Americans are aware of major problems.

The sources of discrepancies between general attitudes and personal experiences thus emerge from conflicting channels of information. The media emphasize the extraordinary cost escalation of medical care, and the public clearly recognizes it as a major national problem. But in their own experiences, most have insurance linked to their employment or the employment of a family member, and are insulated from high costs. In many instances the insurance involves very small or no premium contributions, and while cost sharing has increased in recent years (Gabel et al. 1991), the out-of-pocket expenditure for medical care for most of the population remains modest relative to income. Household health spending was 5.1 percent of adjusted personal income in 1989 (Levit, Lazenby, Letsch, and Cowan 1991), an increase of 21 percent since 1965 but still within the "modest amount" range for the average individual.

The difficulty is that not all people are average and some face costs that are substantial. The media rightly emphasize the plight of the uninsured, and surveys show considerable compassion for persons in that situation. But the uninsured are a minority, and the problems of access to care they face do not touch most respondents in a personal way. In the abstract, Americans are appalled by the fact that access to health care is determined as much by one's means as one's needs, and most are even willing to pay something more in taxes to remedy the problem. Few, however, are committed to paying the tax increases necessary within our current structure to provide universal access to those now disenfranchised. A 1990 survey found that 72 percent supported comprehensive national health insurance even when a tax increase was required, but that only 22 percent were willing to pay more than $200 per year additional taxes (Blendon and Donelon 1990). As in so many other areas of American life, the people quite readily endorse the goal but resist making the sacrifices necessary when they take into account the more complex configuration of their own competing wants (Etzioni 1991).

This discussion has given considerable attention to the issue of public opinion because, while we must be realistic about what public attitudes signify, the constellation of these attitudes provide a potential opportunity for future reform. The public shares an abstract predisposition toward restructuring, but one not especially notable for affecting concrete personal behavior or political engagement. A national leader who can effectively articulate the issues and make them appealing can draw on this general attitudinal resource to mobilize public opinion toward tangible political objectives. Thus, one can visualize a skillful presidential candidate using the crisis in health care as a basis for a national political campaign, and President Clinton did this to some degree. As gaps in insurance coverage affect ever-larger numbers of people, opportunities will increase for activating the population. In no instance will it be easy to rouse the public, and the opposing political forces will be formidable. But the discomfort the public has about existing health arrangements does present a positive opportunity. Presidential candidates may be cautious in addressing health care reform because general dissatisfaction does not necessarily mean that Americans agree either on the specific remedies needed or on acceptable ways to finance them (Blendon and Donelan 1990).

Presidential leadership would be advantageous, but reform is possible without it. Etheredge (1991) makes a persuasive case that the initiative for health policy reform has shifted to the Congress, and that momentum for change is emerging through the reforms mandated in the Omnibus Budget Reconciliation Act of 1990, the establishment of commissions on hospital and physician payment, and so on, and bipartisan efforts such as the Pepper Commission. Greater presidential interest would help, of course.

THE FUTURE: A FRAMEWORK FOR REFORM

Although American medicine has experimented with planning and regionalization at various points during the past 25 years, the planning process, captured by the strong and aggressive provider community, has typically been given little power and has done little to ensure a rational distribution and allocation of expensive resources. Planning, in a sense, has become a "cost of doing business" that increases the costs of development and expansion without fundamentally altering the configuration of health care. Thus, the planning process has become one more layer of regulation.

American medicine, at this juncture, falls significantly short on each of the three basic goals that have guided health policy considerations over the past quarter century: (1) providing access in reasonable relation to need; (2) moderating the growth of medical care costs; and (3) ensuring uniformly high-quality care. It has yet to give priority to expanding care so that function and quality of life will be maintained not only for the elderly, but also for other populations with chronic diseases and significant disabilities. Extraordinary inequalities in health and health risks by race, class, and ethnicity persist, but the distribution of care is related as much to the ability to pay as it is to need. Prevention remains more rhetoric than reality, and rehabilitation principles, while highly developed in some specialized areas, have not yet entered the mainstream of care. Much is impressive in American medicine, but it is also evident that many of our citizens are outside the system and that we are far from realizing the value we should expect for the money we currently spend. The remainder of the article examines possible options for the future and barriers to their implementation.

Reform of our health care system has again become a salient issue eliciting a large range of proposals (*Journal of the American Medical Association* 1991). Many proposals focus primarily on the uninsured population, while others are aimed at restructuring the entire system. Blendon and Edwards (1991) have characterized these proposals for reform as falling within four generic approaches: (1) requiring employers to provide private insurance with government filling the gap by providing insurance for those who are not employed; (2) giving employers the option of either insuring their workers or paying a tax (the "play or pay" approach), with the uninsured persons being covered by a government program (as in the Massachusetts plan and in a recent proposal by Senator Mitchell and other Democrats for health care reform); (3) using income-related tax credits to induce individuals to acquire private insurance along the lines proposed by Alan Enthoven (managed competition); and (4) developing systems of national health insurance following such models as that of Canada or of western European countries.

Despite the fact that health care reform is again on the national agenda, and that there is much agreement on the obvious problems, all signs suggest little consensus about approaches to change and point to a protracted discussion. The outcomes inevitably will depend on the political process, and, thus for my purposes here, it is more useful to focus on some generic considerations than to spell out in detail my preferred solutions. I begin, however, with my own point of view since it helps the reader understand my perspective in examining other, perhaps more politically viable, alternatives.

The Canadian System

The Canadian system offers attractive features that would effectively address many of the problems we face. These include a federal-state system, universal and comprehensive coverage, portability between jobs and residence, reasonable access without copayment, nonprofit administration involving a single payer, negotiated budgets, and prospective hospital reimbursement. First, as a federal-state system, with the federal government setting national standards and the states having a variety of options for implementation, the Canadian approach fits our political structure and our preference for problem solving at the state level. The national standards of universal and comprehensive coverage would remedy the problems of insurance instability tied to employment, underinsurance, and the problem of the uninsured. The standard of portability between jobs and residence would give individuals more freedom to choose jobs and geographic location independent of worry about maintaining health insurance. The implementation of nonprofit public administration of the system would be likely to reduce the claims bureaucracy substantially, lessen burdens for physicians and patients, and save many billions of dollars. I also concur with the standard that would guarantee reasonable access without copayments and would prohibit extra billing. As I illustrate later on, copayment reduces the demand for care, but not in a particularly rational way. Extra billing is unnecessary if physicians are paid reasonably, and in the American context, that would in all likelihood be the case.

In a recent report on Canadian health insurance, the General Accounting Office concluded that "if the universal coverage and single-payer features of the Canadian system were applied in the United States, the savings in administrative costs alone would be more than enough to finance insurance coverage for the millions of Americans who are currently uninsured" (United States General Accounting Office 1991, 3). The GAO was particularly impressed by how the power of a single payer with authority to negotiate budgets has been able to act on the concept of prospective budgeting of hospitals and thus to foster successful cost containment while providing all Canadians with reasonable access to primary care and generally appropriate services. Fixed prospective budgets are probably our only means ever to gain control over medical care costs; the Canadian way is far more sensible and effective than the clumsy and overregulated incrementalism that characterizes our present path.

Despite my support of a Canadian-type approach, several features strike me as incompatible with American values and not particularly desirable in our context. In Canada, insurance companies are prohibited from selling insurance for services covered by the national plan, undermining any basis for a competing private system. Such a prohibition is consistent with a concept of equity and, according to Hirschman's theory (Hirschman 1970), encourages greater involvement in maintaining and improving the system—what he calls "voice" and "loyalty." In contrast, a private competing system, the theory suggests, encourages "exit" when people become dissatisfied, and thus prompts less effort to keep improving the public arena. Certainly, if the private system grows too large, these results are likely. But a modest private system complementing the public sector not only provides more choice, and allows disaffected and troublesome clients to go elsewhere, but also serves as a comparison to the public system, challenging it to maintain acceptable services. Thus, I support the concept of a parallel, but smaller, private system.

The counterargument to the Canadian approach that will probably be of major concern to many Americans is its strict rationing of patient access to some expensive technologies and treatments except in emergency situations. Adequate data to assess this issue are not available, and claims and interpretations tell us more about the ideologies of proponents than about the facts. In an effort to get more information, the GAO queried specialty directors in Ontario in charge of magnetic resonance instrumentation (MRI), cardiovascular surgery, lithotripsy, and autologous bone marrow transplants. Questions referred to three types of cases, emergent, urgent, and elective. Respondents reported substantial queues, particularly for elective care, and sometimes the wait was very long (United States General Accounting Office 1991, 52–61). Considerable queuing was reported even for urgent cases, defined as usually involving "serious medical conditions for which the patient is monitored and treated while in the hospital." It seems unlikely, given the high expectations of Americans, that they would accept this magnitude of rationing of technology. Following a Canadian approach, however, does not imply a fixed level of access. Access must be structured to go at least part way in responding to the expectations and demands of the population. The challenge is to design a realistic structure for health care that operates within reasonable cost constraints but with sufficient flexibility to respond to population demands and to new knowledge and technology opportunities for significant enhancement of the population's health. The extent of rationing and queuing is ultimately a political decision.

It is essential to recognize that the Canadian insurance system is primarily a financing strategy—that it does not, by itself, address the range of goals discussed earlier in this article. National health insurance systems lock in whatever priorities prevail at the time of their introduction; they may support highly medicalized systems of care that are not particularly responsive to prevention, encouragement of function, or long-term management of chronic disease. In instituting any such system, careful thought must be given to the types of facilities, services, and practitioners to be covered under the plan (Mechanic 1978b). David Rochefort (1992), for instance, has found in his study of mental health services in Canada that the Canadian system has not encouraged particularly responsive or innovative services for the seriously and persistently mentally ill.

Stating the challenge in broad terms begs many questions because ways of defining the value consensus or of ascertaining the most reasonable expenditures are not clear. The health care industry is incredibly complex, involving hundreds of interest groups highly protective of their domains. It is relatively easy to elicit agreement about abstract principles—for example, that everyone should have access to needed health care or that everyone should have health insurance—but consensus breaks down quickly in the face of concrete proposals that make the winners and losers apparent. This explains why efforts to improve systems of care almost always involve significantly increased expenditures; cooperation and consensus are much more likely to be maintained when everyone involved has something to gain. A good example of this was implementation of the Medicare program during the 1960s.

There is widespread agreement that everyone should have access to care, that primary care is needed to monitor health and illness in a continuing way, and that the health care system should give attention to prevention, health maintenance, and rehabilitation. The logic of primary care is that the provider offers a continuity of responsibility in monitoring health needs, and is sufficiently linked into a larger network so that needed referrals are possible (Lewis, Fein, and Mechanic 1976). Primary care is an important enabling factor for appropriate referral and is not expensive relative to the episodic outpatient hospital care typically found among disadvantaged patients. The Canadian system provides such care abundantly, using more physician services per capita than the United States (Fuchs and Hahn 1990). One short-term strategy for system reform would be to expand Medicaid or develop an alternative system to bring more of the disadvantaged into managed care systems that emphasize prevention, outreach services, and continuity of care. Efforts could be made to coordinate Medicaid with other entitlement programs, and thus to expand the traditional range of medical services to respond to special areas of patient need such as any necessary food supplementation, assistance with housing, or help with other social problems.

This was the strategy used when the Health Care Financing Administration launched a demonstration program on an expanded concept of care for the elderly: the social health maintenance organization (SHMO) (Greenberg, Leutz, Greenlick, et al. 1988). The goal is to integrate acute care and necessary long-term care, and to provide community-based care as an alternative to the nursing home. The services include homemaking, personal care, case management, adult day care, and transportation, and patients are covered as well for a broader array of posthospital care than Medicare supports, including some custodial services. The four SHMOs that are part of the demonstration have been in operation for only about five years and have had some start-up difficulties, particularly in the marketing and financial areas (Harrington and Newcomer 1991), but three of the four are now operating without deficits. This is a complicated undertaking but a modest one given the size and complexity of the health care system. We need much broader experimentation with extended care concepts as we begin to engage our system in addressing long-term community treatment of serious chronic illness.

One context for such effort is the care of seriously mentally ill persons in the community. As we have deinstitutionalized our public mental hospitals (Mechanic and Rochefort 1990), putting increasing reliance on general hospitals and other community facilities (Mechanic 1991a), we have been attempting to provide care in the community for seriously ill patients with a broad array of psychiatric, medical, psychosocial, housing, and subsistence needs. The care has been highly fragmented. Efforts are now being made to integrate responsibility and fiscal authority in ways that allow these broad needs to be managed within a single case-management system using such devices as capitation and the development of public mental health authorities (Mechanic 1989b; Mechanic and Rochefort 1990). The need for integration of services is obvious in many other areas of chronic illness as well, including the care of persons with disabilities (Institute of Medicine 1991). Achieving this goal depends substantially on the enabling economic and organizational framework of care.

Alternative and Short-Term Approaches to System Reform

Whatever the advantages of the Canadian model, it is more likely that reform will follow an incremental path by requiring or inducing employers to provide health insurance coverage for their workers and worker dependents. Through this process various gaps in coverage will be closed over time for insured workers, leaving smaller groups of uninsured to be covered by programs for the medically indigent. This latter could be accomplished by expanding eligibility under Medicaid or by developing alternative programs. By itself, extending insurance coverage does not address many of the problems already described, but such coverage expansion would contribute in important ways to improving access to care.

A highly controversial approach is to extend coverage of a basic set of outpatient and inpatient benefits but to exclude the coverage for more discretionary services. This is what the state of Oregon has in mind in expanding eligibility for Medicaid benefits as a trade-off for a more restricted definition of the benefit package (Kitzhaber 1990; Eddy 1991; Dougherty 1991; Hadorn 1991). Although this is not a long-term solution, it is a plausible strategy to provide a stopgap measure during the stalemate over significant national reforms. The Oregon approach has been compromised practically and ethically, however, by exempting aged, blind, and disabled recipients, thus putting the entire rationing burden on poor mothers and children who account for only about 30 percent of the Medicaid budget (Brown 1991). In principle, I am not in sympathy with those who oppose the Oregon proposal and related approaches simply on the basis that they create two classes of care, although I find the selective exemptions disturbing. I prefer a single standard, but the typical alternative is no guaranteed care at all. The United States is a stratified society in almost every institutional sphere, and it is unlikely that we will see a single standard without a universal system. To oppose a rationing approach associated with increased eligibility because we aspire to a more comprehensive alternative is, in my view, not constructive.

Few challenge the notion of a guaranteed basic minimum, but agreement on the boundaries of such an entitlement is difficult to achieve. While agreement may be possible on limitations of very high cost but uncertain interventions such as the transplantation of hearts, lungs, or livers, the concept of what is basic depends substantially on a person's illness, disability, and level of function. Some argue, for example, that services for mental illness, alcohol abuse, and chemical dependency are discretionary, while persons with these problems see such services as central to their needs. Insurance for the treatment of affective disorders and other mental illnesses, for example, is often limited (Mechanic 1989); but depressive illness, and even depressive symptoms short of disorder, cause more pain, suffering, and disability than most common chronic medical conditions (Wells, Stewart, Hays, et al. 1989). Alternatively, one might choose to design benefits in terms of established knowledge of the effectiveness of respective therapies (Brook 1991). Most widely used medical modalities, however, have never been rigorously evaluated, and establishing the needed research efforts would be a massive challenge.

A major function of medical care is to provide reassurance, support, and health guidance. One strategy would be to provide relatively easy access to primary medical care services and associated cognitive services within relatively lenient boundaries, but in systems in which the primary practitioners would have a gatekeeper role, as in the Canadian and British systems. Expensive modalities, in contrast, would be subjected to more rigorous tests of effectiveness, and access would be controlled. Thus, basic consultations concerning acute problems and health maintenance would be routinely available. As the costs of interventions increased, however, the evidential test justifying intervention and payment would be more explicitly established.

The Role of Competition

In recent years it has been argued frequently that many of the obvious cost difficulties have resulted from a lack of competition and an absence of cost consciousness among consumers (Fuchs 1988). Competition is referred to in many ways, and the advocates often convey different conceptions of it.

One idea is that patients at the time of service should face sharing enough of the cost to make them consider carefully the value of the service they are seeking. Coinsurance and deductibles are successful devices for reducing the demand for medical care and requiring consumers to pay more of the bill. Cost sharing, however, reduces the use of appropriate and efficacious care as well as the use of more discretionary services (Lohr, Brook, Kamberg, et al. 1986; Siu, Sonnenberg, Manning, et al. 1986). Unfortunately, the cost-sharing model particularly affects the behavior of lower-income persons who typically have greater needs for care than those who are more affluent. Moreover, most expensive care decisions are made by professionals, not patients, and extensive cost sharing limits the possibility of careful professional appraisal when patients are deterred from seeking care in the first place because of price.

A more promising alternative, at least within our present framework of care, accepts the irrationality of asking sick people to assess the most cost-effective care option, and focuses on developing a system of controlled competition in consumer selection among alternative health care plans. Enthoven's proposals (Enthoven 1980; Enthoven and Kronick 1989) for introducing a serious framework of controlled competition among health care plans are persuasive in theory; however, achieving acceptance of the concept has been difficult, partly because of the complexity of organization it requires. Enthoven's basic idea is that people would receive a health insurance subsidy sufficient to fund a health insurance policy meeting specified standards, selected from among a standard group of policies. Employees choosing more expensive health insurance programs would have to bear the additional costs, and those selecting more economical options would be allowed to keep the savings.

Competition at this level does work but not as well as advocates suggest. There is an extraordinary degree of inertia among consumers, who strongly prefer to retain prior medical relationships if they have been satisfactory (Mechanic 1989a). This explains the slow expansion of prepaid group practices in contrast to the preferred provider organizations (PPOs) that allow more choice. One may anticipate, however, that over time new cohorts will be socialized to receive their care in a managed care framework that offers them cost advantages.

Controlled competition should play some role in the future health care system, but its form will depend on how our system evolves. Certainly, if we continue with an employer-based insurance system, it will be constructive to offer patients meaningful choices and opportunities to save if they select more economical health care options. If such a system is to avoid major deficiencies, the basic health insurance program should be adequate to meet critical health needs, and information about covered services and plan performance must be appropriate, enabling intelligent choices to be made (Mechanic 1989a). In this sense, competition must be carefully regulated. Even if we were to go to a Canadian-type system, diversity and choice within that system would be helpful in shaping services toward consumer preferences in contrast to bureaucratic inclinations.

Containing Costs

Expanding coverage and enlarging the traditional goals of care to include health promotion must be linked to mechanisms that control overuse of expensive facilities, technical procedures, and professional services. Many ways to pay for care are acceptable, but any viable approach requires some way of limiting total expenditures. In the HMO model, the budget, based on capitation payments, sets constraints on expenditures and motivates primary care physicians to be careful gatekeepers regarding the use of expensive modalities. In fee-for-service practice, similar constraints can be achieved through implementing a fee schedule with values established within the context of a budgetary cap. Unlike a straight capitation that affects providers uniformly, the capped fee-for-service still allows individual physicians to increase their volume as much as they wish, but as physicians do this in the aggregate, each physician gets less per patient service. In the long run, any type of cap will do equally well in achieving cost constraint; but various types of caps may have different consequences for ways in which essential services are allocated and for professional morale (Mechanic and Faich 1970).

The simplest constraint, and one likely to be more acceptable to professionals than other types of constraints, is a fixed budget that sets a limit on total expenditures but does not specify the internal allocation of resources, leaving this to provider planning—a system of implicit rationing (Mechanic 1978a). Such an approach satisfies the payer's need to hold expenditures to a predetermined level without involving the payer in the thousands of decisions relevant to criteria for treatment and appropriate use of technology. An implicit rationing approach leaves these decisions to the managers and health professionals involved, honoring their professional and clinical autonomy. Government and other third parties, far removed from the pressures of illness and its complex contingencies, often introduce bureaucratic inflexibilities in unfortunate attempts to become involved in decisions at the micro level.

Implicit rationing, however, has some major weaknesses. It reinforces a highly discretionary system that can introduce considerable variability, responding differentially to patients by condition, social characteristics—even personality. At the local level, professionals are much influenced by their prior training and personal experience, and may make judgments that are less scientifically based than those made by a central authority that draws on the most rigorous research available. In any system of universal insurance, government has a stake in the principle that persons in comparable situations should be treated equally, but if each institution is given its own discretion in the use of available resources, major differences in access to treatment may result.

All systems are mixed systems that vary the balance between explicit directives and implicit processes (Mechanic 1979). Central decision making whether by government authority or insurance program deals typically with issues such as the services covered, coverage or noncoverage of new or experimental procedures and drugs, reimbursable versus nonreimbursable providers, and related matters. The issue lies in determining the appropriate reach of explicit authority. In cases of highly expensive new technologies and of eligibility or coverage rules, explicit authority is essential for establishing an equitable framework of care. It was fully reasonable, for example, for the Health Care Financing Administration to refuse to pay for tissue plasminogen activator (TPA), which cost far more than comparable drugs and showed no evidence of superiority to them. This action infuriated some physicians, but it was a rational and appropriate decision (Mechanic 1989b). Much of the debate about central decision making focuses on the degree of micro management that is justifiable given the data capacities of central management and the variabilities in practice evident among physicians. My own view is that central management must be judicious and constrained because it is likely to be insensitive to the complexities of medical transactions and to the large variability in tastes, preferences, and orientations among patients. Physicians must retain considerable discretion, essential for subtle management of patients who often are diagnosed with complex disease compounded by difficult social complications.

Essential to any fair system of implicit rationing is a budgeting process sensitive to the resource needs of each institution relative to the social and medical characteristics of the populations it is expected to serve. Payment to hospitals based on diagnosis-related groups is in essence a complexly stratified prospective payment plan that seeks to gauge payment according to patient mix. Despite the detail involved, a persistent criticism of Medicare's prospective payment system is that it is insufficiently sensitive to the severity of patient illness, particularly in institutions that serve large numbers of patients with medical problems compounded by socioeconomic disadvantage. Some efforts have been made to supplement payment to institutions that care for many indigent patients, but reimbursement practices are unlikely to address the true costs of such a case mix.

A FRAMEWORK FOR REFORM: THE IDEAL AND THE REAL

It is easy to construct a utopian health care system that has no possibility of implementation. The appealing logic of health systems with universal access; portability of health benefits; orderly relationships between primary, secondary, and tertiary care; broad concern with function and quality of life considerations as well as cure; and prudent expenditure patterns requires no detailed explication. In fact, however, health systems never emerge anew, but are deeply embedded in the traditions, professional patterns, and organizational structures that have gone before. There is little reason to anticipate that future trends in American health care will be any different. Moreover, the size of the health care industry and the magnitude of the vital interests of involved groups make straightforward reform singularly difficult to achieve.

It would be helpful to eliminate employment-based insurance and develop a standard insurance program covering all eligible persons along the lines of the Medicare program or the government-sponsored health insurance plans of other western nations and Canada. The probability, however, is that we will not go this path, however reasonable. A significant number of people are sufficiently content with their current source of insurance; very powerful interests have a stake in building on current mechanisms; and many persons and institutions fear the expected disruptions of moving to an entirely new approach. Thus, it seems likely that we will remedy gaps gradually through employer-mandated approaches, government-created risk pools for the uninsured, and various possible extensions of Medicare and Medicaid. Some of these initiatives will develop through state legislation, but it seems inevitable that the federal government as well will have to engage these problems and provide assistance to states and small employers burdened by the new insurance mandates. Over time, many of the known gaps will be closed, but not without considerable waste and high administrative cost.

In the next decade the focus will remain as much on cost as it is now. Although the PPS has reduced hospital expenditures to some degree below the level expected had intervention not taken place (Russell 1989), government has been persistently unsuccessful in developing a viable approach to cost containment. The commonly used analogy of the balloon, which when pressed in one place bulges elsewhere, describes the situation. Although government has been making an effort over time to gain control over each practice sector—as it is now attempting with respect to physician payment—this remains a slow, awkward, and uncertain process.[2] The provider community is remarkably creative in identifying (and using) loopholes, and we gain control over the system only with great administrative and regulatory cost. Our own history, and experience in other countries, suggests that we might be able to introduce a more streamlined national system if we are willing to spend lavishly, ensuring that existing interests remain comfortable. But this alternative no longer is feasible. Another alternative, approaching such major changes within an economically constrained framework, is likely to encounter enormous resistance. While I hope for something better, I believe we will muddle along for years to come, trying one partial solution or another, and constructively filing some gaps. The world does change, and major dramatic innovations are not impossible. but in all likelihood, the future of health care reform is likely to be more an incremental series of steps than a great leap forward.

The picture is not entirely pessimistic. Any expanded view of the trajectory of health services will reveal some extraordinary changes over the last several decades (Mechanic 1979). Medicare and Medicaid, while organized in an inefficient and costly way, dramatically changed the provision of health services and brought intensive, sophisticated care to many who had never had such access before. These and other federal programs stimulated a health infrastructure and technological capacity that is truly impressive. We have a large and well-trained corps of health professionals who have the capacity to serve our population exceedingly well. In some sense, what we lack most is a sense of discipline and fairness in capitalizing on this capability. Our problem thus resides not with our basic assets but with both the excesses and the deficiencies of their utilization. The challenge is one of organization, and of our political capacity to bring a greater sense of prudence, balance, and equity to the management of our health affairs.

References

Aaron, H. J. *Serious and Unstable Condition: Financing America's Health Care.* Washington, DC: The Brookings Institution, 1991.

Andersen, R., J. Kravits, and O. W. Anderson. "The Public's View of the Crisis in Medical Care: An Impetus for Change in Delivery Systems?" *Economics and Business Bulletin* 24, no. 1 (Fall 1971): 44–52.

Anderson, O. *The Evolution of Health Services Research: Personal Reflections on Applied Social Science.* San Francisco: Jossey-Bass, 1991.

Assistant Secretary For Health. *Healthy People: National Health Promotion and Disease Prevention Objectives.* DHHS Publication no. (PHS) 91-50213. Washington, DC: U.S. Government Printing Office, 1990.

2. The current debate about implementation of the new physician payment arrangements under Medicare highlights the importance of building and institutionalizing trust. The medical community cooperated in developing these arrangements on the assumption that the payment system would be used to redistribute payment among procedures and specialities, but not to reduce the amount of payment. HCFA, anticipating selective volume increases during the phase-in period, proposed cuts in fees to cover these costs. Physicians felt betrayed. HCFA might have been technically correct, but it responded in a manner that violated prevalent understandings and undermined trust.

______. *Healthy People: The Surgeon General's Report of Health Promotion and Disease Prevention.* DHEW (PHS) Publication no. 7955071. Washington, DC: U.S. Government Printing Office, 1979.

Ball, R. M., and T. N. Bethell. *Because We're All in This Together.* Washington, DC: Families U.S.A. Foundation, 1989.

Blendon, R. J., and K. Donelan. "The Public and the Emerging Debate over National Health Insurance." *New England Journal of Medicine* 323, no. 3 (July 1990): 208–12.

Blendon, R. J., and J. N. Edwards. "Caring for the Uninsured: Choices for Reform." *Journal of the American Medical Association* 265, no. 19 (15 May 1991): 2563–65.

Blendon, R. J., and H. Taylor. "Views on Health Care: Public Opinion in Three Nations." *Health Affairs* 8, no. 1 (Spring 1989): 149–57.

Brook, R. "Health, Health Insurance, and the Uninsured." *Journal of the American Medical Association* 265, no. 22 (12 June 1991): 2998–3000.

Brown, L. D. "The National Politics of Oregon's Rationing Plan." *Health Affairs* 10, no. 2 (Summer 1991): 28–51.

Bunker, J. P., D. S. Gomby, and B. H. Kehrer. *Pathways to Health: The Role of Social Factors,* Menlo Park, CA: Henry J. Kaiser Family Foundation, 1989.

Cherlin, A. J., F. F. Furstenberg, Jr., P. L. Chase-Lansdale, K. E. Kiernan, P. K. Robins, D. R. Morrison, and J. O. Teitler. "Longitudinal Studies of the Effects of Divorce on Children in Great Britain and the United States." *Science* 252 (7 June 1991): 1386–89.

Dougherty, C. J. "Setting Health Care Priorities: Oregon's Next Steps: A Conference Report." *Hastings Center Report* 21, no. 3 (May-June 1991): 1–11.

Dubos, R. *Mirage of Health.* New York: Harper & Brothers, 1959.

Dutton, D. B. "Social Class, Health, and Illness." In *Applications of Social Science to Clinical Medicine and Health Policy.* Edited by L. H. Aiken and D. Mechanic. New Brunswick, NJ: Rutgers University Press, 1986.

Eddy, D. "What's Going On in Oregon?" *Journal of the American Medical Association* 266, no. 3 (17 July 1991): 417–20.

Eisenberg, J. "Economics." *Journal of the American Medical Association* 265, no. 23 (19 June 1991): 3113–15.

Enthoven, A. *Health Plan: The Only Practical Solution to the Cost of Medical Care.* Reading, MA: Addison-Wesley, 1980.

______. "Health Tax Policy Mismatch." *Health Affairs* 4, no. 4 (Winter 1985): 5–14.

Enthoven, A., and R. Kronick. "A Consumer Choice Health Plan for the 1990s. Part 1 and 2." *New England Journal of Medicine* 320, nos. 1 and 2 (1989): 29–37, 94–101.

Etheredge, L. "Negotiating National Health Insurance." *Journal of Health Politics, Policy and Law* 16, no. 1 (Spring 1991); 157–67.

Etzioni, A. "Too Many Rights, Too Few Responsibilities." *Society* 28, no. 2 (January-February 1991): 41–48.

Fox, D. M. *Health Policies, Health Politics: The British and American Experience 1911–1965.* Princeton, NJ: Princeton University Press, 1986.

Fox, D. M., and D. C. Schaffer. "Health Policy and ERISA: Interest Groups and Semipreemption." *Journal of Health Politics, Policy and Law* 14, no. 2 (Summer 1989): 239–60.

Frank, J. D., and J. B. Frank. *Persuasion and Healing,* 3rd ed. New York: Schocken Books, 1991.

Freeman, H., K. J. Kiecolt, and H. M. Allen, II. "Community Health Centers: An Initiative of Enduring Quality." *Milbank Quarterly* 60, no. 2 (Spring 1982): 245–67.

Fuchs, V. "The 'Competition Revolution' in Health Care." *Health Affairs* 7, no. 3 (Summer 1988): 5–24.

______. "The Growing Demand for Medical Care." *New England Journal of Medicine* 279, no. 4 (25 July 1968): 190–95.

Fuchs, V., and J. S. Hahn. "How Does Canada Do It?: A Comparison of Expenditures for Physicians' Services in the United States and Canada." *New England Journal of Medicine* 323, no. 13 (27 September 1990): 884–90.

Gabel, J., S. DiCarlo, C. Sullivan, and T. Rice. "Employer-Sponsored Health Insurance, 1989." *Health Affairs* 9, no. 3 (Fall 1990): 161–75.

Geiger, J. "Community Health Centers: Health Care as an Instrument of Social Change." In *Reforming Medicine's Lessons of the Last Quarter Century.* Edited by V. W. Sidel and R. Sidel. New York: Pantheon, 1984.

Greenberg, J., W. Leutz, M. Greenlick, J. Malone, S. Erwin, and D. Kodner. "The Social HMO Demonstration: Early Experience." *Health Affairs* 7, no. 3 (Summer 1988): 66–79.

Hadley, J., E. P. Steinberg, and J. Feder. "Comparison of Uninsured and Privately Insured Hospital Patients: Condition on Admission, Resource Use and Outcome." *Journal of the American Medical Association* 265, no. 3 (16 January 1991): 374–79.

Hadorn, D. C. "The Oregon Priority-Setting Exercise: Quality of Life and Public Policy." *Hastings Center Report* 21, no. 3 (May-June 1991): 11–16.

Harrington, C., and R. J. Newcomer. "Social Health Maintenance Organizations' Service Use and Costs, 1985–89." *Health Care Financing Review* 12, no. 3 (Spring 1991); 37–52.

Health Insurance Association of America. *Source Book of Health Insurance Data.* Washington, DC: HIAA, 1990.

Himmelstein, D. U., and S. Woolhandler. "Cost without Benefit: Administrative Waste in U.S. Health Care." *New England Journal of Medicine* 314, no. 7 (13 February 1986): 441–45.

Hirschman, A. O. *Exit, Voice, and Loyalty: Responses to Declines in Firms, Organizations, and States.* Cambridge, MA: Harvard University Press, 1970.

Institute of Medicine. *Disability in America: Toward a National Agenda for Prevention.* Washington, DC: National Academy Press, 1991.

Jajich-Toth, C., and B. W. Roper. "Americans' Views on Health Care: A Study in Contradictions." *Health Affairs* 9, no. 4 (Winter 1990): 149–57.

______. "Basing Policy on Survey Data: Proceed with Caution." *Health Affairs* 10, no. 2 (Summer 1991): 170–72.

Journal of the American Medical Association. Special Edition: "Caring for the Uninsured and Underinsured." vol. 256, no. 19 (1991).

Kark, S. L., and A. Steuart. *A Practice of Social Medicine.* Edinburgh: ETS Livingstone, 1962.

Kemper, P., R. Applebaum, and M. Harrigan. "Community Care Demonstrations: What Have We Learned?" *Health Care Financing Review* 8, no. 4 (Summer 1987): 37–52.

Kitzhaber, J. A. "The Oregon Model." In *The Richard and Linda Rosenthal Lectures.* Washington, DC: Institute of Medicine, 1990.

Law, S. *Blue Cross: What Went Wrong?* New Haven, CT: Yale University Press, 1974.

Leventhal, H., T. R. Prohaska, and R. S. Hirschman. "Preventive Health Behavior across the Life Span." In *Prevention in Health Psychology.* Edited by J. C. Rosen and L. J. Solomon. Hanover, NH: University Press of New England, 1985.

Levit, K. R., H. C. Lazenby, C. A. Cowan, and S. W. Letsch. "National Health Expenditures, 1990." *Health Care Financing Review* 13, no. 1 (Spring 1991): 29–54.

Levit, K. R., H. C. Lazenby, S. W. Letsch, and C. A. Cowan. "National Health Care Spending, 1989." *Health Affairs* 10 (1991): 117–30.

Lewis, C. E., F. Fein, and D. Mechanic. *A Right to Health: The Problem of Access to Primary Medical Care,* New York: Wiley-Interscience, 1976.

Lohr, K. N., R. H. Brook, C. J. Kamberg, G. A. Goldberg, A. Leibowitz, J. Keesey, D. Reboussin, and J. P. Newhouse. *Use of Medical Care in the RAND Health Insurance Experiment: Diagnosis- and Service-Specific Analyses in a Randomized Controlled Trial.* Publication no. R-3469HHS. Santa Monica, CA: RAND Corporation, December 1986.

Luft, H. *Health Maintenance Organizations: Dimensions of Performance.* New Brunswick, NJ: Transactions Publishers, 1987.

Marmor, T. R. *The Politics of Medicare.* Chicago: Aldine, 1973.
McCord, C., and H. P. Freeman. "Excess Mortality in Harlem." *New England Journal of Medicine* 322, no. 3 (18 January 1990): 173–77.
Mechanic, D. "Approaches to Controlling the Costs of Medical Care: Short-Range and Long-Range Alternatives." *New England Journal of Medicine* 298, no. 5 (2 February 1978a): 249–54.
______. "Considerations in the Design of Mental Health Benefits under National Health Insurance." *American Journal of Public Health* 68, no. 5 (May 1978b): 482–88.
______. "Consumer Choice among Health Insurance Options." *Health Affairs* 8, no. 1 (Spring 1989a): 138–48.
______. *Future Issues in Health Care: Social Policy and the Rationing of Medical Services.* New York: Free Press, 1979.
______. *Medical Sociology.* 2d ed. New York: Free Press, 1978c.
______. *Mental Health and Social Policy.* 3rd ed. Englewood Cliffs, NJ: Prentice Hall, 1989b.
______. "Promoting Health." *Society* 27, no. 2 (January-February 1990): 16–22.
______. "Recent Developments in Mental Health: Perspectives and Services." *Annual Review of Public Health* 12 (1991a): 1–15.
______. "Some Dilemmas in Health Care Policy." *Milbank Quarterly* 59, no. 1 (Winter 1981): 1–15.
______. "Sources of Countervailing Power in Medicine." *Journal of Health Politics, Policy and Law* 16, no. 3 (Fall 1991b): 485–98.
______. "Strategies for Health Promotion." Proceedings of the Second International Conference of Health Behavior Sciences, Tokyo, Japan, Japan Academy for Health Behavioral Research, September 21–29, 1991c.
Mechanic, D., and L. H. Aiken. "Access to Health Care and Use of Medical Care Services." In *Handbook of Medical Sociology.* 4th ed. Edited by H. Freeman and S. Levine, Englewood Cliffs, NJ: Prentice Hall, 1989.
______. "Caring and the Structure of Health Care Services." Paper presented at the Conference on the Caring Physician. Center for Advanced Study in the Behavioral Sciences, Palo Alto, CA, 1991.
Mechanic, D., and R. Faich. "Doctors in Revolt: The Crisis in the National Health Service." *Medical Care* 8, no. 6 (November-December 1970): 442–55.
Mechanic, D., and D. Rochefort. "Deinstitutionalization: An Appraisal of Reform." *Annual Review of Sociology* 16 (1990): 301–27.
National Center for Health Statistics. *Health, United States, 1990.* Hyattsville, MD: Public Health Service, 1991.
Office of National Cost Estimates. "National Health Expenditures, 1988." *Health Care Financing Review* 11, no. 4 (Summer 1990): 1–54.
Office of Technology Assessment. *Neonatal Intensive Care for Low Birth Weight Infants: Costs and Effectiveness.* Publication no. OTA-HCS-38. Washington, DC: U.S. Government Printing Office, 1987.
______. *Technology and Aging in America.* Publication no. OTA-BA264. Washington, DC: U.S. Government Printing Office, 1985.
Pauly, M. V. "Review of 'Caring for the Disabled Elderly'." *Health Affairs* 7, no. 4 (Fall 1988): 169–72.
Payer, L. *Medicine and Culture: Varieties of Treatment in the United States, England, West Germany, and France.* New York: Henry Holt, 1988.
Pepper Commission. *A Call for Action: Final Report of the U.S. Bipartisan Commission on Comprehensive Health Care.* Washington, DC: U.S. Government Printing Office, 1990.
Report of the Secretary's Task Force on Black and Minority Health, 1985. Washington, DC: U.S. Government Printing Office, 1985.
Rice, D., and J. Feldman. "Living Longer in the United States: Demographic Changes

and Health Needs of the Elderly.'' *Milbank Quarterly* 61, no. 3 (Summer 1983): 362–96.

Rivlin, A. M. ''Agreed: Here Comes National Health Insurance.'' *New York Times Magazine* (21 July 1974): 8.

Rivlin, A. M., and J. M. Wiener. *Caring for the Disabled Elderly: Who Will Pay?* Washington, DC: The Brookings Institution, 1988.

Robert Wood Johnson Foundation. *Medical Education in Transition: The Sciences of Medical Practice.* Princeton, NJ: Robert Wood Johnson Foundation, 1992.

Rochefort, D. ''Canadian Mental Health Services: A Comparative Analysis of Trends and Policy Issues.'' Paper presented at the 20th Anniversary Conference of the Association for Canadian Studies in the United States, Boston, MA, 1992.

Rosenberg, C. E. *The Care of Strangers: The Rise of America's Hospital System.* New York: Basic Books, 1987.

Russell, L. B. *Is Prevention Better Than Cure?* Washington, DC: The Brookings Institution, 1986.

______. *Medicare's New Hospital Payment System: Is it Working?* Washington, DC: The Brookings Institution, 1989.

Russell, M. A. H., J. A. Stapleton, P. H. Jackson, P. Hajek, and M. Belcher. ''District Programme to Reduce Smoking: Effect of Clinic Supported Brief Intervention by General Practitioners.'' *British Medical Journal* 295, no. 6608 (14 November 1987): 1240–44.

Russell, M. A. H., C. Wilson, D. Taylor, and C. D. Baker. ''Effect of General Practitioners' Advice against Smoking.'' *British Medical Journal* 2, no. 6184 (28 July 1979): 231–35.

Siu, A. L., F. A. Sonnenberg, W. G. Manning, F. Goldberg, E. S. Bloomfield, J. P. Newhouse, and R. H. Brook. ''Inappropriate Use of Hospitals in a Randomized Trial of Health Insurance Plans.'' *New England Journal of Medicine* 315, no. 20 (13 November 1986): 1259–66.

Somers, A. R. ''Insurance for Long-Term Care: Some Definitions, Problems, and Guidelines for Action.'' *New England Journal of Medicine* 317, no. 1 (2 July 1987): 23–29.

Somers, H. M., and A. R. Somers. *Doctors, Patients, and Health Insurance.* Garden City, NY: Anchor-Doubleday, 1961.

Sonnefeld, S. T., D. R. Waldo, J. A. Lemieux, and D. R. McKusick. ''Projections of National Health Expenditures through the Year 2000.'' *Health Care Financing Review* 13, no. 1 (Fall 1991): 1–27.

Starr, P. *The Social Transformation of American Medicine.* New York: Basic Books, 1982.

Stevens, R. *In Sickness and In Wealth: American Hospitals in the Twentieth Century.* New York: Basic Books, 1989.

Svarstad, B. ''Patient-Practitioner Relationships and Compliance with Prescribed Medical Regimens.'' In *Applications of Social Science to Clinical Medicine and Health Policy.* Edited by L. H. Aiken and D. Mechanic. New Brunswick, NJ: Rutgers University Press, 1986.

Thomas, L. ''On the Science and Technology of Medicine.'' *Daedalus* 106, no. 1 (Winter 1977): 35–46.

United States General Accounting Office. *Canadian Health Insurance: Lessons for the United States.* Publication no. GAO/HRD-91-90. Washington, DC: GAO, 1991.

Waitzkin, H. *The Second Sickness: Contradictions of Capitalist Health Care.* New York: Free Press, 1983.

Warner, K. E. ''Health and Economic Implications of a Tobacco-Free Society.'' *Journal of the American Medical Association* 258, no. 15 (16 October 1987): 2080–86.

Weissert, W. G. ''A New Policy Agenda for Home Care.'' *Health Affairs* 10, no. 2 (Summer 1991): 67–77.

Wells, K. B., A. Stewart, R. D. Hays, A. Burnam, W. Rogers, M. Daniels, M. S. Berry, S. Greenfield, and J. Ware. ''The Functioning and Well-being of Depressed Patients:

Results from the Medical Outcomes Study.'' *Journal of the American Medical Association* 262, no. 7 (18 August 1989): 914–19.
Woolhandler, S., and D. U. Himmelstein. ''The Deteriorating Administrative Efficiency of the U.S. Health Care System.'' *New England Journal of Medicine* 324, no. 18 (2 May 1991): 1253–58.

Does Health Insurance Make a Difference?

Roger Herdman, *Assistant Director, OTA Health and Life Sciences Division*
Clyde Behney, *Health Program Manager*

INTRODUCTION

Health insurance coverage has been deemed to be an essential element of gaining access to health services. And the receipt of health services is often critical to maintaining and improving health. Yet, in 1990, an estimated 34.4 million individuals, or 15.7 percent of the U.S. population under age 65, were uninsured either all or part of the year (157,159). In addition, an unknown number of Americans were "underinsured": without adequate health insurance coverage. The large number of individuals without insurance raises two concerns: whether lack of coverage is associated with inequitable use of services; and, if so, whether such inequities result in differences in health outcomes.

This background paper reviews and evaluates the available literature linking health insurance coverage with the utilization and process of health care services and with individual health outcomes. The review was requested by the Senate Committee on Labor and Human Resources, and is part of a broader study on health insurance requested by that committee and endorsed by the Ranking Minority Member of the House Committee on Ways and Means Subcommittee on Health and by the House Committee on Energy and Commerce.

U.S. Congress, Office of Technology Assessment, *Does Health Insurance Make a Difference?—Background Paper*, OTA-BP-H-99 (Washington, DC: U.S. Government Printing Office, September 1992).

In this background paper, the term *health insurance* is used broadly, to include both private health insurance coverage and public coverage (including Medicaid, the State/Federal health care financing program for low-income persons). Private health insurance coverage is distinguished from public coverage whenever the data allow. *Utilization* of care is measured by counting particular health service events (e.g., a hospital stay or visit to a physician or other health care provider). The *process* of health care refers to the content and quality of an episode of health care—in other words, what actually happens—when services are received. Examples include the number and types of medical procedures employed, and patient satisfaction. *Health outcomes* are defined here in terms of health status (e.g., perceived health status, stage of sickness, death).

This background paper focuses on the mainstream medical care system (e.g., care provided by physicians for the diagnosis and treatment of overtly somatic [physical] illnesses). It does not examine access to services typically provided outside the mainstream medical care system (e.g., mental health or substance abuse problems, dental or oral health care, nutrition counseling). This background paper makes no attempt to explicitly address the potential effects of insurance-related variations in utilization, process, or outcomes of care on overall national health expenditures.

The chain of events linking insurance coverage to the receipt of health care and to patients' health outcomes is long, complex, and often indirect. Many factors other than insurance status have important effects on patterns of care and on health. Even if insurance does lead to greater use of health services, the impact of the services on health status may be minimal relative to other factors. For example, many have raised questions about the appropriateness of, or need for, a substantial portion of the health care delivered in the United States (e.g., 19,43,117). On the other hand, timely and effective health services can save, and improve the quality of, lives. Almost none of the available research on access and effectiveness analyzes the entire linkage from insurance coverage to utilization to health outcomes. Thus, this literature review had to rely upon building several bridges among available literatures. These literatures focus on relationships:

- between health insurance coverage and utilization of care;
- between health insurance coverage and the process of care when it is received; and
- between health insurance coverage and health outcomes.

The literature review in this background paper is limited to studies published since 1980 that addressed the topics of possible relationships between insurance coverage (or lack of it) and the use, process, or health outcomes of care. The focus is on studies that made some attempt to adjust methodologically for at least some potential alternative explanations for findings (e.g., patient's preexisting health status, income level, site of care). The literature synthesis focused first on whether studies found a relationship between insurance coverage and access to health care or between insurance coverage and health outcomes; then a subset of studies with the most recent data was used to examine the magnitude of the relationships.

KEY FINDINGS

Does health insurance make a difference? Research conducted in the last decade supports the common-sense notion that having or lacking health insurance coverage is related to gaining access to services, to the types, quality and intensity of the care that is delivered, and, logically, to patient health. Although the findings are not completely consistent, the research suggests the following:

- *Uninsured Americans* may be up to 3 times more likely than *private insured individuals* to experience a lower health care utilization rate, potentially inadequate health care, and adverse health outcomes.

- Publicly funded programs such as Medicaid have been developed to improve access to care for those individuals who do not have private coverage, and the available evidence suggests that *individuals with public coverage* may be slightly better off than those who are *uninsured.* When the health experiences of uninsured individuals have been compared with those of publicly covered individuals, uninsured Americans have been found to be up to 1.3 times more likely than publicly insured individuals to experience a lower health care utilization rate, and 1.5 times more likely to experience potentially inadequate health care.

- Publicly covered patients may be worse off than privately insured patients. *Publicly covered patients* are up to 2.5 times more likely than *private insured patients to* experience potentially inadequate health services, and up to 4 times more likely to experience an adverse health outcome.

Specific studies reviewed by OTA find that:

- Lack of insurance coverage may prevent individuals from seeking care. Studies show that uninsured individuals are less likely than privately insured individuals to have a usual source of care (64,73,118), use preventive services (124,189), visit a physician (99), and be hospitalized (31,99). Uninsured individuals are more likely to report that they have not received needed care (3,64).

- Consistent with individuals' self-reports about delaying the receipt of needed care, uninsured patients have been found to be up to 4 times as likely as insured patients to require both avoidable hospitalizations and emergency hospital care (e.g., 61,179). Some evidence suggests that uninsured patients may be up to twice as likely to be at risk of dying when they reach the hospital door (17,61).

- Even if the seeking or receipt of care is not delayed, uninsured patients who are hospitalized have been found to be half as likely as insured patients to receive certain high-cost (but not necessarily more appropriate and effective) procedures (61,129,177,183).

IMPORTANT CAVEATS AND OVERALL CONCLUSIONS

Despite the preponderance of findings showing an association among health insurance, access to care, and health status, some analyses have found no evidence of an independent relationship between insurance coverage and specific aspects of access and health (e.g., 27,60,119,177). Other analyses find that relationships among insurance coverage, access, and health vary by illness and medical procedure (179,183,189), by age, sex, or racial grouping (61), or by hospital (46). There is still considerable question about the nature of the measures used to gauge use, process, and outcomes of health care. There is considerable variability in study results. A range of results is not what would be expected if: insurance coverage was the sole determinant of health care delivery (and health); if public programs typically provided poorer financial coverage (or health care) than private coverage; if uninsured, privately insured, and publicly covered populations were homogeneous; and if measures were perfect. "Noncoverage" factors undoubtedly play some part in access to care and in patient health (e.g., 120,152,153,154,155).

Researchers typically acknowledge that alternative explanations for observed findings cannot be ruled out, and they continue to caution that results of existing studies cannot be viewed as definitive, given existing research approaches (e.g., 61,107,179). Use of prospective designs and better controls could make future studies more informative. Such studies may become more feasible as the health insurance environment continues to change. Given the variation and limitations in methods and data, and the lack of a complete theoretical model to explain the relationships, however, the level of consistent results is impressive. **For now, existing research supports common-sense notions and anecdotal evidence that availability of third party payment for health care can be important, in particular to gaining access to care and to the way care is delivered.**

ORGANIZATION OF THE BACKGROUND PAPER

The next section of this background paper provides supporting details about the literature review and synthesis conducted by OTA and its contractors. A variety of appendices, prepared by OTA, provide background information. Appendix A lists outside experts who contributed to the development of this background paper. Appendix B is a glossary of terms and abbreviations. Appendix C provides a conceptual framework for viewing the interrelationships among insurance coverage, access to and utilization of health services, the process of care, and individual health outcomes, and discusses general methodological issues in research on insurance status, access, and outcomes. Appendix D provides background information on the characteristics of individuals with and without insurance and information about what insurance coverage provides. Appendix E lists important methodological details on the multivariate research studies examined in this review. Appendix F consists of a brief overview of findings from the RAND Health Insurance Experiment.

The contractor paper which served as the basis for the review of the empirical literature on relationships among insurance coverage, utilization, process, and health outcomes (178) is available from OTA.

What Health-Care Crisis?

America's medical care is second to none—and available to all.

Fred Barnes

Bill and Hillary Clinton have contributed heavily to a national myth. Mrs. Clinton, as boss of the administration task force plotting to overhaul America's health-care system, refers routinely to "the health-care crisis." Her husband uses the same phrase ("Our government will never again be fully solvent until we tackle the health-care crisis," Clinton declared in his State of the Union address on February 17). And he goes one step further. "A lot of Americans don't have health insurance," he told a group of schoolkids February 20 during a nationally televised children's town meeting at the White House. "You know that, don't you? A lot of Americans don't have health care."

The press also trumpets the crisis theme. *Parade,* the popular Sunday supplement, emblazoned its February 28 cover with this headline: "THE GROWING CRISIS IN HEALTH CARE." The result is that the American people, despite their personal experiences, now believe there actually is a health-care crisis. Most opinion polls show roughly three-quarters of Americans are satisfied with the availability and quality of the health care they receive. Yet, in most polls, 60 to 70 percent feel the health-care system is failing and needs significant, if not radical, reform.

There is no health-care crisis. It's a myth. If millions of seriously ill Ameri-

---

Senior editor of the *New Republic.* The American Spectator, May 1993.

cans were being denied medical care, that *would* be a crisis. But that's not happening. Everyone gets health care in this country—the poor, the uninsured, everyone. No, our health-care system isn't perfect. There isn't enough primary care—regular doctor's visits—for many Americans. Emergency rooms are often swamped. The way hospitals and doctors are financed is sometimes bizarre. Health care may (or may not) be too costly. But it's the best health care system in the world—not arguably the best, but the best. Its shortcomings can be remedied by tinkering, or at least by less-than-comprehensive changes. An overhaul of the sort Hillary Clinton envisions is not only unnecessary, it's certain to reduce, not expand, the amount of health care Americans receive (price controls always lead to less of the controlled commodity). Then we really will have a health-care crisis.

You don't have to take my word that there's no crisis now and that health care here is the world's best. There's solid evidence. Let's examine four key aspects of the health care debate: access, false measures of quality health care, true measures, and how America's system compares with those of other industrialized democracies (Canada, Germany, Japan, Great Britain).

ACCESS

Will someone please tell Bill Clinton that having no health insurance is not the same as having no health care? The uninsured get health care, only less of it than the insured. Being uninsured means "one is more likely to use emergency-room care and less likely to use office, clinic, or regular inpatient care," said Richard Darman, President Bush's budget director, in congressional testimony in 1991. "This is not to suggest that this is desirable. It is not." But it *is* high-quality health care.

Doctors in emergency rooms are specialists. In fact, they have a professional organization, the American College of Emergency Physicians. Its motto is: "Our specialty is devoted to treating everyone in need, no questions asked." Turning away patients isn't an option. Federal law (section 9121 of the Consolidated Omnibus Budget Reconciliation Act of 1985) requires medical screening of everyone requesting care at a hospital emergency room. If treatment is needed, it must be provided. What this adds up to is "universal access" to health care in America, as one head of a hospital board told me.

It's no secret how much health care the uninsured get. The American Hospital Association estimated in 1991 that hospitals provide $10 billion in uncompensated care annually. Another study found that the 16.6 percent of the nonelderly population who are uninsured—36.3 million people—accounted for 11 percent of the nation's personal health-care expenditures in 1988. They had 37 percent fewer sessions with doctors and 69 percent fewer days in the hospital. There's a reason the uninsured get less health care, beyond the fact most work in low-paying jobs without health insurance. The uninsured tend to be young, thus healthy. According to a new poll by Frederick/Schneiders, 39 percent are 18–29 years of age and another 25 percent are 30–39. By the way, the elderly (65 and up), who require more medical care, are covered. Ninety-nine percent are eligible for Medicare.

To make sure we really have universal access, I checked on how victims of the most recent epidemic, AIDS, are treated. These are the folks doctors are supposed to be leery of dealing with.

What if a penniless AIDS patient showed up at, say, the Whitman-Walker Clinic in Washington, D.C.? That patient, even if indigent, gets treatment. When the time comes (T-cell count below 500), the patient is started on AZT, which costs about $5,000 a year. Later, the patient gets expensive, experimental drugs: DDI, DDC, D-4T. The drugs are paid for mostly by federal funds. There's also doctor care, painkillers, laboratory work. To prevent infections or complications, the patient is treated with prophylaxis.

A friend of mine volunteered to help an indigent, bedridden AIDS patient. He was amazed at the level of care. "It was an endless supply of extremely sophisticated drugs, an elaborate IV system [to feed the patient], and eventually a five-day-a-week home help nurse," my friend said. "Sometimes we had so much medicine, we had to throw it away. There was never a sense we'd be left in the lurch." The patient had no insurance. He lived with a boyfriend, but the boyfriend was not required to pay for any of the care. The federal and city governments—the taxpayers—footed the bill. The American Medical Association says "lifetime medical care" for a single AIDS patient costs $102,000.

FALSE TESTS

Judging by the two most common measures of health, life expectancy at birth and the infant mortality rate, health care in the United States is not the best or even among the best. In 1990, life expectancy in America was 72 years for males, 78.8 for women. This put the U.S. behind Canada, France, Germany, Italy, Japan, and Great Britain, among others. On infant mortality, the U.S. fared still worse, ranking nineteenth in 1989 with a rate of 9.7. (The infant mortality rate is the number of deaths of children under one year of age, divided by the number of births in a given year, multiplied by 1,000.) Finland, Spain, Ireland, East Germany, and Italy finished higher.

What's wrong with these measures? Just this: they're a reflection of health, not the health-care system. Life expectancy is determined by much more than the quality of a nation's health care. Social factors affect life expectancy, and this is where the U.S. runs into trouble. "Exacerbated social problems . . . adversely affect U.S. health outcomes," noted three Department of Health and Human Services officials in the fall 1992 issue of *Health Care Financing Review.* "The 20,000 annual U.S. homicides result in per capita homicide rates 10 times those of Great Britain and 4 times those of Canada. There are 100 assaults reported by U.S. emergency rooms for every homicide. About 25 percent of spinal cord injuries result from assaults." And so on. The incidence of AIDS is even more telling. Through June 1992, there were 230,179 reported AIDS cases here, two-thirds of whom have died. Japan, where life expectancy is four years longer for men than in the U.S. and three years longer for women, has had fewer than 300 AIDS cases. Once social factors have played out, the U.S. ranks at the top in life expectancy. At age 80, when most people are highly dependent on the health-care system, Americans have the longest life expectancy (7.1 years for men, 9.0 for women) in the world.

The infant mortality rate (IMR) is also "reflective of health and socioeconomic status and not just health care," wrote four Urban Institute scholars in the summer 1992 issue of *Health Care Financing Review.* And there are measurement problems. Many countries make no effort to save very-low-birth-weight infants. They aren't recorded as "live born" and aren't counted in infant mortality statistics. In contrast, American hospitals make heroic efforts in neonatal intensive care, saving some infants, losing others, and driving up the IMR. "The more resources a country's health-care system places on saving high-risk newborns, the more likely its registration will report a higher IMR," according to the Urban Institute scholars.

Social factors probably have a bigger impact. A poverty rate twice Canada's and Germany's, a rash of drug-exposed babies, a high incidence of unmarried teenage pregnancy—all lead to low-birth-weight infants and affect the IMR. "Infant mortality rates of babies born to unmarried mothers are about two times higher than the rates of babies born to married mothers," the scholars write. The point is not that America's high IMR is excusable, but that it's grown to abnormal levels in large part because of factors unrelated to the quality of health care.

Not only that. The entire medical system bears the brunt of social and behavioral problems that are far worse in the U.S. than in other industrialized democracies. "We have a large number of people who indulge in high-risk behavior," says Leroy L. Schwartz, M.D., of Health Policy International, a non-profit research group in Princeton, New Jersey. Behavioral problems become health problems: AIDS, drug abuse, assaults and violence, sexually transmitted diseases, etc. "The problem is not the health-care system," says Dr. Schwartz. "The problem is the people. Every year the pool of pathology in this country is getting bigger and bigger. We think we can take care of everything by calling it a health problem." But we can't.

REAL TESTS

While primary and preventive care are important, the best measure of a health-care system is how well it treats the seriously ill. What if you've got an enlarged prostate? Your chances of survival are better if you're treated here. The U.S. death rate from prostate trouble is one-seventh the rate in Sweden, one-fourth that in Great Britain, one-third that in Germany. Sweden, Great Britain, and Germany may have higher incidences of prostate illness, but not high enough to account for the wide disparity in death rates.

An ulcer of the stomach or intestine? The death rate per 100,000 persons is 2.7 in the U.S., compared to 2.8 in the Netherlands, 3.1 in Canada, 4.9 in

Germany, 7.6 in Sweden and 8 in Great Britain. A hernia or intestinal obstruction? The American death rate is 1.7. It's 2 in Canada, 2.7 in Germany, 3 in the Netherlands, 3.1 in Great Britain, and 3.2 in Sweden. Can these be attributed solely to varying incidences of ulcers and obstructions? Nope.

I could go on, and I will. The overall death rate from cancer is slightly higher in America than in Sweden or Germany, but lower than in Canada, the Netherlands, and Great Britain. But for specific cancers, the U.S. has the lowest death rate: stomach cancer, cervical cancer, uterine cancer. Only Sweden has a lower death rate from breast cancer. The U.S. also has the second lowest death rate from heart attack. No matter what the disease—epilepsy, hypertension, stroke, bronchitis—the U.S. compares well. For a country with a heterogeneous population and large pockets of pathology, this is remarkable. Life expectancy for American males at 65 is 14.7 years, only a tad less than Canada (15), Sweden (14.9), and Switzerland (14.9), more homogeneous countries with fewer social problems. (I'm grateful to Dr. Schwartz for all these figures.)

Another measure that's important is the proliferation of new technology. "Major medical technology has had a profound impact on modern medicine and promises even greater impact in the future," wrote Dale A. Rublee, an expert in cross-national health policy comparisons for the AMA's Center for Health Policy Research, in *Health Affairs*. He compared the availability of six technologies—open-heart surgery, cardiac catheterization, organ transplantation, radiation therapy, extracorporeal shock wave lithotripsy, and magnetic resonance imaging—in the U.S., Canada, and Germany in 1987. "Canada and Germany were selected because their overall health-care resources are fairly comparable to the United States," Rublee wrote. The U.S. came out ahead in every category, way ahead in several. In MRI's, the U.S. had 3.69 per one million people, Germany 0.94, Canada 0.46. For open-heart surgery, the U.S. had 3.26, Canada 1.23, Germany 0.74. For radiation therapy, the U.S. had 3.97, Germany 3.13, Canada 0.54. Small wonder that, as Rublee put it, "American physicians, with a universe of modern technology at their fingertips, are the envy of the world's physicians."

RIVAL SYSTEMS

Canadian politicians get special health care privileges, moving to the head of waiting lists or getting treatment at the elite National Defence Medical Centre. But that wasn't sufficient for Robert Bourassa, the premier of Quebec. He came to the National Cancer Institute in Bethesda, Maryland, for diagnosis, then returned to the U.S. for surgery, all at his own expense.

The Canadian health-care system has many nice attributes, but speedy treatment isn't one of them. Ian R. Munro, M.D., a Canadian doctor who emigrated to the U.S., wrote in *Reader's Digest* last September of a young boy in Canada who needed open-heart surgery to free the blood flow to his lungs. He was put on a waiting list. He got a surgery date only after news reports embarrassed health officials. After waiting two months, he died four hours before surgery. This was an extreme case, but waiting is common in the Canadian system, in which the government pays all costs, including set fees for private doctors. A study by the Fraser Institute in 1992 found that 250,000 people are awaiting medical care at any given time. "It is not uncommon for patients to wait months or even years for treatments such as cataract operations, hip replacements, tonsillectomies, gallbladder surgery, hysterectomies, heart operations, and major oral surgery," according to Edmund F. Haislmaier, the Heritage Foundation's health-care expert. Canada has other problems: health costs are rising faster than in the U.S., hospital beds and surgical rooms are dwindling, and doctors are fleeing (8,263 were practicing in the U.S. in 1990).

The Japanese model isn't any better. When Louis Sullivan, M.D., President Bush's secretary of health and human services, visited Japan, he was surprised to find medical care matched that of the U.S.—the U.S. of the 1950s. Japan has universal access and emphasizes primary care at clinics, financed mostly through quasi-public insurance companies. The problem is price controls. "Providers seek to maximize their revenue by seeing more patients," wrote Naoki Ikegami, professor of health at Keio University in Tokyo. "This dilutes the services provided."

Patients receive assembly-line treatment. "In outpatient care, a clinic physician sees an average of 49 patients per day [and] 13 percent see more than 100," Ikegami said. For the elderly, a survey found, the average number of doctor's visits for a six-month period was 17.3 (3.6 here) and the length of visits was 12 minutes (30 in the U.S.). Like Canada's queues, this is an extraordinarily inefficient way to dispense care. Patients return repeatedly to get the same care that in the U.S. is given in a single visit.

Japanese doctors also prescribe and sell drugs. Not surprisingly, they sell plenty. Thirty percent of the country's health expenditures are for drugs (7 percent in the U.S.). In Japan, wrote Ikegami, "no real incentives exist to maintain quality." The one exception is specialists at Japan's teaching hospitals. To avoid queues, patients pay bribes of $1,000 to $3,000 to be admitted to a private room and treated by a senior specialist.

Germany also has strict fees for doctors, with predictable results. Annual doctor's visits per capita are 11.5 (5.3 here), a figure exceeded only by Japan (12.9). In other words, price controls are as inefficient in Germany as in Japan. Hospitals face perverse incentives, too. The government pays a fixed rate per day, regardless of the patient's illness or length of stay. So hospitals pad their billings by keeping patients for unnecessarily long recuperations, which compensates for the losses they incur taking care of critically ill patients.

Then there's Great Britain, home of the National Health Service. Officials take great pride in having reduced the number of patients waiting more than two years for medical attention. In 1986, the number was 90,000; in 1991, 50,000. In April 1992, it was down to 1,600. Sounds great, but there's a catch. The number of patients waiting six months or less grew by 10 percent. The overall drop in waiting lists was only three percent. And this was achieved, a survey by the National Association of Health Authorities and Trusts found, chiefly because of a 13 percent hike in NHS spending in 1991, not increased efficiency. The good news in Great Britain is that private insurance is allowed and 6.6 million Brits have it. Insurance firms encourage beneficiaries to have an operation or other treatment in a private hospital. Sure, the company pays, but it knows that once a patient has experienced care in a private hospital, he'll never go back to the socialized medicine of NHS. And he'll keep buying health insurance. Private hospitals, anxious to fill empty beds, have their own come-on. At Christmas, they offer discount prices for operations.

In truth, the U.S. has little but painful lessons to learn from the health-care experience of other countries. There's practically nothing to emulate. On the contrary, foreign health officials, Germans especially, now look at the incentives in the American medical system as a way to remedy problems in their health care systems. Hillary Clinton and health policy wonks should stop apologizing for our system.

They won't. The existence of a few health care problems, chiefly the lack of proper primary care for several million Americans, allows them to declare a crisis and go on wartime footing. Liberals love this. Hillary's task force meets in private, keeps the names of its members secret, obsesses over leaks, spurns the advice of outsiders (doctors, Republicans). The problem that emerges is sure to dwarf the problem. If enacted, it will make the problem worse. This is a common phenomenon in Washington. Some people never learn.

In 1991, an American official addressed Russian health experts in Moscow. He bemoaned that many Americans get care at emergency rooms and occasionally wait six or eight hours. To the American's shock, the Russians erupted in laughter. In Russia, with twice as many doctors per capita as the U.S., a wait of six to eight hours represented unusually fast service.

Problems with Expanding Medicaid for the Uninsured

Jeffrey A. Buck,
Health Care Financing Administration
Mark S. Kamlet,
Carnegie Mellon University

Recently, a multiplicity of proposals has been put forth for addressing the problems of those without health insurance. Estimates place 31 to 33 million Americans in this category at any particular time (Congressional Budget Office 1991; Moyer 1989). Although the uninsured are not a new phenomenon, the issue has become more important as a result of rising medical costs, declining health insurance coverage, and the increasing problems of uncompensated care (Brown 1989; Friedman 1989; Kilpatrick et al. 1991).

Proposals for addressing the situation are wide-ranging, encompassing everything from a recommendation for a Canadian-style national health system (Himmelstein et al. 1989) to an outline for a predominately private one (Butler and Haislmaier 1989). Many proposals, however, seek to minimize disruptions to the existing health care system. They generally recommend increasing both employer health plans and the public financing of care for those who are unemployed or not potentially covered as a dependent of an employee.

Expanding the Medicaid program is frequently viewed as the chief means of extending public health coverage to the uninsured poor. Medicaid offers some important advantages for this purpose. First, it has an administrative structure

Journal of Health Politics, Policy and Law, Vol. 18, No. 1, Spring 1993.

already in place that can handle large numbers of beneficiaries. Second, it is oriented to the health needs of the poor. Finally, all states participate in the program and are fiscally committed to its support.

Despite the potential advantages of Medicaid expansion, serious problems remain to be addressed if it is to be successful. Current analyses of Medicaid expansion for the uninsured have generally ignored these problems. Instead, they have focused on the merits of particular recommendations and their associated costs.

One problem is the fiscal impact that Medicaid expansion will have on states. The size and range of these impacts call into question current financing arrangements for the program. Additionally, if Medicaid is to be a major element of a comprehensive national system of health care, differences between the program and private plans must be resolved. Otherwise, individuals may experience major disruptions in moving from one form of coverage to another or find themselves with significant incentives for choosing Medicaid in situations where they are eligible for other plans. Resolving the differences is also necessary if economies are to be fully realized in both sectors.

In this article, we examine a sample of proposals for the uninsured that include recommendations to enlarge the Medicaid program. In choosing proposals for review, we have selected among those whose recommendations for Medicaid expansion retain fundamental features of the program. Such features include shared federal and state financing of the program, state administration of benefits, and at least some state flexibility in determining eligibility, payment rates, and scope of benefits. Some proposals that may be labeled Medicaid reform, such as the bill for the Health-America Act, S. 1727, 102d Cong., 1st Sess. (1991), or the recommendations of the Pepper Commission (1990), in fact would so fundamentally change the program as to create a new one.

In this paper, we discuss first the similarities and differences among the selected expansion proposals and go on to present estimated costs of commonly made recommendations. We then illustrate the fiscal problems that these will cause for states. Finally, we outline major differences between Medicaid and private plans, presenting options for addressing each of the issues identified.

PROPOSAL FEATURES

The selected proposals and their major features are summarized in Table 1. They represent the kinds of recommendations made by major interest groups with different perspectives on the problems of the uninsured, including those of providers (American Medical Association [AMA] 1990), insurers (Health Insurance Association of America [HIAA] 1989), and Medicaid program administrators (American Public Welfare Association [APWA] 1988). Also presented in the table is the proposal of the Health Policy Agenda for the American People ([HPA] 1989), a coalition of public and private sector organizations.

Under the current Medicaid program, states must include all those who qualify for Aid to Families with Dependent Children (AFDC), nearly all those covered by the Supplemental Security Income (SSI) program, and certain other low-income groups (e.g., pregnant women and children). States may also cover various other low-income individuals at their option. Medicaid's focus on specific groups means that nearly half of the non-elderly below the poverty level are not eligible (Holahan and Zedlewski 1990). In response to this situation, all of the expansion proposals recommend uncoupling eligibility for Medicaid from eligibility for categorical assistance and replacing this with a single national income eligibility standard. The AMA proposal, however, would adjust this standard for each state by taking into account differences in each state's cost of living.

In addition to expanding basic eligibility, the APWA, HIAA, and HPA proposals would allow additional groups not meeting the initial income standard to participate in the program. HIAA and HPA would require "medically needy" programs in all states. These programs allow individuals not initially eligible for Medicaid coverage to become so by applying their medical expenses against their income to meet eligibility standards. Thirty-five states plus the District of Columbia had such programs in1989 (Health Care Financing Administration [HCFA] 1991a).

The current Medicaid program requires states to include certain basic services and offers them the option of including others. All but the HIAA proposal would change these provisions. The AMA and HPA proposals would retain all or nearly all of the current mandatory benefits plus require several more, such as dental services. In contrast, the APWA proposal would eliminate more than half of the number of existing mandatory benefits (e.g., home health services) but add others, such as well child care.

The HIAA proposal also would permit individuals and families with incomes between 100 percent and 150 percent of the poverty level to purchase a limited package of benefits. The APWA proposal would allow similar purchases of the complete benefit package for the unemployed with incomes above 75 percent of the poverty level. Both of these provisions would be accomplished through payment of an income-related premium, with Medicaid paying the balance up to some income limit. For Medicaid-eligible individuals who are employed, the HIAA proposal would allow states to pay the employee's out-of-pocket expenses associated with employer-offered plans. In contrast, the APWA proposal would expand the ability of states to impose cost sharing on Medicaid beneficiaries with incomes above the minimum standard.

Finally, the HPA proposal contains two provisions relating neither to benefits nor eligibility. The first would change the current cost-sharing formula by which the federal government determines what proportion of a state's Medicaid expenditures it reimburses. The second provision seeks to increase provider participation in the program, primarily by raising payment rates. We discuss both of these issues in detail below.

ESTIMATED COSTS OF PROPOSALS

Some of the recommendations would be costly. Estimates vary according to the particular data sources used; they also differ because of different assumptions about variables such as other program characteristics, eligibility requirements, and enrollment behavior, particularly of those with existing group insurance (Holahan and Zedlewsky 1990; Holahan et al. 1990; Needleman et al. 1990; Thorpe et al. 1989). Accordingly, estimates of the most important recommendations, those eliminating Medicaid's link to categorical program eligibility and establishing a national income eligibility standard, vary widely. The estimate of the total increase in costs for a national eligibility standard established at 100 percent of the poverty level ranges from $9 billion (Thorpe et al. 1989) to as much as $15 billion (Holahan et al. 1990: 17).

Estimates have not been published of the costs of the specific benefit packages outlined in the proposals we review here. However, some have been made of the additional expenditures that would be incurred if all states had a minimum package equal in actuarial value to the package now provided by a median state. If such a package were to be imposed on current beneficiaries, costs would be expected to increase by nearly $5 billion (Needleman et al. 1990: 151). If such a requirement were to be imposed after the eligible population had expanded under a noncategorical income standard, increased costs could range from $16–22 billion (Thorpe et al. 1989). Using a different methodology, though, Holahan et al. (1990: 21) place this figure at about $6 billion.

Some estimates have been made of other recommended features. A universal medically needy program for noninstitutionalized persons could add $2 billion to the program without any other changes (Needleman et al. 1990: 146). Raising physician payment rates to Medicare levels would be expected to increase expenditures by nearly $2 billion, if no other changes were made, and over $7 billion, if applied after a noncategorical income standard (Holahan et al. 1990: 19; Thorpe et al.1989). The latter amount could increase by an additional $3–4 billion if hospitals were reimbursed at the level of incurred costs (Thorpe et al. 1989).

Finally, one estimate has been made of the "buy in" recommendation. Such a feature would allow those with incomes immediately above the eligibility standard to obtain Medicaid coverage through the payment of an income-related premium. This provision has been viewed as one means of extending benefits to the uninsured at minimal cost. Nevertheless, it appears that such an option would be as expensive as any of the others presented here. If a third of persons with incomes between 100 and 185 percent of the poverty level took advantage of such a proposal by paying a premium equal to 5 percent of their income, and if a $250 family deductible and 20 percent coinsurance were imposed, such a provision could cost nearly $21 billion (Needleman et al. 1990: 177). Because of the low income of the target population, only about $3 billion would be generated by premium payments, for a net cost of $18 billion.

STATE FISCAL EFFORT AND EQUITY

In presenting the costs as we have just done, we do not mean to analyze specific proposals but to illustrate their potential total expense. Such costs affect both federal and state budgets. Estimates provided by the Urban Institute suggest a total increase of $20 billion for the two most commonly recommended changes—establishing a national categorical income standard at 100 percent of poverty and standardizing benefits at the median level (Holahan et al. 1990). Such an amount would represent a 37 percent increase in fiscal year 1989 Medicaid expenditures (Health Care Financing Administration 1990b). Of this sum, 56 percent, or $11 billion, would be the federal share, with the remainder falling to the states to fund. This amount is equivalent to a 1.2 percent increase in fiscal year 1989 federal tax revenues.

Knowing the effect of proposals on the total Medicaid budget, however, serves as a poor guide for gauging their effects on individual states. First, states vary significantly in their current AFDC (and, therefore, Medicaid) eligibility standards. To take the extremes, in 1989 Alabama's standard for a family of three was 14 percent of the poverty level, while Alaska's was 77 percent (National Governors' Association 1989: PC7). States also differ in their inclusion of optional eligibility groups. Thus, a national standard of 100 percent of the poverty level would require a much bigger change in some states than others.

A second reason concerns each state's income distribution. For any given national income standard, states have widely different percentages of their population that qualify for it. For instance, the 1980 census indicates that 7.9 percent of Wyoming's population falls below the poverty level while the corresponding figure for Mississippi is triple this, at 23.9 percent (U.S. Bureau of the Census 1989:452).

A third factor is differences in service costs and utilization. In 1988, for example, the average Medicaid expenditure for an AFDC adult in South Carolina was $1,433, while that in Ohio was $3,046 (Health Care Financing Administration 1988). Medicaid daily inpatient costs averaged $329 in Kansas in 1986, while they averaged $672 in California (Health Care Financing Administration 1987). These differences not only reflect varied utilization and practice patterns but also input costs. To take one comparison, physicians' input costs are estimated to be two-thirds higher in Alaska than in Arkansas (Welch et al. 1989).

Implications for Expansion Proposals

Generally, proposals for Medicaid expansion have ignored state fiscal impact issues despite the genuine dilemma that they pose for implementation. Only the AMA proposal touches on this area, by recommending that a national income eligibility standard be adjusted for state differences in cost of living. As described above, however, such differences are only one factor contributing to variations in state fiscal burden.

Three areas should be addressed in examining solutions for the fiscal problems of Medicaid expansion. First, the overall percentage of federal participation in the program should be evaluated. If Medicaid is to be a major part of a national health care system, financing should reasonably balance the fiscal burden of the program between states and the federal government. Second, indices other than state per capita income should be examined as a basis for compensating states based on their ability to pay. Finally, methods of reflecting the actual fiscal burden of a state's program need to be identified.

Failure to address these issues will likely have serious consequences. Fiscal stress resulting from Medicaid expansions enacted in the 1980s have already resulted in states eliminating some optional services or eligibility groups, or reducing the scope of benefits (U.S. General Accounting Office 1991). Indigent services to non-Medicaid groups have been reduced. These actions resulted from changes in net state Medicaid spending that increased Medicaid's net share of state revenues by *less than 1 percent* over a five-year period (U.S. General Accounting office 1991). In contrast, the least impacted of the states we have illustrated (Wisconsin) would experience spending increases more than twice this level, presumably over a shorter period of time. Further, we have illustrated these impacts for only two of the expansion recommendations. Others could increase the estimated amounts by 50 percent or more (see section on estimated costs).

COMPARISON TO PRIVATE PLANS

In addition to ignoring state fiscal issues, proposals for Medicaid expansion have overlooked differences with private insurance plans. These differences will become more important as ways are sought to create a system of health care financing that provides some source of coverage for all Americans. Failure to address them could seriously disrupt care for those moving between Medicaid and other plans. For those working poor who might be eligible for both Medicaid and an employer-sponsored plan, the incentives to move out of private plans could greatly expand the Medicaid population beyond desired levels. Additionally, Medicaid restrictions on the use of cost control methods could make an expanded program more expensive than it need be. Finally, a Medicaid program that is part of a comprehensive health care system will need to justify methods of payment and service organization that differ significantly from other sectors. Proposals for Medicaid expansion need to address these problems and suggest solutions to them.

There are five important areas of difference between Medicaid and private health insurance: benefits, cost sharing, managed care, cost containment, and provider payment. In each area, we will contrast Medicaid with private insurance plans and discuss applicable elements of the expansion proposals. For some, an expanded Medicaid program may benefit from becoming more like the private sector, while for others the opposite may be preferable.

Benefits

It is not possible to make detailed comparisons between Medicaid and private health insurance benefits, because state Medicaid programs and private plans vary widely and administrators and surveyors define terms in different ways. Nevertheless, by comparing state Medicaid information collected by the Health Care Financing Administration (1990a) with that of private plan surveys conducted by the HIAA and the Bureau of Labor Statistics (Sullivan and Rice 1991; U.S. Department of Labor 1990) we can make some general characterizations.

If services offered by 50 percent or more of state Medicaid programs are contrasted with those for 50 percent or more of private employees with coverage, the most important observation is that Medicaid enrollees have a much richer package of benefits than private employees. A majority of states cover the following services under Medicaid that are not covered for a majority of people in employee plans: dental care, vision care, personal care, rehabilitative services, and extended nursing home care. Further, unlike Medicaid beneficiaries, an employee must wait an average of nine months before receiving coverage for a preexisting condition.

Certainly, the more extensive coverage of Medicaid partly reflects a concern that the poor could not purchase any kind of health care without having some kind of coverage. It may also indicate that some of the groups within the Medicaid population (e.g., those with physical disabilities) have special needs. There would be little disagreement with such arguments, were Medicaid to continue to be limited to current groups. However, the reasoning becomes much weaker if the recommendations to uncouple Medicaid from categorical eligibility and to increase the income limit were to be implemented.

Under such circumstances, issues of economy and perceived equity become more important. A richer benefit package not only limits the degree to which Medicaid may be expanded for a given level of resources. Because low-income workers could qualify for both Medicaid and employer-offered health insurance, more generous benefits could create incentives for them or their dependents to abandon employer coverage in favor of Medicaid. Finally, as greater numbers receive such benefits, political opposition to the program might increase from those with less generous private coverage.

Accordingly, proposals for the uninsured must assess the trade-offs between benefit generosity and eligibility expansion. Only the AMA proposal for a standard benefit package appears to fully recognize this problem. It would restrict federal funding to a group of benefits substantially more limited than that now provided by most states. The other proposals would either establish a more generous package (HPA) or limited benefits only for groups above a particular income level (APWA and HIAA).

Cost Sharing

Generally, state Medicaid programs are severely restricted in their ability to impose cost sharing on beneficiaries. For instance, the categorically needy generally cannot be charged premiums, and significant numbers of services (e.g., child or emergency services) cannot be subject to copayments or deductibles for most eligibility groups. Where cost sharing is permitted, states may usually charge only nominal amounts (e.g., a $0.50 copayment on each drug prescription).

Limits on cost sharing in Medicaid probably stem from concerns for the low-income population that uses medical care, as well as from Medicaid's origin in an era when first-dollar coverage in private indemnity plans was common. This situation has changed, however. Although the percentage of consumer expenditures for health care paid out of pocket declined in the seventies, this trend reversed in the eighties. Such expenditures are now increasing at a real annual rate of 4.8 percent (Short 1988). Currently, an average employee in a conventional plan has an annual deductible of about $200 and a family deductible of $450. Most also have a coinsurance rate of 20 percent (Sullivan and Rice 1991).

The best evidence about the possible effects of increasing cost sharing for the Medicaid population comes from the RAND Health Insurance experiment (Lohr et al. 1986). This study examined the effects of different levels of coinsurance on utilization and health status. It found that coinsurance affected outpatient utilization primarily by reducing the probability of visits, rather than their intensity. This effect was strongest for poor children. Although the overall effect of cost sharing on general health outcomes was minimal, the differences that were detected were more concentrated in the study's low-income group. This group contained many individuals with incomes above the federal poverty level, who might reasonably be included in a Medicaid expansion.

While this evidence does not strongly support increased cost sharing in an expanded Medicaid program, neither does it justify continuing current restrictions. Imposing premium payments would discourage an expansion of the covered population unless it was done involuntarily, such as through an income tax surcharge. Increasing the use of deductibles and coinsurance, on the other hand, offers the possibility of greater Medicaid expansion through the reductions such requirements produce in per capita expenditures. Only the APWA proposal recommends such a change. Such proposals merit consideration, not only to allow limited resources to reach more people, but again to reduce incentives for individuals to leave existing plans with cost sharing for an expanded Medicaid program.

Managed Care

Another area in which Medicaid differs significantly from the private sector is in the use of managed care, an area not addressed by any of the expansion proposals. In 1990, 20 percent of Americans with employer-sponsored coverage were enrolled in HMOs (Sullivan and Rice 1991). Another 18 percent participated in PPOs or point-of-service plans, which often include capitation or other financial incentives for providers to limit unnecessary utilization (Sullivan and Rice 1991; Hoy et al. 1991). In contrast, Medicaid enrollment in capitated plans is only about a quarter of this level (Health Care Financing Administration 1991b). In 1990, about 8 percent of Medicaid beneficiaries participated in an HMO-type system (federally or state-qualified HMO, or a prepaid health plan, and less than 1 percent in some sort of partial capitation arrangement (primarily a health insuring organization).

Several explanations exist for this difference. First, states must seek waivers of some regulations and meet other requirements to be able to establish capitated plans within their Medicaid programs. As of 1990, twenty-two state Medicaid programs had no capitated plans of any kind (Health Care Financing Administration 1991b). Second, even when such requirements have been met, HMOs may be reluctant to participate in such programs. Negative perceptions of the Medicaid population, their rate of turnover, difficulties in marketing to this group, and concerns about contracting with state government all have been cited as contributing to this situation (Congressional Research Service 1988; Spitz and Abramson 1987). Finally, when capitated plans are available, Medicaid enrollees have few incentives to participate in them, and states are limited in their ability to mandate such participation (Congressional Research Service 1988: 424; Welch and Miller 1989).

Even if fuller use were to be made of managed care in Medicaid, it is not certain what the outcomes would be. Within Medicaid, managed care has been expected to reduce expenditures by decreasing beneficiaries' reliance on multiple health care providers and emergency room care. At the same time, improvement in access and service quality has been sought through identifying a single source of care and guaranteeing adequate physician participation (Freund and Hurley 1987; Long and Settle 1988).

Regarding the first goal, some studies have shown significant savings from Medicaid managed care programs, while others have documented none, or found increased expenditures (Freund et al. 1989; Welch 1990). Findings concerning effects on access and quality of care also have been inconsistent (Freund et al.1989; Hohlen et al. 1990; Hurley et al. 1989; Ware et al. 1986). Nevertheless, in the absence of clear evidence to the contrary, expansion proposals should strongly consider allowing state Medicaid programs the same freedom to use managed care as the private sector.

Cost Containment

Medicaid expansion proposals also have not addressed the differences between Medicaid and private plans in the use of cost containment strategies. Private fee-for-service/indemnity plans have increased their use of such methods in recent years (Gabel et al. 1989; Sullivan and Rice 1991). Seventy-nine percent of conventional employer plans now require preadmission certification for inpatient care (Sullivan and Rice 1991). Half or more also utilize concurrent utilization review, mandatory second opinions, and case management for large claims and mental health services.

The use of such strategies can lower costs. Studies of preadmission certification and concurrent utilization review in the private sector, for instance, have shown significant reductions in admissions and days of care (Scheffler et al. 1991; Wickizer et al. 1990). Indemnity plans that use cost containment strategies are experiencing lower premium increases than those that are not (Woolsey 1990).

Cost containment has also been employed by state Medicaid agencies, in particular, preadmission certification, concurrent utilization review, and mandatory second opinions. Nevertheless, agencies may not be using such strategies as extensively as the private sector or in ways that produce similar results.

Surveys of employers indicate that hospital preadmission certification and case management of large (or potentially large) medical claims are the most effective cost containment methods (Geisel 1990a, 1990b). When used in the private sector, preadmission certification is generally mandatory and conducted by insurance companies, often using personnel who are not physicians.

In contrast, Medicaid regulations merely require that the need for hospital admission be certified by a physician. Only about 60 percent of states responding to a survey of cost containment strategies said that they had a formal preadmission certification program (Lindsey 1989). Of these, the majority contracted with peer review organizations (PROs) as the authorizing agency. Medicaid and Medicare regulations encourage PROs to be constituted primarily of physicians. They also discourage insurance companies that may perform such functions in the private sector from qualifying for PRO status. 42 C.F.R. § 462.107 (1991). Lastly, many Medicaid preadmission certification programs exempt different types of admissions from review and a majority will still reimburse a hospital if a patient is admitted without advance approval (Lindsey 1989).

Case management of large medical claims is a more recent cost containment measure used by the private sector. Under this strategy, patients generating or predicted to generate large claims are identified and assigned to a case manager. The case manager then helps plan the most cost-effective treatment and assists in obtaining necessary care. Again, such programs are often conducted by insurance companies or specialized managed care firms.

Although state Medicaid agencies are increasing their use of case management programs, the nature of such programs generally differs from that of the private sector. This is partly due to the lack of specific goals and definitions in the applicable Medicaid regulations (Spitz and Abramson 1987). As a result, there are a variety of types of case management programs (Hurley and Freund 1988). Some of these are really managed care strategies that place providers at partial financial risk (see section on managed care). Others, however, have sought to better coordinate care while also performing a gatekeeping function through limiting access to a single point of entry. This is often done by assigning enrollees to individual physicians who agree to serve as a primary provider, often in return for an enhanced fee. Limited information is available about such programs but they may only change utilization patterns while not affecting or actually increasing associated expenditures (Hohlen et al. 1990; Hurly et al. 1989; Long and Settle 1988).

Notwithstanding their effectiveness or lack of it, Medicaid case management programs are unlike those in the private sector in two fundamental respects. First, they have not limited their focus to high-cost cases. Second, they have generally used providers rather than third parties as case managers, reducing incentives for providing certain kinds of cost-effective care. These differences mean that they are unlikely ever to reproduce results that may be obtained by private plans, without substantially changing their current characteristics and focus.

Expansion proposals should explicitly consider the advantages of increasing the use of cost containment strategies in the Medicaid program. Alternatively, they should determine if practices in use for the current Medicaid population are desirable for an expanded, noncategorical one, or if those in use by the private sector merit continuing under a national system of health coverage.

Provider Payment

Only the HPA proposal addresses the remaining major area of difference between Medicaid and private sector plans: levels of provider payment. In 1986, for instance, inpatient revenue averaged $539 per day, while Medicaid costs per inpatient day averaged $490 (American Hospital Association 1986; Health Care Financing Administration 1987). A survey of three states found that 1987 Medicaid payments for twenty diagnosis-related groups (DRGs) averaged from $964 (26 percent) to $2,150 (51 percent) lower per DRG than the Medicare payment (U.S. General Accounting Office 1990b: 20). Probably as a result of these differences, it is estimated that Medicaid payments fully covered costs in only 12.7 percent of hospitals in 1989 (Fraser et al. 1991).

Most of the interest in this area, however, has focused on payments to physicians. Medicaid physician spending declined in constant dollars from 1979 to 1984, and fees declined relative to Medicare (Cohen 1989). This trend was accompanied by a general shift in Medicaid payment methodology from a "customary, prevailing, and reasonable" basis, such as that used in Medicare, to one using a fee schedule that can be independent of prevailing charges. Perhaps as a result, a 1984 study found that half of states paid less than 80 percent of Medicare levels, with the lowest under 40 percent (Holahan 1984). A more recent investigation yielded similar results, with state Medicaid fees averaging 64 percent of Medicare-allowed charges (Physician Payment Review Commission 1991).

Because of differences in payment rates, concerns have been expressed about whether services are available to Medicaid beneficiaries to the same extent as they are for those with private coverage. Only a small percentage of hospitals appear to discourage the admission of Medicaid patients (Schlesinger et al. 1987). In contrast, studies generally have found a positive relationship between Medicaid fee levels and physician participation (e.g., Held and Holahan 1985). Whether low fees have led to decreases in needed services, though, is not well established. One study found a minimal reduction in some physicians' participation (Perloff et al. 1986) while another actually found an increase (Mitchell 1990). Others have suggested that fewer physician office visits may be offset by increases in other types of care (Cohen 1989; Long et al. 1986).

Congress recently increased requirements for states to demonstrate that they provide services within the Medicaid program equivalent to that for the general population. Social Security Act §§ 1902(a)(30)(A), 1926 (1991). This legislation makes it clear that increased fees should be the chief means of achieving this goal. Nevertheless, other factors also influence provider participation (e.g., payment delay), meaning that states may be able to increase participation through other means (Perloff et al. 1986).

It is possible that current state Medicaid reimbursement policies represent reasonable efforts to promote economical medical care for their beneficiaries. Under an expanded program, though, increased numbers would be covered by such policies. Many would experience major disruptions in continuity of care in the transition from such programs to private ones with very different payment rates. For this reason, expansion proposals need to recommend solutions for this problem. Such recommendations might result in higher Medicaid rates, or identify areas in which private plans should reduce theirs.

SUMMARY

Medicaid offers some important advantages for extending health care coverage to the uninsured poor, including an existing administrative structure and strong fiscal support by states. Medicaid expansion proposals commonly advocate eliminating categorical eligibility for the program and establishing a single national eligibility standard based on income. Another frequent recommendation is to create a new set of mandatory benefits, usually to reduce disparities between state programs.

Those advocating Medicaid expansion for the uninsured have focused on the desirability of particular proposal features. To a lesser degree, they also have estimated the cost of their recommendations. Unfortunately, these efforts have ignored important problems that must be addressed before realistic Medicaid expansion can be accomplished.

The most serious of these problems is the fiscal impact that Medicaid expansion would have on states. The current federal Medicaid matching formula fails to reflect either a state's Medicaid burden or its capacity to pay for the program. Under it, states would have to increase their revenues proportionally much more than the federal government to pay for expansion. Equally important, the fiscal impacts would not be uniformly distributed, with some states required to increase revenues proportionally more than three times as much as others. Contrary to common opinion, the degree of fiscal impact would have little relationship to a state's Medicaid program generosity.

Medicaid expansion proposals also have overlooked important differences between the program and private insurance plans. Compared to a majority of private plans, Medicaid offers a richer benefit package and requires little or no cost sharing from beneficiaries. It also uses managed care and cost containment strategies much less than the private sector. Generally, it reimburses providers less than other payers.

These differences pose serious obstacles to Medicaid expansion. The more generous benefits that Medicaid offers could create adverse migration incentives for those eligible for both Medicaid and an employer-sponsored plan. Medicaid restrictions on cost sharing, managed care, and cost containment strategies limit potential program economies. Differences in payment rates will raise issues of perceived equity and continuity of care.

Medicaid expansion proposals must address these fiscal and structural problems if they are to succeed. Most important, they need to acknowledge the fiscal problems that Medicaid expansion will create for states and how the Medicaid matching formula contributes to them. Solutions to these problems will almost certainly require changes in current financing arrangements.

There are a variety of possible solutions to the structural problems associated with Medicaid expansion. How desirable each is partly depends on changes expected for other parts of the health services system. Nevertheless, a general goal for Medicaid expansion proposals should be to reduce the differences between the Medicaid program and private sector plans. This may ultimately prove to be more important than any action to reduce state program disparities. Both Medicaid and the private sector may have to change.

Although the fiscal and structural problems of Medicaid expansion require solution, they do not argue against the desirability of such expansion. Rather, they should be viewed as resulting from a change in the program's original purpose of providing medical assistance to welfare recipients. Despite its difficulties, Medicaid has generally fulfilled this purpose. In proposing a new and larger role for the program, its governing assumptions may need to change. Doing so may allow Medicaid to meet new objectives.

References

Advisory Commission on Intergovernmental Relations, 1990. *1988 State Fiscal Capacity and Effort*. Report No. M-170. Washington, DC: Advisory Commission on Intergovernmental Relations.

American Hospital Association. 1986. *National Hospital Panel Survey Reports*. Chicago: American Hospital Association.

American Medical Association. 1990. *Health Access America.* Chicago: American Medical Association.

American Public Welfare Association. 1988. *Investing in Poor Families and their Children: A Matter of Commitment*. Washington, DC: American Public Welfare Association.

Brown, E. R. 1989. Access to Health Insurance in the United States. *Medical Care Review* 46 (4): 349–85.

Butler, S. M., and E. F. Haislmaier. 1989. *A National Health System for America.* Washington, D.C.: Heritage Foundation.

Cohen, J. W. 1989. Medicaid Policy and the Substitution of Hospital Outpatient Care for Physician Care. *Health Services Research* 24 (1): 33–66.

Congressional Budget Office. 1991. *Selected Options for Expanding Health Insurance Coverage*. Washington, D.C.: U.S. Government Printing Office. July.

Congressional Research Service, 1988. *Medicaid Source Book: Background Data and Analysis*. Washington, D.C.: U.S. Government Printing Office.

Fraser, I., J. Narcross, and P. Kralovec. 1991. Medicaid Shortfalls and Total Unreimbursed Hospital Care for the Poor, 1980–1989. *Inquiry* 28 (Winter): 385–92.

Freund, D. A. and R. E. Hurley. 1987. Managed Care in Medicaid: Selected Issues in Program Origins, Design, and Research. *Annual Review of Public Health* 8:137: 137–63.

Freund, D. A., L. F. Rossiter, P. D. Fox, J. A. Meyer, R. E. Hurley, T. S. Carey, and J. E. Paul. 1989. Evaluation of the Medicaid Competition Demonstrations. *Health Care Financing Review* 11 (2): 81–97.

Friedman, E. 1989. Hospital Uncompensated Care: Crisis? *Journal of the American Medical Association* 262 (21): 2975–77.

Gabel, J., S. DiCarlo, S. Fink, and G. de Lissovoy. 1989. *The Health Insurance Picture in 1988.* Washington, D.C.: Health Insurance Association of America.

Geisel, J. 1990a. Firms Assess Value of Cost Control Tools. *Business Insurance,* 5 February, pp. 1, 23.

______. 1990b. Poll Rates UR Tools on Ability to Cut Cost. *Business Insurance,* 19 February, pp. 67–68.

Health Care Financing Administration. 1988. *Statistical Report on Medical Care: Eligibles, Recipients, Payments, and Services.* Baltimore, MD: Health Care Financing Administration.

______. 1990a. *Medicaid Services State by State.* HCFA Publ. No. 02155-91. Baltimore, MD: Health Care Financing Administration.

______. 1990b. *Quarterly Statement of Expenditures for the Medical Assistance Program.* Baltimore, MD: Health Care Financing Administration.

______. 1991a. *Medicare and Medicaid Data Book, 1990.* HCFA Publ. No. 03270. Baltimore, MD: Health Care Financing Administration.

______. 1991b. *Report on Medicaid Managed Care Enrollment.* Baltimore, MD: Medicaid Managed Care Office.

Health Care Financing Administration, Office of the Actuary. 1987. Unpublished data on incurred inpatient hospital cost per day. Baltimore, MD: Health Care Financing Administration.

Health Insurance Association of America. 1989. *Proposal for Financing Health Care for Americans.* Washington, D.C.: Health Insurance Association of America.

Health Policy Agenda for the American People. 1989. *Including the Poor.* Chicago, IL: American Medical Association.

Held, P. J., and J. Holahan. 1985. Containing Medicaid Costs in an Era of Growing Physician Supply. *Health Care Financing Review* 7 (1): 49–60.

Himmelstein, D. U., S. Woolhandler, and the Writing Committee of the Working Group on Program Design. 1989. A National Health Program for the United States: A Physicians' Proposal. *New England Journal of Medicine* 320: 102–8.

Hohlen, M. M., L. M. Manheim, G. V. Fleming, S. M. Davidson, B. K. Yudkowsky, S. M. Werner, and G. M. Wheatley. 1990. Access to Office-based Physicians under Capitation Reimbursement and Medicaid Case Management. *Medical Care* 28 (1): 59–68.

Holahan, J. 1984. Paying for Physician Services in State Medicaid Programs. *Health Care Financing Review* 5 (3): 99–110.

Holahan, J., and S. Zedlewski. 1990. *Insuring Low-Income Americans: Is Medicaid the Answer?* Washington, DC: Urban Institute.

Holahan, J., S. Zedlewski, and C. Winterbottom. 1990. *Estimating the Cost of Medicaid Eligibility and Benefit Uniformity.* Working Paper No. 3836-04. Washington, D.C.: Urban Institute.

Hoy, E. W., R. E. Curtis, and T. Rice. 1991. Change and Growth in Managed Care. *Health Affairs* 10 (4): 18–36.

Hurley, R. E., and D. A. Freund. 1988. A Typology of Medicaid Managed Care. *Medical Care* 26 (8): 764–74.

Hurley, R. E., D. A. Freund, and D. E. Taylor. 1989. Gatekeeping the Emergency Department: Impact of a Medicaid Primary Care Case Management Program. *Health Care Management Review* 14 (2): 63–71.

Hutchison, T. 1990. The Medicaid Budget Tangle. *State Legislatures*, March, pp. 15–19.

Kilpatrick, K.E., M. K. Miller, J. W. Dwyer, and D. Nissen. 1991. Uncompensated Care

Provided by Private Practice Physicians in Florida. *Health Services Research* 26 (3): 277–302.
Lindsey, P. A. 1989. Medicaid Utilization Control Programs: Results of a 1987 Study. *Health Care Financing Review* 10 (4): 79–92.
Lohr, K. N., R. H. Brook, C. J. Kamberg, G. A. Goldberg, A. Leibowitz, J. Keesey. D. Regoussin, and J. P. Newhouse. 1986. *Use of Medical Care in the RAND Health Insurance Experiment*. No. R-3469-HHS. Santa Monica. CA: RAND.
Long, S. H., and R. F. Settle. 1988. An Evaluation of Utah's Primary Care Case Management Program for Medicaid Recipients. *Medical Care* 26 (11): 1021–32.
Long, S. H., R. F. Settle, and B. C. Stuart. 1986. Reimbursement and Access to Physicians' Services under Medicaid. *Journal of Health Economics* 5:235–51.
Mitchell, J. B. 1990. Physician Participation in Medicaid Revisited. Paper presented at the meeting of the American Public Health Association, New York, NY, 30 September–4 October.
Moyer, E. M. 1989. A Revised Look at the Number of Uninsured Americans. *Health Affairs* 8 (2): 102–15.
National Governors' Association. 1989. *Catalogue of State Medicaid Program Changes: 1989*. Washington, D.C.: National Governors' Association.
Needleman, J., J. Arnold, J. Sheils, and L. S. Lewin. 1990. *The Health Care Financing System and the Uninsured.* Washington, D.C.: Lewin/ICF.
Office of Management and Budget. 1990. *Budget of the United States Government, Fiscal Year 1991*. Washington, D.C.: Government Printing Office.
Pepper Commission (U.S. Bipartisan Commission on Comprehensive Health Care). 1990. *A Call for Action*. S. Prt. No. 101-114. Washington, D.C.: U.S. Government Printing Office.
Perloff, J. D., P. R. Kletke, and K. M. Neckerman. 1986. Recent Trends in Pediatrician Participation in Medicaid. *Medical Care* 24 (8): 749–60.
Physician Payment Review Commission. 1991. *Physician Payment under Medicaid.* Report No. 91-4. Washington, D.C.: Physician Payment Review Commission.
Scheffler, R. M., S. D. Sullivan, and T. H. Ko. 1991. The Impact of Blue Cross and Blue Shield Plan Utilization Management Programs, 1980–1988. *Inquiry* 28 (Fall): 263–75.
Schlesinger, M., J. Bentkover, D. Blumentahl, R. Musacchio, and J. Willer. 1987. The Privatization of Health Care and Physicians' Perceptions of Access to Hospital Services. *Milbank Quarterly* 65 (1): 25–58.
Short, P. F. 1988. Trends in Employee Health Benefits. *Health Affairs* 7 (3): 186–96.
Spitz, B., and J. Abramson. 1987. Competition, Capitation, and Case Management: Barriers to Strategic Reform. *Milbank Quarterly* 65 (3): 348–70.
Sullivan, C. B., and T. Rice. 1991. The Health Insurance Picture in 1990. *Health Affairs* 10 (2): 104–15.
Swartz, K., and T. D. McBride. 1990. Spells without Health Insurance: Distributions of Durations and Their Link to Point-in-Time Estimates of the Uninsured. *Inquiry* 27 (3): 281–88.
Thorpe, K. E., J. E. Siegel, and T. Dailey. 1989. Including the Poor: The Fiscal Impacts of Medicaid Expansion. *Journal of the American Medical Association* 261 (7): 1003–7.
U.S. Bureau of the Census. 1989. *Statistical Abstract of the United States: 1989*. (109th ed.). Washington, D.C.: U.S. Government Printing Office.
U.S. Department of Commerce. 1990. *State Government Tax Collections, 1989*. Report No. GF-89-1. Washington, D.C.: U.S. Government Printing Office.
U.S. Department of Labor, Bureau of Labor Statistics. 1990. *Employee Benefits in Medium and Large Firms, 1989*. Bulletin No. 2363. Washington, D.C.: U.S. Government Printing Office.
U.S. Department of the Treasury, Office of State and Local Finance. 1985. *Federal-State-Local Fiscal Relations*. Washington, D.C.: U.S. Government Printing Office.

U.S. General Accounting Office. 1983. *Changing Medicaid Formula Can Improve Distribution of Funds to States*. Report No. GGD-83-27. Washington, D.C.: U.S. Government Accounting Office.

______. 1990a. Medicaid Formula: Fairness Could Be Improved. Statement of Janet L. Shikles before the Subcommittee on Human Resources and Intergovernmental Relations Committee on Government Operations, House of Representatives, 7 December.

______. 1990b. *Medicare: Comparative Analyses of Payments for Selected Hospital Services*. Report No. HRD-90-108. Washington, D.C.: U.S. General Accounting Office.

______. 1991. *Medicaid Expansions: Coverage Improves but State Fiscal Problems Jeopardize Continued Progress.* Report No. HRD-91-78: Washington, D.C.: U.S. General Accounting Office.

Ware, J.E., Jr., R. H. Brook, W. H. Rogers, E. B. Keeler, A. R. Davies, C. D. Sherbourne, G. A. Goldberg, P. Camp, and J. P. Newhouse. 1986. Comparison of Health Outcomes at a Health Maintenance Organisation with Those of Fee-for-Service Care. *Lancet* 1 (3 May): 1017–22.

Welch, W. P. 1990. Giving Physicians Incentives to Contain Costs under Medicaid. *Health Care Financing Review* 12 (2): 103–12.

Welch, W. P., and M. E. Miller. 1989. Mandatory HMO Enrollment in Medicaid: The Issue of Freedom of Choice. *Milbank Quarterly* 66 (4): 618–39.

Welch, W. P., S. Zuckerman, and G. Pope. 1989. *The Geographic Medicare Economic Index: Alternative Approaches*. Working Paper No. 89–2. Baltimore: Office of Research and Demonstrations, Health Care Financing Administration.

Wickizer, T. M., P. J. Feldstein, J. R. C. Wheeler, and M. C. McDonald. 1990. Reducing Hospital Use and Expenditures through Utilization Review: Findings from an Outcome Evaluation. *Quality Assurance and Utilization Review* 5 (3): 80–85.

Woolsey, C. 1990. Health Plan Rate Hikes Moderate at Midyear. *Business Insurance*. 20 August, pp. 1, 29–30.

The History and Principles of Managed Competition

Alain C. Enthoven

To understand the procompetition movement and the idea of managed competition, one must first understand the history of the noncompetitive system we have today. The word *competition* as used by economists, if not qualified by some phrase indicating the contrary (such as *nonprice competition*), means price competition. When there is price competition, suppliers compete to serve customers who are using their own money or are otherwise motivated to obtain maximum value for money. *Price competition* does not mean that price is the only factor influencing the customer's choice. Quality and product features also enter in. It simply means that price is one of the factors. Perhaps *value-for-money competition* would be a more apt phrase. One of the striking features of the U.S. health care economy to date is how little value-for-money competition there is.

Charles Weller has described our traditional system of fee-for-service, solo (or small, single-specialty group) practice, free choice of provider, and payment by a remote third party as "guild free choice."[1] The principles of this system and their economic consequences are as follows: (1) Free choice of doctor by the patient, which means that the insurer has no bargaining power with the doctor; (2) free choice of prescription by the doctor, which prevents the insurer from applying quality assurance or review of appropriateness; (3) direct negotiation between doctor and patient regarding fees, which excludes the third-party payer,

Health Affairs Supplement 1993

1. C. D. Weller, " 'Free Choice' as a Restraint of Trade in American Health Care Delivery and Insurance," *Iowa Law Review* (July 1984): 1351–1392.

who would be likely to have information, bargaining power, and an incentive to negotiate to hold down fees; (4) fee-for-service payment, which allows physicians maximum control over their incomes by increasing the services provided; and (5) solo practice, because multispecialty group practice constitutes a break in the seamless web of mutual coercion through control of referrals that the medical profession has used to enforce the guild system.[2]

These principles dominated the U.S. health care system until well into the 1980s, and their effects are still important today. They were enforced by legislation (for example, guild principles were built into all state insurance codes until the 1980s and into Title XVIII of the Social Security Act), boycotts (for example, by doctors against hospitals contracting with health maintenance organizations [HMOs]) professional ostracism (for example, from county medical societies and hospital staffs), denial of medical staff privileges and harassment.[3] Blue Cross and Blue Shield were created, respectively, by hospital associations and medical societies as chosen instruments to apply the guild principles to health care financing. For example, hospitals subsidized Blue Cross plans by giving them discounts. Only in fairly recent years have providers been forced to yield controlling positions on Blue Cross and Blue Shield boards.[4] Commercial insurance companies offered coverage based on the casualty insurance model. They comfortably accepted the guild principles because they were and, with a few important exceptions, remain financial intermediaries with expertise in underwriting risk, not in organizing, managing, or purchasing medical care.

Employers also fit into this model. A few attempted to contract selectively with doctors for the care of their employees. But for the most part, this was beaten down by organized medicine.[5] An overwhelming majority of employers offered traditional "guild free choice" coverage of either the Blue Cross/Blue Shield or the commercial variety because that was all there was. The typical pattern was virtually 100 percent employer-paid coverage. This pattern spread rapidly because health insurance was an attractive fringe benefit, it was cheap, it was tax deductible to the employer and tax free to the employee, employment groups could buy coverage at much less than the cost of individual coverage, and employer-paid health benefits were a great source of bargaining prizes for unions. In the minds of many employees, fee-for-service coverage fully paid by the employer became normal, an entitlement. Employment-based insurance spread to small employers. Roughly half of the privately employed labor force is either self-employed or in groups of 100 or fewer. This added another element of noncompetition: Such

2. A. C. Enthoven, *Theory and Practice of Managed Competition in Health Care Finance* (1987 Professor Dr. F. de Vries Lectures, North-Holland/American Elsevier, 1988).
3. L. G. Goldberg, and W. Greenberg, "The Emergence of Physician-Sponsored Health Insurance: A Historical Perspective," in *Competition in the Health Care Sector: Past, Present, and Future*, ed. W. Greenberg (Germantown, Md.: Aspen, 1978); and J. G. Smilie, *Can Physicians Manage the Quality and Costs of Healthcare? The Story of the Permanente Medical Group* (New York: McGraw Hill, 1991).
4. Weller, " 'Free Choice' as a Restraint of Trade."
5. Goldberg and Greenberg, "The Emergence of Physician-Sponsored Health Insurance."

groups are too small to offer individual employees a choice of health care plans. I return to this point later.

When HMOs entered the scene in large numbers in the 1970s and employers were required to offer them, employers usually agreed to pay HMO premiums in full as long as they did not exceed the cost of the traditional coverage. Thus, HMOs were placed in the noncompetitive system created by the guild model. Medicare and Medicaid also adopted the dominant guild model. Section 1801 of the Social Security Act prohibits any federal interference in the practice of medicine; section 1802 is entitled "free choice by patient guaranteed."

All of this created a system dominated by the cost-increasing incentives of fee-for-service payment combined with the cost-unconscious demand of insured patients. This in turn inspired greatly increased numbers of people to choose careers in medicine, especially in high paid specialties. This was fueled by federal grants to induce medical schools to expand. This open-ended, cost-unconscious demand, combined with large increases in federal funding for biomedical research, led to a huge outpouring of costly new medical technologies.

Finally, most well-functioning markets contain an adequate supply of information to assist purchasers in making decisions. In health care, there is no regulation to require the uniform production of health outcomes information. In fact, providers have been active and successful in political activities to block access to such information.[6]

MANAGED COMPETITION DEFINED

Managed competition is a purchasing strategy to obtain maximum value for money for employers and consumers. It uses rules for competition, derived from rational microeconomic principles, to reward with more subscribers and revenue those health plans that do the best job of improving quality, cutting cost, and satisfying patients. The "best job" is in the judgment of both the sponsor, armed with data and expert advice, and informed, cost-conscious consumers. The rules of competition must be designed and administered so as not to reward health plans for selecting good risks, segmenting markets, or otherwise defeating the goals of managed competition. Managed competition occurs at the level of integrated financing and delivery plans, not at the individual provider level. Its goal is to divide providers in each community into competing economic units and to use market forces to motivate them to develop efficient delivery systems.

Managed competition is price competition, but the price it focuses on is the annual premium for comprehensive health care services, not the price for individual services. There are several reasons for this. First, the annual premium encodes the total annual cost per person. It gives the subscriber an incentive to choose the health plan that minimizes total cost. Second, it is the price that people

6. S. J. Singer, "Problems in Gaining Access to Hospital Information," *Health Affairs* (Summer 1991): 148–51.

can understand and respond to most effectively, during the annual enrollment, when they have information, choices, and time for consideration. Third, sick, nonexpert patients and their families are in a particularly poor position to make wise decisions about long lists of individual services they might or might not need. They need to rely on their doctors to advise what services are appropriate and on their health plans to get good prices. For economical behavior to occur, doctors must be motivated to prescribe economically. Managed competition is compatible with selected copayments and deductibles for individual services that can influence patients to do their part in using resources wisely and that are price signals patients can understand and to which they can respond.

Sponsors and Managed Competition

To understand managed competition, one must begin with the concept of a sponsor. Markets for most goods and services are normally made up of suppliers on one side and individual purchasers on the other. This is not the model that actually works in most of private health insurance in the United States, and, in my view, this model is not workable at the individual level in health insurance, for a number of reasons.

First, insurers have strong incentives to group their customers by expected medical costs and to charge people in each group a premium that reflects their expected costs. This practice is known as experience rating or underwriting. The consequence is that those people having high predicted medical costs face high premiums. Many sick people find such premiums unaffordable and may go without insurance, taking their chances that they will receive free care. Second, healthy individuals face strong incentives to ride free, that is, to go without insurance or with minimal coverage until they get sick, at which point they seek to buy comprehensive coverage. Consumers are more likely than insurers to know more about their prospective medical needs. Third, partly because of the behaviors induced by these incentives and partly because of high marketing costs to reach individuals or small groups, the administrative costs of individual health insurance policies are very high—40 percent of medical claims or more. This creates more of an incentive for relatively healthy people to go without insurance. Rather than bearing the risks and expenses of covering individuals who are sick, even at a high price that would cover their expected costs, most insurers choose not to cover them at any price. Fourth, health insurance contracts are extremely complex and difficult to understand and administer. Insurers deliberately make them even more complex to segment markets and to make it difficult for consumers to compare prices.

The model of private health insurance that works—the one that covers most employed people—is group insurance with a sponsor. Most sponsors are employers, but the federal Medicare program and labor/management health and welfare trusts are also sponsors. Examples of large employers that offer their employees such a multiple choice of health care coverage include the federal government;

many states, including California, Wisconsin, and Minnesota; and Stanford University. While some HMOs and some PPI carriers compete for unsponsored individuals, most of their business is in sponsored groups. Sponsors set the rules for competition among them.

Sponsors Establish Rules of Equity

The sponsor has several important functions in managed competition. First, through contracts with the participating health plans, it establishes and enforces principles of equity such as the following: (1) Every eligible person is covered or at least is offered coverage on terms that make it attractive, even for persons with low expected medical costs, and at a moderate financial cost. Health plans accept all eligible persons who choose them. (2) Every eligible person has subsidized access to the lowest-priced plan meeting acceptable standards of quality and coverage. Persons choosing a plan priced above the lowest-priced plan must pay full premium difference with their own money. (3) Coverage is continuous; that is, once a person is enrolled, coverage cannot be canceled (except for nonpayment of premium or serious noncompliance with reasonable norms of patient behavior). Moreover, everyone can reenroll during the annual enrollment period. (4) Community rating (or limited departures from it) is established, whereby the same premium is paid for the same coverage regardless of the health status of the individual or small group. (This might be blended with, for example, age rating if it is felt that pure community rating requires excessive subsidies of the old by the young.) (5) No exclusions or limitations are placed on coverage for preexisting conditions. Obviously, some of these principles may have to be compromised with other practical considerations, depending on the circumstances.

Sponsors Select Participating Plans

The freedom of the sponsor in selecting participating plans will depend on the circumstances. A private employer will have more freedom of action than a public employer. And a public employer will be able to exercise more freedom than will a health insurance purchasing cooperative (HIPC) that serves as the gatekeeper for much or all of the market in a geographic area.

Sponsors Manage Enrollment Process

In managing enrollment, the sponsor should serve as the single point of entry to all participating health plans. Subscribers notify the sponsor of their choice of plan (probably through the employer), and the sponsor notifies the health plan. This is normal in large employment groups but, unfortunately, is not the usual practice with such public programs as Medicare and Medicaid. The purpose is to create an institutional embodiment of the principle that health plans take all who apply and to obviate what would otherwise be a large set of opportunities for screening and selecting applicants. The sponsor must define the enrollment procedures, such as giving each subscriber an annual opportunity to switch plans. It also must establish procedures to enroll newcomers and to deal with changes in address or family composition. The sponsor also should prepare informative materials about the benefits covered, the characteristics of the health plans and locations of their providers, and the quality controls in place. The sponsor establishes contractual payment terms with participating employers and individuals. And the sponsor runs a clearinghouse for the money.

Sponsors Create Price-elastic Demand

Next, the sponsor must seek to create price-elastic demand. (A seller faces inelastic demand if the seller can increase revenue by raising price, and elastic demand if the seller increases revenue by reducing price.) For there to be an incentive for health plans to cut price, demand must be so elastic that the additional revenue gained exceeds the additional cost of serving more subscribers. Managed competition is about creating such price elasticity.[7] The following are some of the main tools for accomplishing this.

(1) *Employer/sponsor contributions*. The key point here is that the sponsor's contribution to the premiums must not exceed the price of the lowest-priced plan. An essential component of managed competition is that it must always be possible for the lowest-priced plan to take business away from higher-priced plans by cutting premiums more. The lowest-priced plan must be able to widen the gap between its price and the next lowest by cutting price. Premiums of course are quoted in the context of annual enrollments. The sponsor sets its contribution after the health plan have submitted their quotes.

(2) *Standardized coverage contract*. Standardization should deter product differentiation, facilitate price comparisons, and counter market segmentation. There are powerful reasons for as much standardization as possible within each sponsored group. The first is to facilitate value-for-money comparisons and to focus comparison on price and quality. The second is to combat market segmentation—the division of the market into groups of subscribers who make choices based on what each plan covers (such as mental health or vision care) rather than on price. The third is to reassure people that it is financially safe to switch plans for a lower price with the knowledge that the lower-priced plans did not realize savings by creating hidden gaps in coverage. The fourth is that biased risk selection can reduce demand elasticity for health plans that enroll a favorable mix of risks.

(3) *Quality-related information*. People will be reluctant to switch from Plan A to Plan B to save $20 per month if they have no information that Plan B is safe

7. A. C. Enthoven, "Why 'Competition' in Health Care Has Failed: What Would It Take to Make It Work?" (The 1992 Clemens Lecture, St. John's University, Collegeville, Minnesota, 17 September 1992).

for their health. The Jackson Hole Group proposes creation of a national Outcomes Management Standards Board that would set standards for outcomes reporting.[8] Sponsors should play a role in making such information accessible to the local market. Sponsors are also the appropriate agencies to survey their sponsored populations regarding experience with health plans and to publish the results for consumers.

(4) *Choice of plans at individual level.* Sponsors should structure the market to offer annual choice of plan at the individual subscriber level, not the employment group level. Limitation of choice to the group level is a major barrier to price-elastic demand. (Effective managed care plans are linked to specific doctors. Because some people have strong attachments to their doctors, it is much harder to persuade a whole group to change plans and doctors to obtain lower premiums than to allow individuals who are willing to change to choose to do so.)

There are other opportunities for sponsors to exercise ingenuity in making demand curves for health plans more price elastic. For example, an alert sponsor might create a system to inform all patients of primary care physicians who contract with more than one health plan about which plan has the lowest premium so that patients can switch to the lowest-priced plan covering their doctor's services. Combined with standardized benefits, this could greatly increase people's willingness to switch plans to save money.

Finally, current income and payroll tax laws create a heavy tax on cost containment. These laws must be changed so that a health plan that cuts its premium by a dollar sees the full dollar transmitted to the subscriber, as an incentive to select that plan. This gives the health plan the full marketplace reward (more subscribers) for cutting price. Thus there must be a limit on tax-free employer contributions at a level that does not exceed the premium of the lowest-priced plan. This is beyond the scope of the sponsor and is mentioned here only for the sake of completeness.

Sponsors Manage Risk Selection

Finally, in managed competition, the sponsor must manage the problem of biased risk selection. The goal here is to create powerful incentives for health plans to succeed by improving quality and patient satisfaction, not by selecting good risks and avoiding bad ones. This is a crucial and complex issue. Here I describe the general outlines without getting into technical detail.

Joseph Newhouse has noted that in the RAND Health Insurance Experiment, the 1 percent of patients with the highest costs in a given year accounted for 28

8. P. M. Ellwood, A. C. Enthoven, and L. Etheredge, "The Jackson Hole Initiatives for a Twenty-First Century American Health Care System," *Health Economics* 1 (1992): 149–168. The Jackson Hole Group is an informal collection of health industry leaders, public officials, and health services researchers that started meeting in the mid-1970s in Paul Ellwood's living room in Jackson Hole, Wyoming.

percent of total costs on average.[9] Most of these patients could not be identified in advance. But such concentration suggests that it could be very profitable for a health plan to find ways to avoid enrolling or retaining such patients.

To accomplish the goal of managed risk selection, the sponsor should follow a coordinated strategy with the following elements.

(1) *Single point of entry.* Subscribers notify the sponsor of their choice and the sponsor notifies the health plan. The health plan must accept all enrollees. This should be combined with continuity of enrollment; that is, patients cannot be dropped from enrollment, and they must be allowed to reenroll during the periodic open enrollment in the plan of their choice.

(2) *Standardized coverage contract.* Coverage contract features can be a powerful tool for selecting risks.

(3) *Risk-adjusted premiums.* The general idea is as follows. Health risks are likely to fall differently among the different plans, either by design or by accident. The characteristics of the population enrolled in the different plans (for example, age, sex, family composition, retiree or disability status, and diagnosis) should be measured and translated into estimates of expected relative medical costs, independent of plan. Each plan can be assigned a relative risk index, for example, 1.01 for a plan with unfavorable selection that makes its expected costs 1 percent above the whole group average. Then a dollar value is assigned to one percentage point of risk. For example, that might be 1 percent of the premium of the lowest-priced plan or the average-priced plan. This is a policy choice; there is no single mathematically correct answer. Surcharges are then applied to premiums of plans that received favorable selection; subsidies are given to plans that received unfavorable selection, to compensate for risk selection. This takes selection out of the competition.[10]

The natural starting point is the available demographic variables (age, sex, family composition, and retiree status). Unfortunately, these do not explain much of the variation in individual annual expenditures. Newhouse found that of the total variation in individual expenditures, only about 15 percent is explainable even with complete knowledge of patient characteristics.[11] Demographic variables might explain two to three of the fifteen percentage points.

There is research under way to develop better risk-adjustment models, based on diagnostic information. It turns out to be much harder than one might think to turn available diagnostic information into good "risk adjusters." For example, among patients diagnosed in one year to have breast cancer or human immunodeficiency virus (HIV), there will be a very wide variation in medical costs the next year. But it seems reasonable to suppose that diagnosis-based models eventually

9. J. Newhouse, "Rate Adjusters for Medicare under Capitation," *Health Care Financing Review* (1986 Annual Supplement): 45–56.

10. For recent literature, see M. C. Hornbrook, "Risk-Based Contributions to Private Health Insurance," *Advances in Health Economics and Health Services Research* (Greenwich, Conn.: JAI Press, 1991).

11. Newhouse, "Rate Adjusters for Medicare."

will be available. Another approach may be to fund treatment of some conditions by fixed payments per case outside the capitation payments, or to use specific capitation payments on behalf of people with very costly diseases such as acquired immunodeficiency syndrome (AIDS).

In the Jackson Hole proposal, sponsors are the final arbiters of risk selection. An interesting paper by Harold Luft casts the sponsor in the role of expert mediator among health plans that are in a "zero sum game" over risk selection.[12] This suggests periodic face-to-face meetings with the marketing directors of all participating health plans, with the sponsor serving as honest broker. If Plan A is skimming, that hurts the other plans. The sponsor should lead a discussion on how risk selection can be defined, measured, and compensated for. This is an ongoing process, not a single event.

Since the sponsor must be seen as an impartial broker, not a biased participant, it should not have its own plan. Medicare's management of competition among HMOs has been seriously impaired by the Health Care Financing Administration's (HCFA's) preoccupation with protecting fee-for-service Medicare, which HCFA considers to be "its plan" to be protected from HMOs. Similar problems occur in the private sector.

(4) *Monitoring of enrollment patterns*. Sponsors should monitor voluntary disenrollments for evidence of risk-selecting behavior. With a brief questionnaire, sponsors can ask people why they switched plans. The box to watch would be one such as "They told me Plan B was better at treating my kind of cancer."

(5) *Monitoring of specialty care and quality*. Sponsors need to examine the quality of tertiary care arrangements and also monitor access to specialty care. A good way to avoid enrolling diabetics is to have no endocrinologists on staff in the county. A good way to avoid cancer patients is to have a poor oncology department. HMO regulation now monitors such aspects. These are subtle matters in which judgment must be applied.

HEALTH INSURANCE PURCHASING COOPERATIVES

Large employers of, say, 10,000 or more employees in one geographic area have the size needed to perform the functions of sponsorship with reasonable effectiveness, especially if they collaborate with other large employers. But over 40 percent of the employed population is in groups of 100 or fewer workers. Such groups (and even much larger ones) are too small to spread risks. Thus we observe wide variations—tenfold and more—in the premiums paid by small groups, depending on their claims experience. They also cannot achieve economies of scale in administration. Thus administrative expense reaches 35 percent of claims in groups of five to nine and 40 percent in groups of one to four, compared with

12. H. S. Luft, "Compensating for Biased Selection in Health Insurance," *The Milbank Quarterly* 64, no. 4 (1986): 566–589.

5.5 percent in groups of 10,000 and more.[13] Small groups cannot acquire needed information and expertise to function effectively in this market. In theory, agents and brokers perform this function. In practice, agents and brokers have their own interests, related to the commissions carriers pay, and they lack competence regarding quality or value of medical care.

The Jackson Hole initiative proposes to solve these problems by establishment of a new national system of sponsor organizations—HIPCs—to function as a collective purchasing agent on behalf of all small employers and individuals in a geographic area.[14] HIPCs are designed to correct the problems of market failure in the small-group market and to cut employers' administrative burdens to a minimum (for example, administering for them the requirements of mandated continuity of coverage and public subsidies). They provide a solid basis for determining the competitive costs of covering uniform benefits that could be used to establish a tax-exclusion limitation for each market area.

HIPCs would be nonprofit membership corporations whose boards would be elected by participating employers. HIPCs would contract with participating employers and would accept all qualifying employment groups in their area. They would not be allowed to exclude groups or individuals because of health status. HIPCs would manage competition, applying business judgment in determining the numbers and identities of competitors, and would carry out all the sponsor functions described above.

HIPCs would select the participating health plans. Some would favor a rule that a HIPC must offer all health plans that achieve federal certification and that wish to be offered in the HIPC's territory. Whether or not market forces would resolve the problems arising from this arrangement is a debatable proposition about which reasonable people can differ. I would prefer to see HIPCs have some authority to select and drop health plans. The presumption should favor competition. Thus it would make sense for a HIPC to encourage participation by all provider groups in the territory, but some discretion might be appropriate for the following reasons. First, federal qualification and state regulation do not guarantee financial solvency. Second, many "managed care" plans offer overlapping provider networks (that is, many providers contracting with many plans). Some overlap may not be undesirable. But too many carriers all offering essentially the same set of providers can add to administrative costs and weaken the sponsor's purchasing power with providers. As noted above, managed competition seeks to motivate providers to create efficient delivery systems. Third, HIPCs should be able to drop health plans that persistently achieve very low market penetration. Fourth, HIPCs should be able to drop carriers that are persistently uncooperative with the HIPC's risk management program.

13. "Private Health Insurance: Options for Reform," House Ways and Means Committee on Health, 101st Cong., 2d sess., Committee Print 101-35 (Washington: U.S. Government Printing Office, 1990).

14. Ellwood et al., "The Jackson Hole Initiatives."

HIPCs would administer health benefit contracts. The HIPC should act like a competent, effective employee benefits office serving beneficiary inquiries and complaints. It should interpret the contracts for beneficiaries, stand behind patients in disputes with health plans, and resolve disputes on terms that are fair to beneficiaries. This should be much more efficient than taking disputes to litigation. The HIPC also should monitor what is happening in the health care settings. It should survey consumer experience and make the information available for consumers. It should investigate complaints and should aggregate complaint data to identify problem areas.

HIPCs should not bear risk. Health plans should bear all risk for medical expenses, for several reasons. First, if HIPCs were to bear risk, we would have a whole new class of risk-bearing entities that would have to be capitalized and regulated, and we have more than enough of them now. Second, HIPCs should be unbiased, honest brokers among risk-bearing entities. Third, providers—doctors and hospitals—must be at risk for the cost of care to give them powerful incentives to reduce cost.

Finally, HIPCs could contract with government agencies to cover publicly sponsored populations, such as Medicaid, the otherwise uninsured, and public employees.

Creating HIPCs means that persons and groups with low health care costs in a given year share in the costs of persons and groups with high costs. If given a choice, people expecting low costs are not likely to do so voluntarily. Once the HIPC is operating at a large scale, there will be important benefits for small employers, even those with good health risks—including economies of scale, stable rates, competition, and individual choice of plan. But to get HIPCs going and to prevent a spiral of adverse selection, there must be compelling incentives or legal requirements for all small employers to participate. In the Jackson Hole initiative, small-group participation in a HIPC would be a condition for exclusion of employer contributions from employees' taxable income.

One large and successful HIPC is the health benefits program of the California Public Employees Retirement System (CalPERS). CalPERS arranges coverage and manages competition for more than 870,000 people who are employees, retirees, and dependents of the state and more than 750 public agencies, some of which have as few as two employees. CalPERS offers each subscriber a choice of plan: twenty-three HMOs, four preferred provider organizations (PPOs) offered to employee association members, and a statewide PPO.

ROLE OF ORGANIZED SYSTEMS OF CARE

Managed competition is not based on a mere hope that the market will somehow generate better models of care. It is based on demonstrations of successful, high-quality, cost-effective, organized systems of care that have existed for years. To date, the strongest evidence of their economic superiority relates to prepaid multispecialty group practices. For example, the RAND Health Insurance Experiment found that Group Health Cooperative of Puget Sound cared for its randomly assigned patients for a cost 28 percent below that for comparable patients assigned to a fee-for-service plan whose care was paid for entirely by insurance or with 25 percent coinsurance (up to an annual out-of-pocket limit of $1,000).[15] The evident marketplace success of Kaiser Permanente, now serving over 6.5 million people, reinforces this finding. Successful large-scale HMOs based on individual practice styles have merged in recent years. These HMOs carefully select participating physicians and arm physicians and management with strong information systems about practice patterns. These models can expand rapidly, and they offer a practice style that is familiar to many doctors and patients. While we do not have proof of their efficacy in the form of a randomized controlled trial, we do know that some of them now compete effectively with Kaiser Permanente and Group Health Cooperative.

Compared to the traditional fee-for-service model, there are many things such organizations can do—and, if appropriately motivated, will do—to improve quality and cuts cost. (1) Fee-for-service has created a costly adversarial relationship between doctors and players. Organized systems can attract the loyalty, commitment, and responsible participation of doctors. They can align the incentives of doctors and the interests of patients in high-quality, economical care by appropriate risk-sharing arrangements. (2) Fee-for-service has failed to create accountability for health outcomes and the outcomes information systems doctors need to evaluate and improve practice patterns. Organized systems can gather data on outcomes, treatments, and resource use; evaluate practice patterns; and motivate doctors to choose economical practices that produce good outcomes.

(3) Fee-for-service "free choice" leaves patients to make remarkably poorly informed choices of doctor. Organized systems select doctors for quality and efficient practice patterns, monitor performance, and take corrective action where needed. (4) Fee-for-service has left us with excess supply in many specialties. Organized systems can match the numbers and types of doctors to the needs of enrolled populations. (5) Fee-for-service has left us with major excesses in hospital beds, high-tech equipment, and open-heart surgery facilities. At least some systems can match all resources used to the needs of the enrolled population.

(6) Our present system is characterized by major misallocations of resources. Organized systems can allocate all resources—capital and operating—across the total spectrum of care, including less costly settings. (7) Fee-for-service has little or no capability to plan and manage processes of care across the total spectrum (inpatient, outpatient, office, and home); organized systems do. (8) Organizations that integrate financing and delivery, and doctors and hospitals, can practice total quality management/continuous quality improvement, the powerful management philosophy employed by the most successful world-class industrial companies.[16]

15. Manning et al., "A Controlled Trial of the Effect of a Prepaid Group Practice."
16. D. Berwick, A. B. Godfrey, and J. Roessner, *Curing Health Care* (San Francisco: Jossey-Bass, 1990).

This cannot be done effectively with doctors who are in fee-for-service practice in several hospitals and are attached to none.

(9) Fee-for-service has led to a costly and dangerous proliferation in facilities for such complex procedures as open-heart surgery. Such surgery done in low volumes has higher costs and higher death rates than when done in high volumes.[17] Organized systems concentrate open-heart surgery in regional centers with low mortality rates and low costs. Such regional concentration in the most cost-effective hospitals could save a great deal of money. (10) Systems can organize ongoing technology assessment and facilitate a rational response to the results. (11) HMOs emphasize prevention, early diagnosis and treatment, and effective management of chronic conditions. Traditional third-party coverage is usually based on the casualty insurance model: It pays very generously for costly inpatient episodes but not for the preventive services and management of chronic conditions that can reduce the need for inpatient care. Organized systems can use systematic management processes to make sure these services are actually delivered, not merely covered. And they can be held accountable for their enrolled populations.

WHY COMPETITION?

Why attempt to bring about these changes through competition and market forces? Why not expect the government simply to order them? First, we have an extremely wasteful and inefficient system that has been bathed in cost-increasing incentives for over fifty years. We badly need a radically more efficient system. That will mean closing hospitals and putting surgeons out of work. As Charles Schultze has written, "Under the social arrangements of the private market, those who may suffer losses are not usually able to stand in the way of change. As a consequence, efficiency-creating changes are not seriously impeded."[18] Government controls, on the other hand, tend to freeze industries in place. Thus we find it extraordinarily difficult to close an unneeded school or air base. Government action is constrained by what Schultze calls the rule to "do no direct harm."

Second, to offset the expenditure-increasing effects of an aging population and an expanding array of medical technologies, we need to foster a process of continuing productivity improvement and of development of cost-reducing technologies. Only ongoing competition to provide value for money can do this. Third, as medical technology and social and economic conditions of the population change, we need a health care system that is flexible and can come up with entirely new ways of organizing and delivering care. Fourth, we need and want a system that is user-friendly. Government monopoly public service agencies are notoriously user-unfriendly.

Fifth, our society needs to make cost/quality trade-off judgments. These

---

17. H. S. Luft, J. Bunker, and A. C. Enthoven, "Should Operations Be Regionalized?" *The New England Journal of Medicine* (20 December 1979): 1364–1369.

18. C. L. Schultze, *The Public Use of Private Interest* (Washington: The Brookings Institution, 1977); and Enthoven, "Consumer Choice Health Plan."

should be made by consumers who are using their own money at the margin. For example, given a choice, many might prefer a much less costly style of care, based on limited access in tightly controlled facilities, with more use of physician-extenders, and so on. They might have other worthy uses for their money, such as their children's education. Others may be happy to pay more for wider access and greater convenience. (Note that under managed competition, consumers would be exercising this preference with their own net after-tax dollars, not with pretax dollars and substantial tax subsidies for the more costly choice as happens today.) In this country we are now spending nearly 14 percent of gross domestic product (GDP) on health care services. It is altogether possible that a very efficient competitive system could get us back to 9 or 10 percent. This would free up resources that are badly needed for education and other investments in long-term economic growth. In theory, a government-imposed "global budget" might be seen as a way to reduce national health expenditures as a share of GDP. In practice, this would be extremely difficult to do if all of the cost-increasing incentives of fee-for-service, and all of the wastefulness of the present system were to remain in place. The reduced spending would mean care denied to people who need it and a sustained barrage of complaints by health care providers. The global budget would be hard for our government to sustain politically. Finally, competition is the way to achieve a system that is driven by the informed choices of consumers who are responsible for the cost consequences of their choices. A government-controlled system is driven by political forces.

WHY UNIVERSAL COVERAGE?

Today, millions of Americans either have no health care coverage or have coverage that will disappear or become extremely costly when they need it. Nobody defends the proposition that people without coverage or money to pay should go without necessary medical care or should be allowed to suffer, be disabled, or die for lack of reasonable care. For this reason our society has developed a complex patchwork of institutions to care for and finance the care of the uninsured. These institutions are extremely wasteful and often unfair, permitting preventable medical bankruptcies and disabilities. They lead to delayed care, which can often mean serious and costly illness that could have been prevented by early treatment. They lead to care in costly settings—particularly, hospital emergency departments—when care could have been delivered at much lower cost in the primary care physician's office. They permit epidemics of communicable diseases that could have been prevented. They generate requirements for costly eligibility determinations. They lead to cost shifting from those who do not pay and those who provide free care to those who do pay for health insurance. They lead to the closing of hospital emergency departments, which are the major point of entry for patients who cannot pay. This, in turn, deprives whole communities of an important resource.

By putting market pressure on providers to cut costs, market reforms promoting competition—if not accompanied by universal coverage—could exacerbate access problems. (This would be true of any serious cost containment program.) It would be more humane, economical, and rational simply to adopt a policy providing coverage to virtually everybody through an integrated financing and delivery organization that provides primary and preventive care as a part of a comprehensive benefit package.

A necessary condition for universal coverage is that everybody who can contribute to financing the system must do so. A system of universal coverage will not work if everybody is covered, but only those who voluntarily choose to do so pay for it. Such a system would be destroyed by free riders.

Universal contributions might be achieved in a variety of ways that are compatible with managed competition: (1) a requirement that employers and full-time employees jointly buy coverage ("employer mandate"), combined with payroll taxes on part-time employees and taxes on nonpoor nonemployed (such as early retirees), with revenues used to subsidize purchase of coverage for them through a HIPC; (2) a requirement that every household buy coverage through a HIPC or pay an equivalent tax ("individual mandate"), with subsidies to assist low-income households; and (3) payroll taxes or more broadly based taxes.

MANAGED COMPETITION OR TOP-DOWN GLOBAL BUDGETS?

The level and growth of tax-supported and tax-subsidized national health expenditures is an appropriate object of public concern. Excessive growth in these expenditures, relative to other priorities, crowds out other programs important to our nation's future. Managed competition offers the most powerful force for reducing national health expenditures. That is, it makes economical decisions about health resource use in everybody's personal interest—an almost complete reversal of the cost-increasing incentives that drive the present system. However, as is the case with any other policy, there is no guarantee that managed competition will automatically hold spending growth to acceptable levels, even if implemented optimally as I have proposed here. Patients would be insured, thus not using their own money when demanding care. The health insurance and health services industries have an extensive history of market imperfections, not all of which will be corrected by managed competition. Very costly technologies might emerge. And directly or indirectly (through tax subsidies), government pays about half the bill.

What should government do if national health expenditure growth is excessive under managed competition? "Top-down," government-imposed global budgets are not likely to work well. Such global budgets today would have to be imposed on sectors such as hospitals, doctors, and pharmacies and enforced by price controls. The most plausible candidate for price controls would be Medicare payment methods and volume performance standards, which penalize sectors that increase volume by offsetting reductions in next year's prices. Such controls block efficiency-improving reallocations across sectors, such as doctors working harder to keep people out of the hospital. They create a "tragedy of the commons," penalizing the most economical doctors. They leave all of the cost-increasing incentives in place and even intensify them as providers struggle to maintain target incomes.

Top-down global budgets, if imposed on capitation rates of integrated financing and delivery organizations, would avoid some of the worst inefficiencies and disincentives. But they would focus the whole health services industry on political efforts to raise or maintain the ceiling as a percentage of gross national product (GNP). The British refer to the likely behavior as "shroud waving." Regulatory authorities are held responsible for the economic survival of the regulated entities. Hospital rate regulators are notoriously unwilling to force unneeded or inefficient hospitals to close. Insurance rate regulators are responsible for the solvency of insurers. So such regulation becomes cost reimbursement. Only impersonal market forces can close down unneeded, inefficient activities. Thus the history of such regulation is that it does not really lower cost to consumers.

Moreover, regulatory authorities are not czars. They must observe the due process requirements of the Administrative Procedures Act and the Fifth Amendment. They must hold hearings, consider arguments, and base conclusions on evidence—all of which can be costly. Such global budgets would raise a whole maze of paradoxes and conundrums: Would they be equal per capita across states, and if unequal, on what basis? How would one deal with high- versus low-cost states? Could one justify locking Massachusetts and Arkansas, with a nearly two fold difference in per capita spending, into the same percentage rate of increase forever? Who decides?

Finally, for managed competition to work well, the managed care industry must make a great deal of investment in corporate restructuring, service expansion, and information and reporting systems, all of which are much less likely to appear attractive if government threatens to set prices and expropriate the return on investment.

How then should government respond? The answer is that the managed competition framework gives government a number of tools to use to influence the outcome. First, government could define as the "global budget" the lowest capitation rate in each HIPC, multiplied by the number of people residing in each HIPC area, added up over all HIPCs. These would be market-determined global budgets and would encompass all publicly supported and tax-subsidized national health expenditures. Government could then decide on a public policy that sets a target for this global budget relative to GNP. If the global budget grows faster than the target, the president and Congress should direct the National Health Board to develop and implement a set of targeted interventions designed to reduce health spending based on solid and current data. The list might include, for example, reducing covered benefits; raising copayments and deductibles (except for the poor); removing from coverage and inclusion in the uniform effective covered benefit package those drugs and other technologies of very high cost in relation to the benefits produced (with protection against tort litigation for providers who comply); antitrust action against local cartels; and possibly taxing the excess of premiums over the premiums of the low-cost benchmark plan in each area. In other words, government should examine the causes of excess spending and apply specific remedies, rather than trying to sweep the problems under the carpet of a national global budget.

WHAT MANAGED COMPETITION IS NOT

Managed competition is not a lot of things it has been called by people who do not understand it or who prefer central governmental controls to decentralized markets. (1) Managed competition is not a free market. A free market does not and cannot work in health insurance and health care. If not corrected by a careful design, this market is plagued by problems of free riders, biased risk selection, segmentation, and other sources of market failure. Managed competition uses market forces within a framework of carefully drawn rules. (2) Managed competition is not merely a ''voucher'' system (giving people a certificate and seeing if they can find insurance). In managed competition, sponsors work actively to perfect the market. Everyone is given an opportunity to enroll. (3) Managed competition is not deregulation. It is new rules, not no rules. (4) Managed competition is not what we have had for the past ten or fifty years.

(5) Managed competition is not forcing everyone into large clinic-style HMOs or other types of care they do not like. On the contrary, managed competition emphasizes the importance of individual (not employer) choice of plans. Many systems and styles would be able to compete effectively, including familiar solo doctor styles in some selective individual practice models. However, managed competition does make people bear the economic consequences of their choices. (6) Managed competition is not a reduction in the quality of care. On the contrary, far more often than not, quality and economy in medical care go hand-in-hand. The correct diagnosis done promptly, and the appropriate procedure done by someone very proficient, without errors or complications, is best for the patient and the payer. Competing managed care plans would have powerful incentives to improve the quality of care.

(7) Managed competition is not blind faith in an untested economic theory. We know that some types of managed care can cut cost substantially. We know that there are wide variations in costs for many procedures and that the best producers have the lowest costs. We know that when given responsible choices and information, most people choose value for money. We know that HIPC-like arrangements work well. All of the pieces of the managed care/managed competition model are in actual successful practice somewhere. The challenge is to put these best practices together into one complete managed competition system. The rest is extrapolation based on generally accepted principles of rational economic behavior. All reform proposals must rely on similar extrapolation. (8) Managed competition is not just the latest buzzword that anybody should feel free to appropriate. It has been explained, developed, and debated in the academic literature

for more than a decade.[19] Also, managed competition does not exist in Canada. Managed competition is not just a grab bag of ideas that sound good. It is an integrated framework that combines rational principles of microeconomics with careful observation and analysis of what works.

(9) Managed competition is not a panacea. Its authors do not claim that it can solve America's problems of racism, poverty, homelessness, the frail elderly, and others. It cannot be counted on to bring comprehensive care to Nome, Alaska. Managed competition is aimed at care for the 90 to 95 percent of Americans whose medical needs can be met by programs that look like prevailing employment-based coverage. For most Americans managed competition can mean higher-quality care at a much lower cost, organized and delivered in a much more coherent and satisfactory way. Special programs, usually publicly sponsored, will be needed for special populations. If managed competition is successful, more public money will be available for them.

(10) Managed competition will not take until the year 2010 to transform health care financing and delivery in this country. It does not depend merely on the steady growth of existing prepaid group practices. In response to managed competition, thousands of hospitals and their medical staffs could quickly form integrated organizations and begin accepting capitation contracts. Many individual practice and network HMOs could expand very rapidly. And Blue Cross and/or Blue Shield plans must now have statewide preferred provider networks in existence in practically every state.

MANAGED COMPETITION AND THE AMERICAN WAY

The managed competition idea attracted widespread support in 1992, in recognition of the urgent need to do something serious about costs and as an alternative to federal price controls. Paul Tsongas adopted it as his health platform during his presidential bid. In developing its proposal, the Bush administration began with a managed competition model.[20] Unfortunately, for political reasons, they withdrew some of the essential features needed to make it effective, especially the limit on tax-free employer contributions to employee health care and the powerful tax incentive needed to motivate small employers to join HIPCs. In April 1992 the sixty-member Conservative Democratic Forum (CDF) in the

19. A. C. Enthoven, *Health Plan: The Only Practical Solution to the Soaring Cost of Medical Care* (Reading, Mass.: Addison-Wesley, 1980); A. C. Enthoven, "Managed Competition in Health Care and the Unfinished Agenda," *Health Care Financing Review* (1986 Annual Supplement): 105–119; A. C. Enthoven, "Managed Competition: An Agenda for Action," *Health Affairs* (Summer 1988): 25–47; Enthoven, *Theory and Practice of Managed Competition in Health Care Finance*; A. C. Enthoven and R. Kronick, "A Consumer Choice Health Plan for the 1990s: Universal Health Insurance in a System Designed to Promote Quality and Economy," *The New England Journal of Medicine* (5 and 12 January 1989): 29–37 and 94–101; and A. C. Enthoven and R. Kronick, "Universal Health Insurance through Incentives Reform," *Journal of the American Medical Association* (15 May 1991): 2532–2536.

20. *The President's Comprehensive Health Reform Program* (The White House, 6 February 1992).

House of Representatives announced its support for the Jackson Hole initiative. The CDF introduced a bill, the Managed Competition Act of 1992, in September 1992.[21] A similar bill was introduced in the Senate and drew bipartisan support. In October 1992 presidential candidate Bill Clinton said, "Managed competition, not price controls, will make the budget work and maintain quality."[22]

Managed competition is compatible with a variety of ways of financing universal coverage—from a tax-financed approach as in the proposal of California Insurance Commissioner John Garamendi and my 1977 proposal to the Carter administration, to an employer/employee mandate plus an individual mandate and subsidies for the nonemployed as in the Jackson Hole initiative, to an individual mandate.[23] Thus, it can appeal to liberals, whose main concern is universal access, and to conservatives, who have strong preferences for decentralized private markets and against centralized governmental power.[24]

Like any serious reform proposal, attempts to enact a national managed competition model will be controversial. Some of the most powerful congressional leaders distrust market mechanisms and prefer direct government price controls. Many of the specific features of managed competition will be opposed by private-sector interests seeking to hold onto the present market imperfections that favor them. However, recent months have seen considerable movement among the private sector toward support of real managed competition as it becomes apparent that government will be forced to act decisively to contain costs.

In the coming debate, managed competition has the important advantage that it is compatible with strong American cultural preferences, as articulated by Alexis de Tocqueville, for limited government, voluntary action, decentralized decision making, individual choice, multiple competing approaches, pluralism, and personal and local responsibility.[25]

---

21. The Managed Competition Act of 1992, H.R. 5936, 102d Cong., 2d sess., 15 September 1992.
22. Press release, Clinton/Gore '92 Committee (Little Rock, Arkansas, 8 October 1992).
23. J. Garamendi, "California Health Care in the 21st Century: A Vision for Reform" (Sacramento: California Department of Insurance, February 1992); and Enthoven, "Consumer Choice Health Plan: A National Health Insurance Proposal."
24. P. Starr, *The Logic of Health-Care Reform* (Knoxville, Tenn.: Whittle Direct Books, 1992).
25. A. de Tocqueville, *Democracy in America* (New York: Aflred A. Knopf, 1948).

A Bridge to Compromise: Competition Under a Budget

Paul Starr and Walter A. Zelman

In some minds the word compromise raises the specter of compromised principles and corrupt bargains. But in a democracy compromise is not merely unavoidable; it is a source of creative invention, sometimes generating solutions that unexpectedly combine seemingly opposed ideas.

The American political process clearly has not worked any such magic in health care reform. Three-quarters of a century after the first proposals for universal health insurance, we are still short some thirty-six million people; more than ever, rising costs strain public budgets and the private economy. Even as political leaders and interest groups have acknowledged the gravity of these problems, they have been unable to bridge their differences. To be sure, we have had compromises in health reform before—generally weak ones that gave each side only a little of what it wanted. The question now is this: Can our politics produce a *strong* compromise to restructure the system, extend insurance to all, and bring costs under control?

Our purpose is to set forth the outlines of one such strong compromise: universal coverage through insurance purchasing cooperatives, managed competition, and global budgeting. This approach—managed competition under a cap—may not satisfy dedicated free-market or single-payer advocates, yet it should have broad appeal. To conservatives it offers consumer choice and competition among private health plans. To liberals it offers coverage for all at community

Health Affairs Supplement 1993.

rates, with comprehensive benefits, and with an emphasis on consumer protection and information. And to the public at large it promises to break the gridlock in health system reform to achieve broad economic and social objectives.

The debate over health policy has been plagued by a misleading polarization between "competition" and "regulation." Managed competition, we are told, exemplifies a competitive strategy; global budgeting, a regulatory strategy. This antinomy poses a false choice. With new rules and institutions in the market, we can—and almost certainly will—have both. Managed competition does not just "release" the forces of the market; it reconstructs the market. And even without global budgeting, managed competition involves much new insurance market regulation. Moreover, with its emphasis on capitated health plans, managed competition provides a better platform for global budgeting than exists in the current system.

The model we offer is consistent with the principles that President Bill Clinton endorsed during his campaign: "competition within a budget" and "universal coverage . . . privately provided, publicly guaranteed."[1] In line with his approach, the federal government would require employers to cover their workers, who would also have to share the cost; public financing would help to make coverage affordable for the unemployed and for low-income households as well as low-wage employers. The specifics in the model presented here are our own. However, the framework and many details reflect an extended conversation over the past year among analysts trying to break through false ideological dichotomies. This paper distills from that dialogue the essential features of reform, as we understand them: the framework of managed competition, the roles of purchasing cooperatives and employers, a method for financing universal coverage, and a national budgeting process.

This approach recognizes that the imperatives of reform are moral and economic in equal degree. The moral imperative is to achieve equal access to care and protection against financial destitution for the millions now uninsured or underinsured. The economic imperative is to slow the rise in health costs, which have consumed an additional 1 percent of gross national product (GNP) every thirty-five months for the past twelve years.

The two sides of the problem are inseparable. Runaway costs put coverage out of reach for more people and make universal insurance seem unaffordable, while the continued exclusion of millions from basic coverage and care makes the system's failings and excesses morally unacceptable. Cost containment itself has become a moral issue, as ballooning medical costs have crowded out other needs from governmental and household budgets alike. Health care reform used to be a specialized (if not special) interest; now it has become a precondition for America's economic health—and reputation for decency.

1. Clinton/Gore National Campaign, "Controlling Costs and Guaranteeing Care for All—The Clinton/Gore Health Care Plan" (Little Rock: 24 September 1992).

THE FRAMEWORK OF MANAGED COMPETITION

Managed competition under a cap, as we envision it, involves new relations between the federal government and the states, between the public and private sectors, and between health care finance and health service delivery. The federal government would establish the framework of the new system but allow the states flexibility in implementing it. Under federal law, all American citizens would be guaranteed the right to a comprehensive set of benefits, defined in general terms by legislation and interpreted and adjusted over time by a National Health Board. The federal government would require all individuals and all employers, except perhaps the very smallest, to share the cost of health insurance. All—except, most likely, employees of large firms—would obtain coverage through new regional health insurance purchasing cooperatives (HIPCs).

These purchasing cooperatives—the central innovation in this model—would neither deliver health care nor pay providers. Rather, they would contract with varied private health plans, including health maintenance organizations (HMOs), preferred provider organizations (PPOs), and one free-choice-of-provider option. The plans would be paid by capitation (although many plans would pay their physicians by other methods, including both salary and fee-for-service). Once a year, the HIPC would give every consumer an opportunity to choose a plan under the following principles of managed competition.

(2) *Open enrollment.* Any HMO, insurer, or other plan that wanted to do business with the regional HIPC would have to take all who apply—no medical underwriting or any other device for risk selection would be allowed. To prevent plans from marketing only to the healthy, the purchasing cooperative would conduct the enrollment process.

(2) *Standard, comprehensive benefit package.* The plans would compete on the same benefit package. If allowed to vary the package, the plans might well use those variations for risk selection purposes—limiting benefits, such as alcoholism treatment, that attract high-risk groups and extending benefits that attract low-risk groups. A uniform benefit package will enable consumers to make clear-cut choices based on the price and quality of plans. It also will strengthen the hand of the HIPC in negotiations with plans, since plans will no longer have the excuse of complex benefit variations for higher prices. This standard package must not be minimal or barebones, but a mainstream package broadly acceptable to the public.[2]

(3) *Routine quality measurement.* Federal legislation should specify uniform standards for the plan to report data on quality of care, including outcomes of treatment. The purchasing cooperatives would publish such data to help consumers in their choice of plans. They would regularly survey consumers for satisfaction and complaints, oversampling vulnerable groups, such as people with disabil-

2. See L. A. Bergthold, "Benefit Design Choices under Managed Competition," in this volume of *Health Affairs*.

ities and those living in low-income areas, to monitor whether they are receiving the services for which the plans are contractually responsible.[3]

(4) *Contribution pegged to the low-cost benchmark plan.* For any given enrollee, the purchasing cooperative would pay no plan more than it pays the benchmark plan—that is, the plan providing the uniform benefit package at the lowest price and a satisfactory standard of care. Consumers who choose other plans would pay the marginal difference in cost.

(5) *Community-rated premiums charged to the enrollees, risk-adjusted premiums paid to the plans.* The plans would charge consumers the same; premiums would not be higher for those who are older or for people with disabilities or preexisting conditions. However, the purchasing cooperatives would risk-adjust the overall payments to plans—that is, they would estimate differences in average risk among the plans' enrolled populations, adjusting upward payments to plans attracting higher-risk subscribers and adjusting downward payments to plans enrolling lower-risk subscribers.[4] The techniques for risk adjustment would be prescribed by the National Health Board.

Purpose of the Framework

The purpose of this framework is to encourage consumers to make quality-conscious as well as cost-conscious decisions and to encourage plans to serve both high-risk and low-risk populations. The cost of any plan should depend not on the kinds of subscribers it attracts, but on the quality and efficiency of its services. Today, with little information about quality of care, many people judge quality by price—they think a more expensive plan is better. But indicators of quality may well show that less expensive plans have equally good outcomes (perhaps better) and thereby encourage people to respond to price competition. Much the same reasoning is behind the requirement of a uniform benefit package. Such a package is vital to give consumers enough confidence to respond to price and, thereby, to give plans sufficient incentive to compete on price to get more enrollment.

Although the framework of managed competition appears to change only the method for purchasing insurance, it also is designed to encourage the integration of health insurance and health care provision into the same organizations (the health plans). The more integrated the plans, the better able they will be to control cost and quality. Thus, the new system will tend to alter the organization of services, not just the flow of funds. The method here is reform of finance; the true objective is reform of styles of medical practice and structures of management to promote a more conservative, cost- and quality-conscious framework of medical decision making.

3. For more on these functions, see S. Sofaer, "Informing and Protecting Consumers under Managed Competition"; and A. L. Hillman, W. R. Greer, and N. Goldfarb, "Safeguarding Quality in Managed Competition," both in this volume of *Health Affairs*.

4. See J. C. Robinson, "A Payment Method for Health Insurance Purchasing Cooperatives," in this volume of *Health Affairs*.

HIPCs themselves would have important effects. First, they would reduce sharply the costs of insurance administration in the small-group market (currently twenty-five cents of every premium dollar for firms between twenty-five and forty-nine employees). This would not only permit lower rates for small groups—especially those that have suffered from experience rating—but also would mean more health benefit for every dollar spent.

Moreover, the purchasing cooperatives would open up choices in health plans that many consumers have never had before. Currently, some employers are imposing managed care, often depriving employees of a choice of plan or physician. The purchasing cooperatives, in contrast, can make available a diverse array of plans, thereby restoring a liberty that employer-based insurance is now threatening.

Managed competition, however, does not merely make alternatives available; it is designed to clarify the true economic consequences of choice at several levels. The system implicitly asks consumers whether plans other than the benchmark plan are worth the extra cost. It confronts the plans with their relative performance within a region. And since regional HIPCs will have separate rates, those HIPCs with higher costs will have an incentive (especially under the pressure of global budgeting) to learn from best-practice regions. In short, this approach to reform creates not only a competitive environment, but a learning environment that links quality and cost-effective performance.

Balancing Federal and State Control

The balance between federal and state control needs to be carefully calibrated to achieve these ends while allowing for diversity and experimentation. On the one hand, the federal government would set the ground rules for the system, establish global budgets, assess new technologies, develop practice guidelines, and have other continuing responsibilities, such as support for training, medical research, and public health. The states, on the other hand, would be given direct authority to supervise the purchasing cooperatives and license health plans. As we conceive them, the HIPCs most likely would be state-chartered public corporations; their boards would be designed to represent the purchasers—that is, consumers and employers in their region.[5]

This approach builds in flexibility because HIPCs could be adapted to different conditions. Yet, states could seek federal approval to opt out of the national program in favor of defined alternatives, including use of the HIPCs as single payers, as long as they met federal budget targets and provided no less than the guaranteed benefits. The expected pattern, however, would be not to preserve private health plans, but to increase competition among them.

5. In separate papers in this volume, we discuss the legal and organizational structure of the purchasing cooperatives and a plan for their national development. W. A. Zelman, "Who Should Govern the Purchasing Cooperative?"; and P. Starr, "Design of Health Insurance Purchasing Cooperatives," in this volume of *Health Affairs*.

SOME DIFFERENCES IN APPROACH

Although the approach taken here owes a great deal to earlier managed competition proposals, it also differs significantly from some of them—most notably in its integration of global budgeting and emphasis on the central role of HIPCs. Unlike the Jackson Hole Group, we do not call for federal certification of a new category of "accountable health partnerships."[6] At least at first, the purchasing cooperatives would allow managed care plans operating in a region to compete; HIPCs might also be specially charged with facilitating the entry of new managed care plans in many areas.

A Free-Choice-of-Provider Option

We also do not envision restricting the competition to managed care plans. Consumers who want to enroll in a free-choice-of-provider option with fee-for-service payment should be able to do so, as long as they pay the true difference in cost. To minimize that cost, HIPCs should use periodic competitive bidding to select one insurer to operate that plan. Evidence from the federal employees' health system and the Civilian Health and Medical Program of the Uniformed Services (CHAMPUS) suggests that multiple fee-for-service plans raise overall administrative costs and invite risk selection problems.[7] Because the free-choice-of-provider plan under managed competition should be competing only on claims administration (by definition, it has no provider network), there is no reason to have more than one at a time. The competition among fee-for-service insurers can be serial rather than simultaneous.

Competition among managed care plans on the ground rules set by federal law, such as open enrollment and community rating, also will likely produce extensive consolidation. In addition, the purchasing cooperatives should be able to reject plans that do not show the capacity to meet service responsibilities or persistently fail to meet standards. While not opposing federal certification of "accountable health plans" on principle, we think HIPCs and states should be able to develop their own methods for choosing qualified plans. Moreover, implementation of universal coverage and managed competition should not be held up until federal standards are set and individual plans are certified.

Benchmark Plan

Another difference in our approach is the conception of the benchmark plan. Other proposals have emphasized the low-cost plan as the point of reference. That term gives rise to misunderstanding; most people assume that the low-cost plan

6. P. M. Ellwood, A. C. Enthoven, and L. Etheredge, "The Jackson Hole Initiatives for a Twenty-First Century American Health Care System," *Health Economics* 1 (1992): 149–168.

7. U.S. General Accounting Office, *Federal Health Benefits Program: Stronger Controls Needed to Reduce Administrative Costs* (Washington: U.S. Government Printing Office, 12 February 1992).

would offer less coverage when, in fact, the coverage would be the same. In addition, because people judge quality by price, the term *low-cost* may carry some stigma; *benchmark,* on the other hand, avoids that stigma and promotes a concern for quality. Indeed, HIPCs should have authority to evaluate whether a low-cost plan has sufficient capacity and quality to serve as the benchmark in its region.

Flexible Approach to Competition

Unlike some other proponents of managed competition, we do not expect the purchasing cooperatives to rely exclusively on competitive forces. To be sure, where competition exists, the purchasing cooperative should manage it. Where competition can develop, the cooperative should promote it. But where the potential for competition is limited or absent, the states and purchasing cooperatives must be able to use other means to guarantee universal coverage, control costs, and improve quality.

Global Budgets

Moreover, we see the purchasing cooperatives not only as managers and promoters of competition but as a source of countervailing power and a mechanism for carrying out national spending limits. In these respects, too, we differ from advocates of managed competition who oppose any national budget setting. Some may ask why, if we believe competition will work, we also see a need for global budgets. One might as soon ask the designers of a new airplane if their specifications of a second engine demonstrates a lack of confidence in the first. Good designs often build in redundancy. If competition is a complete success, the provisions for global budgets will turn out to be superfluous. But, given past experience, a backup system of cost control seems prudent. Moreover, if employers are going to give up control of health benefits, they are going to expect strong guarantees of cost containment. Global budgets are that guarantee.

EMPLOYEES AND THE PURCHASING COOPERATIVES

Perhaps the single most important choice in the design of managed competition is the role of the purchasing cooperatives. Are HIPCs conceived as a remedy for the small-group market or as a general manager of health plan competition and global budgets? The latter conception would entail mandating all (or all but the largest) employers to participate in the purchasing cooperatives. The higher the proportion of health expenditures passing through the HIPCs, the easier global budgets will be to set and enforce. The principles of managed competition are also more likely to succeed if put into practice by purchasing cooperatives with large populations. The smaller the risk pool, the more likely risk selection is among competing plans. Moreover, even large companies will rarely have the capacity to offer the range of options available through a HIPC.

Wider participation in HIPCs will prevent them from being viewed as residual, second-class pools. It also will facilitate continuity of health care and coordination of coverage, for if large employers are outside the HIPC, they will set up their own provider networks or contract with different managed care plans. Employees will then often face disruption of care and provider relationships when switching jobs between firms in and out of the HIPC. Moreover, families with earners at different firms will often be unable to arrange for care from the same providers if, as seems likely under a reformed system, they are each required to take their own firm's coverage. Responsibility for coverage of dependents will also be difficult to resolve.

Large Firms

If participation in the purchasing cooperative is required only for employers with fewer than a given number of employees (100, 250, 500, and 1,000 are the most frequently mentioned levels), two possibilities arise for larger firms. They will either be barred from HIPCs or be offered HIPCs as an option. Barring larger firms would create several problems. First, large firms with high health care costs, such as the auto companies, will argue that a reformed system excluding them fails to address their concerns. Second, even large employers with low costs may worry that if they are unable to get into the HIPC, private health plans will shift costs from the HIPC population to their own employees. The option of entering the HIPC is the large firm's protection against cost shifting. Finally, if an absolute bar became policy, small firms would be forced out of the HIPC once they expanded beyond the ceiling, disrupting the health care of many employees. Denying employees access to a system that gives them more choice and a better price seems unlikely to be a highly popular policy.

On the other hand, if larger firms can join HIPCs voluntarily, the firms that do so will tend to have higher-than-average costs. The problem of adverse selection will be especially severe if these firms are offered the purchasing cooperatives' community rates. Hence, if the purchasing cooperatives are voluntary for some class of employers, any employer from that class that wants to join must be given a risk-adjusted rated.

The more inclusive the HIPC, the greater will be the reduction in administrative complexity. If myriad employer plans continue to operate, providers still may well face much of the current complexity and cost.

Therefore, on grounds of cost containment, portability and seamlessness of coverage, and simplicity of financing and administration, we prefer to see broad, mandatory employer participation in HIPCs. Hence we urge that the mandatory cutoff point be set as high as is politically feasible: a reasonable goal is the level of 1,000 employees in the bill introduced by the Conservative Democratic Forum.[8] Larger employers should also be given the option to join at risk-adjusted rates.

8. The Managed Competition Act of 1992, H.R. 5936, 102d Cong., 2d sess., 15 September 1992.

Opting Out

If a reformed system is going to assure Americans access to guaranteed benefits (among which we would include choice of a health plan), employers with over 1,000 employees opting out of the HIPC should have to meet the following requirements. (1) Employers opting out should have to offer a benchmark plan to their employees at no greater cost than if they were in the HIPC. In addition to protecting the interests of employees, this rule should restrain employer spending outside the HIPC. (2) All other employer-provided health plans should have to fulfill the same obligations imposed on plans contracting with HIPCs. Self-insurance should not be a route of escape from federal regulations governing the benefit package, uniform data, and other provisions for electronic billing and administrative simplicity. (3) Any employer offering more comprehensive benefits than the standard should be required to offer those benefits in a supplementary package available to all employees whether they subscribe to the benchmark plan or to the employer's other plans. (4) Any employer opting out of the HIPC should have to conduct an annual enrollment allowing employees to choose among the benchmark plan and other plans it offers, and it should follow federal guidelines for risk-adjusting payments to the plans.

The requirement that employers offer a benchmark plan would replace the unevenly enforced federal regulation that employers offer a qualifying HMO. Other regulations on health coverage outside the HIPC would replace the provisions of the Employee Retirement Income Security Act (ERISA) regarding health insurance.

A FRAMEWORK FOR FINANCE

Reform will meet fewer objections if its financing resembles the current, employer-based system of insurance premiums. A tax-based system might well be simpler, more efficient, and more progressive. Nevertheless, converting to a tax-financed system inevitably would create large numbers of losers as well as winners—and the losers would be affluent and powerful. Health care reform is hard enough without stirring upper-income taxpayers to opposition.

Under one option that we have proposed, the regional HIPC would annually declare a community-rated premium based on its benchmark plan (or alternatively on a weighted average of the lowest-cost plans making up at least 30 percent of overall enrollment). Employers would be required to pay a minimum share of that premium—say, 75 percent—for employees and their dependents, although they could choose to pay a larger share (even the entire amount). Employees would pay the remaining portion. To ensure that these premiums were affordable for low-wage employers and low-income employees, both employers' and employees' obligations for the benchmark premium would be capped. The employer's 75 percent share could not exceed a given percentage of payroll—say, 7 percent. The employee's share could not exceed a given percentage of family income—say 2 percent. Governmental subsidies would kick in at those levels.

(The subsidies would not, however, apply to additional premium charges paid for plans more costly than the benchmark plan.) To avoid giving employers an incentive to employ part-time workers, firms would pay a payroll tax on the wages of part-time workers whose premium costs they did not share.

The unemployed, the self-employed, part-time workers, and those out of the labor force would also be required to obtain health coverage through the HIPC. They too would have to pay the community-rated, benchmark premium in their region, but again, governmental subsidies would ease the burden. If their incomes were beneath the poverty level, they would pay nothing. If above poverty, they would pay a fixed percentage—say, 9 percent—of the difference between their income and the poverty line, up to the value of the premium.

To minimize out-of-pocket costs, the federal government could build the subsidies for employees into the tax-withholding mechanism and pay the subsidies for the unemployed and others without jobs directly to the HIPCs. Additional subsidies to the health plans would reduce or eliminate cost sharing at the point of service for subscribers below the poverty level.

In this volume of *Health Affairs,* John Sheils and colleagues report estimates of the public expenditures required under this approach—that is, with premium obligations capped at 7 percent of payroll for all employers, at 2 percent of family income for all employees, and at 9 percent of above-poverty income for all remaining individuals under age sixty-five, including current Medicaid beneficiaries. With low cost sharing and a broad benefit package, the total public subsidies come to $120.3 billion for 1993. Against this cost, however, one must set projected acute care Medicaid spending ($62.6 billion) and the prospective payroll tax on part-time wages ($4.1 billion), leaving approximately $53 billion to be made up in additional revenues. Under a high cost-sharing plan (which we do not favor), the residual revenue needs fall to $42 billion.[9]

Several additional effects of universal coverage would reduce the net cost. Much of the new spending for the uninsured, as well as the higher reimbursement rates for care of current Medicaid beneficiaries, will flow back into the public sector—that is, to public hospitals and clinics now being financed in part by state and local governments. In addition, newly available health insurance benefits at low-wage jobs will encourage movement from welfare to work among many who have remained on welfare because it gives them access to Medicaid. One study suggests that universal coverage could bring about a one-fourth reduction in welfare caseloads.[10] Federal legislation should also encourage the states to achieve economies in the health care component of workers' compensation by merging it into the general health insurance system.[11]

9. J. F. Sheils, L. S. Lewin, and R. A. Haught, "Potential Public Expenditures under Managed Competition," in this volume of *Health Affairs.*
10. R. Moffitt and B. Wolfe, "The Effect of the Medicaid Program on Welfare Participation and Labor Supply," Working Paper no. 3286 (Cambridge, Mass.: National Bureau of Economic Research, 1990).
11. L. C. Baker and A. B. Krueger, "Twenty-Four-Hour Coverage and Workers' Compensation Insurance," in this volume of *Health Affairs.*

States and localities thus could benefit financially from the federal program we have described in four ways: (1) Medicaid's acute care provisions would be folded into universal coverage; (2) "safety-net" spending at public hospitals and clinics for uncompensated care would be sharply reduced; (3) welfare costs would be cut; and (4) substantial savings can be achieved from merging the health care component of workers' compensation into health insurance. The Lewin-VHI study in this volume of *Health Affairs* considers only the first of these. Unpublished estimates by Lewin-VHI of the impact of Sen. George Mitchell's (D-ME) HealthAmerica plan put savings in general assistance, public hospital, and other state and local costs at $10 billion.[12] The low cost-sharing package we favor should cut those costs even more. With these other savings to states and localities taken into account, the net costs to the public sector of the program described above might well fall below $25 billion.

In addition, this approach can easily be modified either to reduce needed revenue or to make the plan more attractive. For example, instead of providing subsidies to all firms to keep their premium obligations within 7 percent of payroll, we could limit the subsidies to small employers (or to those employers who enter the HIPCs). Alternatively, without increasing the subsidies required, we might graduate the cap—say, from 9 percent on larger firms down to 4 or 5 percent on the smallest. And, for small firms only, we might exclude some fixed amount of payroll in calculating the cap—say, $5,000 per employee—thereby reducing premium obligations only for small firms with low average wages.

Yet another possibility would be to exclude entirely the smallest employers—those with five or fewer employees—and treat their owners and workers as if they were part of the self-employed population. (Lewin-VHI estimates the additional public cost of this measure at $2 billion.) There are strong administrative as well as political arguments for this policy. Small businesses start up, close, move, and change names with great frequency. It may be easier for HIPCs to deal with these employees individually. If such a firm bought insurance for its employees, it would have to do so through the HIPC; if it did not, the employees would enter the HIPC individually.

For the additional public revenue required, three possibilities seem to us particularly attractive: a partial reduction in the tax benefits to employer-paid insurance (worth $92 billion in 1993); provider taxes; and the so-called monster cigarette tax of $2 a pack (worth $35 billion a year when fully phased in).[13] While enacting any tax is difficult, each one of these can be designed to improve incentives as well as to raise needed revenue.

GLOBAL BUDGETS UNDER MANAGED COMPETITION

The term *global budgeting* refers to an overall budget limit on health care services, regardless of where the funds originate. In some contexts, global budgeting has

12. Unpublished estimates from Lewin-VHI Health Benefits Simulation Model.
13. Ibid.; and P. Passell, "Doing Well by Doing Good," *The New York Times*, 24 December 1992, D2.

come to mean setting a limit on spending by sector—that is, specific allocations for doctors, hospitals, and so on. This kind of global budgeting risks freezing in place the current composition of expenditures and thereby may retard progressive changes, such as the substitution of lower-cost ambulatory care for inpatient care. Moreover, under this kind of budget, individual physicians would still have incentives to increase service volume and intensity. This is an especially serious problem in the United States because of the bias toward high-cost procedures, the oversupply of specialists, and excess hospital capacity. Given balance billing, inadequate state-level data resources, and the lack of enforcement mechanisms, it is also not clear how such a budget would be carried out. All in all, fee-for-service global budgeting seems a fine recipe for blocking structural reform, heightening conflict, and discrediting the concept of a budget.

Global budgeting through capitated payments to health plans does not suffer from these problems. First, the plans can shift expenditures among different categories of service; indeed, they have an incentive to make exactly the kinds of progressive, cost-saving changes that fee-for-service payment has inhibited. Second, the plans have a strong incentive to enlist their providers in adopting conservative practice patterns to comply with the organizations' budget limits. It is this link between financing and provision that is missing in the fee-for-service insurance system.

The aim of policy should be to use the capitated health plans at the local level to carry out nationally set targets for health care spending. The purchasing cooperatives are clearly suited for connecting the two. But what exactly is the budget that policy should be trying to control? And how can spending caps be consistent with managed competition and some degree of regional and state flexibility?

The budget for a region could be defined in at least four ways: (1) the benchmark premium times the total number of enrollees; (2) total premiums paid to all plans, including out-of-pocket premium payments for higher-cost plans; (3) total spending on covered benefits for all eligible individuals (that is, premiums plus out-of-pocket payments for services); and (4) total spending on health care for covered and uncovered services. Of these four budget alternatives, the first has a special significance because it identifies government, employer, and individual obligations. All other spending would be with out-of-pocket (preferably after-tax) dollars. Thus, if a global budget cap were interpreted as limiting the growth of benchmark premiums, it would focus policy on the mandated core of health spending.

Ordinarily, such a cap should be sufficient. But the HIPCs and national board should keep an eye on the various forms of out-of-pocket spending that might signal a problem—a shift in the composition of HIPC enrollment toward higher-cost plans; escalation in the premiums of higher-cost plans; and potential inadequacies in the benefit package as services evolve.

Under this approach, which might be called benchmark budgeting, the federal government would determine a maximum allowable rate of increase in benchmark premiums each year and set a target for discretionary, aftertax spending. The cap and the target might be set by the president and Congress on the advice of economic advisers and the National Health Board, which would evaluate demographic and technological factors and recent changes in interpretations of benefits. The board might then translate the overall national spending limits into caps and targets for the states, taking account of changes in population and other variables. With these constraints in mind, the HIPCs would then bargain with the health plans.

HIPCs would have various means at their disposal to bring in plans with sufficient capacity at the allowable rate of growth and to achieve the overall target for out-of-pocket spending. Clearly, by virtue of their dominant role as purchasers, they would be in a position to jawbone the plans and effectively impose a rate. But they would also have other means. They could work with the plans to reduce the costs of covered benefits by using those with the lowest costs and best results as models for the others. They could "carve out" some high-cost benefits from all of their contracts and seek competitive bids for a single, globally budgeted provider. They could enter into a state-administered arbitration process with the plans.

If local and state remedies were to no avail, a HIPC could seek a finding from the National Health Board that managed competition and bargaining had failed to keep NIPC premium increases within the allowable range. The board could then adopt any of several measures, ranging from advisory recommendations for improved cost containment to imposition of strict regulatory controls. Conceivably, the board might decertify the HIPC if it found the HIPC's board to be negligent or incompetent. It might also impose onerous controls on provider rates and capital spending. Given the risks to all local parties, HIPCs would have strong incentives to meet the spending cap without calling in federal intervention.

Under an alternative approach, the federal government would merely set targets for HIPC premiums as well as discretionary spending, allowing states and HIPCs to exceed targets but reducing federal subsidies as a penalty. Thus, if states spent above budget goals, premiums would have to rise and states would have to make up the difference between the amount of the guaranteed subsidy and the amount the federal government was paying. Such an approach might seem at first to be much weaker than a strict federal cap on HIPC premium increases. But if the states had to raise new revenue to pay the extra costs, they would, in effect, become the chief enforcers of the cap.

Should the states also be able to reduce the federally mandated benefit package? We favor a relatively comprehensive national standard for the benefit package for several interrelated reasons. Coverage is the key to control; the costs of services not included in the package will be harder to regulate. Also, if limits on high-cost services are imposed, many individuals will turn to government in the end; it is better to require them to carry full insurance in the first place. Moreover, capitated health plans—the linchpins of the new system—work best when they are responsible for providing the full array of medical services. In the capitation context, it makes no sense to exclude routine or preventive medical services or to impose deductibles—techniques of cost control relevant to the conventional fee-for-service model that has, in fact, been unable to control costs. But since fee-for-service will continue, at least for some time, states dependent upon it may need some flexibility on the benefit package, particularly cost sharing.

States may also need contingent authority to regulate rates. As we have suggested, the federal government would establish a set of provider rates that could be used as a backup to managed competition. The presumption would be that rate setting would be approved only when managed competition failed. But, in areas with little effective competition, states or HIPCs might have greater discretionary authority to employ rate regulation, in part to create pressure on providers to develop new delivery systems that might obviate the need for rate setting.

Rate setting would be available in reserve in all regions for the one fee-for-service option. It is important that there be such a plan, and only one such plan, in every HIPC region. An insurer that won the bidding to run the plan would have two options for paying providers. It could negotiate with provider representatives or invoke a government-mandated rate structure in the event of a failure to come to terms. Balance billing should be banned in this plan as in the managed care options; cost containment with balance billing is like building a dam with a gaping hole in the middle.

STRATEGIC CHALLENGES

The introduction of a managed competition system through purchasing cooperatives faces undeniable political and structural impediments. The transitional problems are not primarily, as many believe, the additional public expenditures, which can be held to manageable levels. Rather, the problems stem from the complexity of disentangling present arrangements and the anxieties of so many whose lives and livelihoods are tied to them.

Some of the most legitimate concerns come from groups representing the poor and others dependent on existing programs. Federal legislation should address those concerns by requiring HIPCs to ensure that plans under contract provide accessible services to vulnerable populations. To avoid segregating the poor in the benchmark plan, HIPCs could require that all plans with higher charges accept a specified percentage of low-income individuals at the rate paid to the benchmark plan. In some regions, HIPCs might promote plans that would take service to the poor or to language minorities as their special responsibility. Protecting the "floor" will always be an issue (even under national health insurance systems the poor do not, in fact, get the same services as the elite or even the middle class). This approach would provide the poor with a mainstream level of coverage and vest responsibility for assuring care as well as coverage in a new, consumer-oriented institution—the purchasing cooperative.

Even with universal coverage and integration of Medicaid (other than long-term care), "safety-net" needs will persist. Inevitably, some people, such as illegal immigrants, will not be covered; states and counties might use HIPCs to contract for such care. Moreover, some states now provide benefits to the poor (such as transportation, eyeglasses, and, most important, care for severe, chronic mental illness) that will not be covered under the uniform benefit package. To maintain such services, states now providing them could create a wraparound benefit package for the poor.

We do not foresee requiring current Medicare beneficiaries to move into the new system. Of all groups, the elderly are most wedded to fee-for-service medicine. Yet they might be offered an annual choice through their regional HIPC as an alternative to fee-for-service Medicare, with the inducement of broader coverage, including prescription drugs. Instead of graduating into Medicare, new cohorts of the elderly might remain in the new system. Traditional Medicare would thereby wither away.

Although the strategic challenges of reform are immense, the risks of failure are even greater. Under the pressure of rising costs, the insurance system is unraveling. Many small businesses and individuals can no longer afford the cost; major corporations are dumping their responsibilities for retirees. People who were once comfortably insured now stare at financial ruin. The prospects facing government are not much better. Under current policies, according to the Congressional Budget Office, health costs will hit 18 percent of GNP by the end of the decade, up from 13.6 percent in 1992, and will represent 30 percent of federal outlays (excluding interest), up from 18 percent today.[14] This is nothing short of an economic catastrophe. A combined strategy of managed competition and global cost controls is the best way to avert that disaster and achieve what other Western countries have long had—an economically sustainable system of universal health insurance.

14. Congressional Budget Office, *Projections of National Health Expenditures* (Washington: CBO, October 1992).

Why Managed Competition Won't Work

The medical monster has swollen to much beyond what we can afford, expropriating virtually every resource available for health and for other social agendas as well.

Rick J. Carlson

The U.S. medical industry, since the demise of the Soviet military machine, is the largest single organized system of economic activity in the world. Medical care is our most costly entitlement program. And we can't afford it. But what to do?

Policy initiatives are being tossed around like obscenities at a hockey game; all seek to rein in costs of a galloping medical care system, and all position managed care as the jockey. But "managed competition" won't work. The core reason is that it can't deliver real reform—a health care system that delivers health, not just limitless treatments. In any case it can't cut costs nearly fast enough, if it can cut them at all.

Real reform is not on the agenda. There's no money for real reform because we spend it all on medicine. And since medical care has very little to do with health, cutting costs, even if we can, will have very little to do with anything other than cutting costs.

Healthcare Forum Journal, May/June 1993

"Managing" competition will only change the rules of play for delivery organizations, all of which will continue to deliver the same set of products and services as those now provided. We've had competition in medical care for a long time, and to date it has not reduced costs at all and, tragically, has produced virtually no product innovation. The product of medicine today, after years of competition, is essentially the same product it has always been, just fancier, glitzier, a little less invasive, and a whole lot more expensive.

So managing health care competition is like asking a pro football team to compete on the color and sheen of their uniforms, the sexiness of their cheerleaders, and the size and architectural magnificence of their stadiums, rather than on the game itself. All it will encourage is marginal price competition on the same product.

If you manufacture tires you can marginally reduce the cost of making those tires and pass some or even most of those savings to your customers. Some of this may in fact occur through managed competition, and so over a number of years we may experience some savings as a result—at the margin. But if we truly are going to affect the explosive escalation of costs in medical care, and in the course of doing so create a system that delivers health and not just more units of treatment, what is needed is a new and different tire.

Managed competition will not produce that new and different tire, just the old tire, no better, no worse, though maybe at a slightly lower price. What would it take to produce a new and different tire? Here are my suggestions for initiating real reform:

1. EXPLODE PHYSICIANS' WORM'S-EYE VIEW

Doctors, often to their credit, are trained to control and to focus that control on one person at a time—the patient they're seeing. They aren't trained to work in teams, and they aren't trained to solicit or elicit patient participation. (Not surprisingly, physicians are the only group who conduct their own AA meetings.)

This approach works fine when one or more conditions is met: the problem being treated is somatic (even better when the patient is comatose); when preventive approaches do not seem as obvious and profoundly more cost-effective as they often do; or when the problem appears to have a singular cause and hence can arguably be treated, extirpated, or even sometimes just ameliorated by a targeted intervention: a drug, surgery, or physical therapy.

Our medical care system was born out of the need to treat raging infections, when pain and suffering demanded melioration, and at a time when acute diseases, injuries, and accidents were the norm—not the exception as they are now. Today our health problems have dramatically changed. Most, in fact nearly all, of our health challenges are chronic and multifactorial (having more than one and frequently many causes).

To many doctors trained to see one problem at a time, our current major health challenges are unnerving. They are highly complex, intertwining the physical, emotional/psychological, and social in a skein that's hard to unwind. And their resolution is frequently dependent on the full-faceted involvement of the patient.

It's one thing to deplore the narrow focus of the physician, however understandable and even commendable it might be in the abstract. But we continue to foster and celebrate this finely tuned "one on one" medicine that has long since swollen to much beyond what we can afford, expropriating virtually every resource available for health and, in times of increasingly stringent economic constraints, resources for other social agendas as well.

For example, just after the riots in L.A., in spring 1992, President Bush, in defending his administration's urban policies, pointed out that between 1988 and 1992, federal spending in California on the needs of the inner cities had risen by nearly $70 billion. What he failed to add was that 85 percent of that increase was in Medicaid and Medicare expenditures alone.

We must begin to train physicians better and differently, to create new generations of healers. The ones we have now are largely ineducable in the ways of health that must prevail if we are to both contain rising costs and produce cost-effective and lasting results.

2. DISMANTLE THE REPLICATING ENGINE

No industry has ever even come close to creating demand like medical care has. The US has built a voracious medical replicating engine that can speed up at will, while at the same time laying its own track. It lays track by medicalizing even the most hard-to-reach and sometimes innocent facets of human behavior: first by making the trials and tribulations of living (gambling, sexual behavior, and a variety of other addictions) into problems that are only soluble by the purveyance of more medicine, and second through defining and redefining medicine's turf. Adolescent medicine, as a specialty, for example, arose only as pediatricians ran out of enough younger patients.

It is this second method—supply-creating demand—that is so potent and dangerous. In a series of studies, now approaching classic status, the supply of medical care can be seen to be virtually equal to demand. The original studies, done in New England, compared rates of certain procedures such as tonsillectomies and other surgical interventions among like communities. The rates of these procedures turned out to be proportionate to the number of physicians, particularly surgeons, providing them—and unrelated to differences among patients or communities.

Almost everyone in the medical care business—including all suppliers of equipment, tools, chemicals, software, paper, plastic, new procedures/techniques of treatment, and, yes, even money, mostly risk capital; virtually all providers of care; most managers of delivery systems; nearly all healthcare insurers; and, emphatically, all of us buyers—have the same incentives: more and more medicine.

It is as though someone turned on a giant automatic robot, and forgot to turn it off. Medicine does what it does, sometimes mindlessly, over and over again, unit by unit, almost irrespective of the volume, the alternatives, and the consequences.

The system has gotten loose; King Kong is climbing the Empire State building clutching a claim form.

3. DISCIPLINE THE SPOILED CHILD

The single most potent obstacle to controlling the runaway expansion of medical care is our own inflated expectations—what we, the public, have been educated, really conditioned, to believe helps us.

That conditioning has taken hold with a vengeance: Notwithstanding its excesses, we love the medical care system. We exalt in it and celebrate it. The average American takes pride in its gross inefficiencies, as long as it's available to him or her, whenever needed, in any amount, and at any expense.

We only deplore its excesses for others. Whatever its shortcomings, we seem to want as much of it as we can get—as long as someone else pays for it.

Maybe it's time for the spoiled children of the medical system to exercise a little self-discipline—to question our expectations and curb our exorbitant utilization.

4. TURN THE REWARD SYSTEM UPSIDE DOWN

Definitive research is now available to show that investments in prevention, health enhancement, and self-care are cost-effective. This evidence has been available for more than a few years, so all that's missing now is the political will to force the medical care system to do something other than treat-after-the-fact, treat, treat, and then treat some more.

The sad fact, and one that must be confronted directly, is that our medical care system repetitively rewards excessive and unwarranted treatments, educates our physicians only to treat, and then reductionistically, one patient and one problem at a time.

If ''health status'' is the measure, medicine as it is practiced is absurdly unproductive. There are vastly superior ways to produce health, such as the reduction and elimination of toxins in our environment.

But prevention, even when the research support is convincing, is rarely taught, indifferently practiced, and stintingly rewarded. This state of training and practice cannot be changed in even ten years. It would represent a sea change for medicine, and one that must be promoted now and unrelentingly pursued.

5. HONOR THE CONSUMER

About 80 percent of the health problems people have cannot be decisively treated; either the treatment or the cause or both are equivocal. And so decisions have to be made about the best course of action or whether there's any course of action.

We let physicians make virtually all these decisions. We aren't asked. But we should be. It's our health, and in many cases our decisionmaking may be better.

The evidence for the efficacy of self-help for a wide variety of conditions is impressive. And the case for cost-effectiveness is dramatic, especially if we can keep people from falling hopelessly into the medical care vortex, because then, like Alice, they are often swept worldlessly into a bizarre and disorienting world.

Further, the emerging evidence for consumer ''informed decisionmaking'' is striking. In a recent and celebrated study, when men facing the prospects of prostate surgery were shown an interactive video display offering in-depth information about their options, including self-care, about 60 percent elected to delay or avoid surgery. Since we spend about $3–4 billion a year to provide this surgical intervention, if we could instead provide information to all surgical candidates, we could save $2–3 billion a year. Consumers can be, and probably are, more risk-aversive than their doctors when given full information.

Information about health and disease is the most ''classified'' body of data we have—even more than that for national security. Because of professional training, fear, bias, and institutional complicity, real people have not been entrusted with information about their own health that, if available, could, and probably would, alter many of the choices people make, not only about medical interventions, but about prevention, health enhancement, and self-help.

6. ADMIT THAT WE CAN'T AFFORD IT ANYMORE

Investment for profit does stimulate innovation. Pharmaceutical manufacturers plaintively make this point. But there are two problems with this truism: First, the innovation isn't always the right kind, and second, it doesn't mean that we can afford it.

The pressures and push of billions of dollars of investment capital and the expectations of capital for handsome rates of return feed the development of technologies that fit our existing reimbursement system, enriching its capabilities to treat and cure. But such innovation does not work to our advantage as a population because the targets of investment continue to be procedures and treatments for individuals resulting in arguable health benefits at the margin. Little, if any, monies are allocated to health promotion, the prevention of disease, and self-care tools and technologies. (That has always been the case, and unless the incentives in the system are changed, it is likely to always be the case.)

A byproduct of this investment pattern is that other medical care systems around the world benefit from our largesse. The Canadian system, for example, which operates at a far lower percentage of GNP than we do, feeds off our innovation, and hence, eschews mechanisms for enrichment.

Our problem is that we can no longer afford this pattern of investment. Even if such a model were defensible, the technological innovation resulting from investment capital is one of the major drivers of the medical cost increases. In our society, when a procedure is proven to be efficacious (leaving aside whether it is cost-effective), our political and social ethic dictates that the benefits must be made available to everyone—those who can afford to buy care on their own, those who purchase through insurance, and/or those who are beneficiaries of public programs.

As little as ten years ago, less than 10 percent of all capital available for venture capital investment in the US was directed to the medical care system. Recent estimates suggest that it is now close to 30 percent, which shows that unless investors are unbelievably ignorant about what they're doing with their money, they seem to know a good deal when they see it.

Given that there are probably more winners than losers in this investment game, and assuming further that standard rates of return apply to medical care investments, then what we're really doing is providing investors an opportunity to richly benefit from our fast-expanding medical care enterprise with little commensurate return in value to society.

It has been reliably reported, for example, that gains in the personal shareholdings by key stockholders of the Health Corporation of America over a three-year period in the late Eighties were about 720 percent. Gains like this do not occur just in the for-profit sector. A recent issue of *Modern Healthcare* reported that the income level of the 20 largest nonprofit healthcare systems increased by 24 percent from 1990 to 1991.

What is the justification for sustaining a medical care system that enriches individuals so lavishly when nearly 40 million people lack any insurance at all and when millions of others must rely on under-financed and often shabby public programs?

7. GET RID OF THE INSURANCE INDUSTRY

It doesn't even come close to serving the public interest. It doesn't write insurance; it discriminates against the poor, the lame, the halt, and the sick in order to preserve its premium cash flow so it can make stupid investments in sour real estate deals. And it is extremely costly.

Empire Blue Cross and Blue Shield, the largest but only one of four Blue Cross/Blue Shield plans in New York State, has more administrative and claims processing personnel than all of Canada. Because of the way our medical care system grew like topsy, with virtually no plan, the number of payers has multiplied like cancer cells. Perversely today, the number of payers continues to expand as the number of delivery units for care declines, because of consolidation among providers. Left to nature, it is conceivable that at some point in the future there will be more payers than providers.

The costs of this excess are substantial. Estimates vary, but most analyses suggest that an instant savings of $80–100 billion could be achieved if we moved to a single-payer system such as Canada's.

Why don't we do it? What's the justification for having so many payers (some families in the US have three or four in just one family unit)? The answer usually given—and with a straight face—is "competition": arguably, the costs of medical care are lower because all these insurance companies, while presumably screening for quality, use their spare time to aggressively bargain for the best price.

Unfortunately, there is no evidence that this occurs. Not only do our myriad insurance carriers do little more than listlessly chastise providers for their high charges, they no longer even pretend to "insure." What they really do is assess risk, stratify it by what it's likely to cost, and then avoid taking on the higher-cost "bad" risk. This results in shifting costs to those least able to avoid it: the government, smaller weaker carriers, and, of course, those who can't afford to buy insurance at any price, who then join the ranks of Americans who lack insurance coverage.

Recently added to this pretty picture is a grotesquerie: The Supreme Court has just ruled that self-insured employers—about 80 percent of the bigger ones and about 65 percent overall—can change their benefits "at will," even after covered individuals have received the care for which they presumed they were covered. What this means is that "insurance" not only isn't really insurance because risks aren't spread, but buying it doesn't guarantee that it will do that for which you bought it—namely, pay your bills.

Is there anyone around who thinks we keep insurance carriers in business for any reason other than their lobbying muscle?

What's the alternative? We don't have to socialize healthcare. The delivery system can be left private, with only the financing made public. Yes, this will introduce public inefficiencies to substitute for private degradations.

But ask the people who haven't any insurance about it, and those who fear losing what coverage they have and so are locked into jobs they'd gladly leave (as many as one in five workers, according to a recent estimate).

And then seek out those whose parents have "spent down" their life savings in order to secure Medicaid's meager benefits, and check out the fears of the baby boomer generation about what to do if their parents get sick and dependent.

And while you're at it, ask those whose coverage, bought and paid for, is slashed or eliminated because they've gotten sicker than their employer counted on or have a disease their employer finds distasteful.

So ask all of these folks which they would rather have: the security of coverage through a public financing system, as sloppy as it might be, or taking their chances in a free market for insurance that has red-lined them.

8. FORCE MEDICINE TO BE A SCIENCE

If we have the guts to take on the public financing of medical care, we might also begin to do what professional exhortations, learned journals, and the patrons of a fledgling medical science can't do: Make doctors and hospitals do the right thing.

The lack of good science as a platform for what physicians and hospitals do to us daily is a shock to those who discover how little of medical practice is based on much more than the hopefully astute observations of a handful of patients by a few discerning practitioners. Very little of standard medical practice—probably around 10 percent by best estimates—is based on the kind of research that would justify either reasonable costs or presumed benefits.

The absence of an adequate research base especially confounds attempts to fix global budgets, something that, controversy notwithstanding, virtually everybody agrees could work. In the absence of good science, those procedures that survive under global budgeting pressures are those whose advocates are the best politicians rather than the best scientists and healers.

With the arrival, however, of more and better outcomes research results, we are beginning to put a scientific base under habitual practice. As we do so, we shouldn't be afraid to tell doctors that unless they practice a medicine based on the research evidence—and not on hunch, laziness, and "business as usual"—they won't get paid. Today, with multiple payers matching each other only in efficiency, greed, and wimpishness, doctors and hospitals find it easy to do what they will, and to fall back on "accepted standards of practice"—a living tautology—as an excuse.

So it's time to tell them that from now they will only get paid for what works based on a living science of medicine. What are we afraid of—mistakes?

9. ADVOCATE HEALTHY AGING

One of us turns 50 every six seconds. Today, those over 65 in the United States consume 30–35 percent of all medical care resources, though they number slightly less than 13 percent of our population. Those over 50, representing not quite 30 percent of our population, consume more than 50 percent of all medical care, nearly 65 percent of hospital services, and a like amount for pharmaceutical products.

Between now and the end of this century those over 50 will grow dramatically in absolute numbers by about 18–20 million, while those below 50 will decline by 9 million. The future impact on medical care utilization of this already demanding population is almost terrifying. And it is inexorable.

So far the response has been stark fear. In fact, it's remarkably difficult to find reliable projections of the impact of this older population on demand curves as well as on costs. Most cost projections, as utterly terrifying as they are, don't even factor in the increased utilization that will inevitably result from an older population. Once such utilization factors are taken into account, the numbers are so scary that no one even wants to talk about them. Under these circumstances our society has essentially two responses: panic and constructive change.

To date, panic is winning. But it needn't. The evidence is overwhelming that aging does not have to reflect progressive deterioration of faculties and health status. In fact, many opportunities exist for "healthy aging."

There will always be some whose disease and disability will be progressive and irreversible, and hence very costly to treat. And because there are greater numbers of older persons (and will be on into the next century) these treatment costs are likely to rise no matter what we do. However, the opportunities to engineer programs to encourage persons both attitudinally and behaviorally to take better care of themselves and to improve their own health are enormous and potentially very cost-effective. The alternative is unbearable.

WOULD WE DO IT DIFFERENTLY?

We have been doing the wrong things in medical care for so long that even a reform policy that was exactly right—and managed competition isn't—would have very little chance to achieve the results promised in less than ten years, when, since we aren't likely to do things even close to right, the costs of medical care will have sailed to about $2.5 trillion, or 20 percent of GNP.

There's nothing inherently wrong with spending 20 cents of every dollar on medicine. Sure, medical care may be excessive and wasteful and haughtily unresponsive to us. But if we the American people had the chance to think through the options, based on full disclosure of how, why, and when medicine works, and what the tradeoffs are, what would we do? Would we allocate resources as irrationally and mindlessly as providers do?

We deserve a chance to prove otherwise.

Cost Containment, Access, and American Health Financing: Getting Beyond the Shell Game

WALTER J. JONES
Medical University of South Carolina
BERNARD J. REILLY
Widener University
ROBERT W. BROYLES
Medical University of South Carolina

INTRODUCTION

Since the late 1970s no problem has preoccupied analysts and policy-makers in health care more than cost containment. By 1987, annual expenditures on health care in the U.S. had surpassed $500 billion, consuming between 11%-12% of the Gross National Product (Levit and Freeland, 1988). The rate of increase in the national cost of health care is significantly higher than the Consumer Price Index (Friedland, 1987). Even more alarming, "if current trends continue, total costs will double in six years and triple in twelve years, hitting $1.5 trillion in the year 2000" (National Leadership Commission, 1989).

These clearly unacceptable cost patterns cannot be sustained indefinitely and may inflict enormous damage to the American economy if not properly moderated. As a consequence of these developments, policy analysis in the 1980s was committed to the development of a variety of methods by which the major payers in the health care system (most prominently the federal government, but also insurance companies and employers) could slow the constant increases in price

Journal of Health & Human Resources Administration, Winter 1992.

of health care. The ultimate effectiveness of these efforts is still uncertain, but data since 1983 do not show any significant improvement in cost containment.

Friedland (1987:22–23) suggests that, after adjusting for inflationary presence in the economy, "it is clear that there has not been any real decline in the rate of growth in health care expenditures." Spiraling cost increases have been accompanied by serious increases in the number of citizens who have lost effective access to the health care system. Efforts to control Medicare and Medicaid costs have led to tighter program eligibility requirements, cutbacks in the range of services paid for, and increased deductibles. The combined effect has been to reduce access or entirely exclude many citizens at or near the poverty line (Holahan and Cohen, 1986; Sorkin, 1989). In the private sector, many employers (particularly small businesses) have either reduced or eliminated health insurance coverage for their employees. Consequently, "the rate of noncoverage across the population has been rising since the mid-1970's and continues to rise" (Cholet, 1987:188).

The central theme of this article is that the inflationary pressures in the American health care industry and inequities in access result from the transfer of costs and a failure to establish a unified method of financing the use of services. The American health care system at present uniquely combines the disadvantages of both regulation and deregulation. Much of its behavior is motivated by the worst aspects of both public and private sector decision-making. As a result, policies designed to control costs and ensure access in the United States must address the underlying structural problem of cost shifting and financing within health care in the U.S.

COST SHIFTING IN U.S. HEALTH CARE FINANCE

The current financial structure of U.S. health care evolved in response to changes in public values regarding the status of health care as an economic and social good. When health services were considered a relatively ordinary and affordable economic commodity, the public was willing to leave their purchase to private arrangement (though charity care was available in many areas for the poor).

After World War II, however, a major shift in national sentiment took place. Americans began to appreciate the "social maintenance" functions of adequate health care and the extent to which a healthy society might also develop a high degree of social self-satisfaction, solidarity, and cooperation (Smith and Kaluzny, 1986). As a consequence, a general (if vague) national consensus developed that regarded care as a basic human right. With the establishment of Medicare and Medicaid, the federal government irrevocably entered the health care arena as the largest guarantor of access for the poor and the elderly (Califano, 1986). This increased involvement transformed a fundamentally private sector industry into one in which both producers and consumers of health care services are dependent on public finance. Over forty percent of health care expenditures is now financed by federal, state, or local governmental units (McCue, 1989). As in other modern societies, the U.S. health care system features a dominant role for the public sector.

Unlike most other industrial nations, however, the involvement of the federal government in the U.S. has taken place without any significant centralization of health care finance or administration. American health care is provided through a "nonsystem" of numerous independent but uncoordinated public and private sector agencies. The ultimate reason for this condition lies in the historic and firmly-held American commitment to limited, divided, and decentralized government. The public policies affecting the operations of the "nonsystem" are established through a fragmented and often contentious set of government actors and institutions, usually heavily influenced by pressure exerted by interest groups (Brown, 1983; Jones, 1984; Feldstein, 1988a).

The lack of coordination within U.S. health care profoundly complicates the central tasks of controlling costs and ensuring access. No set of individuals or institutions feels (or is perceived to have) responsibility for medical cost inflation or for financing care for the millions of citizens who cannot afford it. Since the American political and health services systems are both structurally designed to diffuse rather than concentrate authority and accountability, the result is, what might be thought of, a shell game.

The characteristic behavior of the shell game in U.S. health care financing is cost shifting (Califano, 1986). Each policy-making actor has a vested interest in shifting the burdens of controlling costs and ensuring access to some other actor. This dynamic provides a powerful incentive for the federal government, the largest payer, to create health care policies that reduce access to the system for major social groups. "The federal government used to view health care as a social problem. Today it views it almost solely as a budget deficit problem. The shift in perspective is important. Social problems can be left to fester; budget deficit problems require more immediate solutions . . . Since governments provide health care primarily to the elderly and the poor, government deficit-reduction measures systematically dismantle the existing system of paying for health care for these groups" (Thurow, 1985:611).

To the extent that effective cost containment and adequate access for all citizens are what economists call "public goods" (that is, goods from which all members benefit but no one member can be compelled to pay for), cost shifting within the U.S. system of health finance is evidence of serious market failure. Hardin (1968) calls such a situation "the tragedy of the commons." All actors know that they will ultimately be ruined if the public welfare is neglected, but each actor's short-term identifiable costs would exceed benefits if he or she did something to preserve the public commons without the participations of all other actors. So each actor rationally waits for someone else to do something and nothing gets done. The public's responsibility in fact becomes no one's responsibility.

Current efforts to control costs and provide access involve the concurrent application of two approaches. On the one hand, the federal government encourages the development of market mechanisms within the health services sector. On the other hand, the federal government is also steadily developing and implementing broader regulatory controls on selected components of the health care system. Each emphasis has a detailed theoretical foundation and defensible policy logic. In practice, however, the results of applying the combination of the two approaches have been problematic at best (Altman and Rodwin, 1988).

THE MARKET APPROACH

Economists have long proposed using market mechanisms and competitive forces as vehicles to improve efficiency, control costs, and ensure that the mix and quality of services correspond to consumer preferences (Okun, 1975). In health care, the market approach consists of policies designed to encourage consumers, producers, and payers to be cost conscious (Bagley and Sullivan, 1986; Easterbrook, 1987). Competitive pressures are supposed to influence supply decisions so as to improve efficiency, lower costs, and reduce prices. In addition, some argue that increased reliance on the market mechanisms will also lower the demand for health care, which in turn will reduce utilization and costs.

With respect to supply, proponents of market mechanisms suggest that increased competition will induce providers to use resources more effectively and efficiently, thus controlling the cost of care (Arnould and Van Vorst, 1985). In particular, there is an assumption that the financial incentives associated with the growing alternative delivery systems (including such entities as HMOs and PPOs) will induce physicians to control utilization and health expenditures (Inglehart, 1986). Stimulated by federal and state laws (beginning with the Health Maintenance Act of 1973), the number of HMOs, PPOs, and IPOs doubled from 1980 to 1985, with a membership increase of 115% and a 5.8% growth in market share. There are estimates that 80% of the insured population in the U.S. will be enrolled in HMOs and PPOs by the year 2000 (Tobarski, 1990). In contrast, the market share of conventional third-party systems such as Blue Cross and Blue Shield declined by approximately six percent (Guterman *et al.*, 1988).

Unfortunately, the existing evidence only partly supports the claims made by market advocates. As summarized by Luft (1981) and Rosko and Broyles (1988), several studies suggest that alternative delivery systems significantly lower the cost and utilization of health services. However, a portion of the savings may be due to a favorable selection bias. Some alternative systems tend to enroll younger and healthier individuals who require less care, resulting in below average costs (Wilensky and Rossiter, 1986; Rosko and Broyles, 1988). To the extent that selection bias exists, alternative delivery systems solve the cost problem by shifting the burden to other health service entities and reducing access for high risk individuals—the shell game described earlier.

Alternative delivery systems like HMOs may also reduce utilization by *de facto* rationing of health services (Brown, 1983). This rationing may be justified to some extent, given the possibility that traditional fee-for-service arrangements result in overutilization (Califano, 1986). However, such rationing does raise the accompanying issue of the ultimate quality of care provided (Ellwood and Paul, 1986). If the quality of care is adversely affected by cost containment considerations, affected patients will be more likely to require health services later on. This would constitute cost shifting from the present to the future.

In addition to these factors, there are other reasons to suspect that market competition will not be sufficiently effective to control health care costs. A growing body of research suggests that greater market pressures lead providers to engage in nonprice competition for patients, based on perceived quality or patient amenities. For example, hospitals may compete for physicians and payers by conducting elaborate marketing and advertising campaigns; offering more sophisticated equipment and procedures; and/or providing more luxurious rooms and meals (Easterbrook, 1987). Nonprice competition results in an increase in the total cost of care, though a portion of the higher cost would be shifted elsewhere.

Finally, even if the market approach does result in significant price competition and lower costs, it is doubtful that it can be applied in all geographical areas of the United States. Beginning in the early 1980s, the era of greater competition coincides with the steady reduction of health services suppliers in small towns and rural areas (Easterbrook, 1987). In other words, the market approach significantly affects access as well as costs—and not always for the better.

The market approach usually entails a set of policy options designed to alter demand decisions so as to reduce utilization and costs. One of the most prominent targets of market advocates is the current tax-exempt provision of health insurance by employers. It is usually argued that tax-exempt health insurance unfairly discriminates against non-insured workers and in effect subsidizes the consumption of health services by lowering the real cost of health care for recipients (Feldstein, 1988b). Further, advocates contend that the tax exemption should therefore be repealed to reduce "excessive" demand and let the health services market work effectively (Postrel, 1990).

As with supply, however, the body of existing research does not provide unequivocal support for the market approach with respect to demand. The contention that an increase in effective price lowers use is based on the traditional theory of consumer demand. However, previous findings indicate that the demand for health services insurance coverage and utilization is much less elastic than market advocates assume (Rosko and Broyles, 1988). The favorable tax treatment of health insurance is only a secondary explanation of health care cost inflation (Chernick, Holmer, and Weinberg, 1987). To lower demand significantly, prices would have to rise to, and remain, at, *much* higher real levels than at present. Such price increases might indeed lower demand but be so Draconian as to constitute a major public policy problem in and of themselves.

Influential interest groups within the healthcare system can also work against a drop in health services demand in response to price increases, shifting the ultimate sacrifices to other sectors of society (Evans, 1974; Feldstein, 1988a; Rosko and Broyles, 1988). Physicians, for example, can response to any decline in utilization by stimulating demand in order to maintain or increase their desired level of income. Hospitals can respond to policies that lower the demand for certain services by aggressively marketing services not affected by such policies. These efforts probably offset at least some of the decline in demand for services that result from market-dictated price increases.

Using the market approach to reduced health services demand has a final and most serious shortcoming. What happens to those who do not have enough money to enter the marketplace? The burden of demand reduction might well be shifted to those who can least afford it—the tens of millions of uninsured Americans (Ginzberg, 1986; Bayer *et al.*, 1988). These are indications that the negative effects on health resulting from higher prices of care are greater among the poor than on middle or upper class citizens (Wagstaff, 1986). As a result, even ardent advocates of health services competition admit that major efforts are necessary to protect the medically indigent from the darker side of freer markets (Goldsmith, 1984).

None of the above considerations exclude the use of market mechanisms and greater competition within health care to achieve greater efficiency and effectiveness. However, they do suggest that the market approach involves risks as well as benefits. They also indicate that, used by itself, a market approach will not succeed in controlling health care costs without unacceptable consequences and side effects. In practice, the United States has therefore combined increased competition with regulations that attempt to compensate for market defects.

THE REGULATORY APPROACH

The logic of regulation begins where competition in practice leaves off—with market failures as well as successes, with significant costs as well as benefits. Advocates of regulation argue that there are social ideals of equity and justice that will be unacceptably damaged by an unfettered market that all too often degenerates into a Darwinian situation of "survival of the fittest." Their remedy involves controls placed on the functioning of the marketplace, usually developed and administered by government agencies with the assistance of relevant professional associations (Noll and Owens, 1983; Feldstein, 1988a).

Regulation of health services, of course, is not a new development. The post World War II era saw the initiation of a wide range of federal and state government controls over health care, including the development of Certificate of Need (CON) statutes; the 1972 Social Security Amendments (which introduced Professional Service Review Organizations or PSROs); and finally the National Health Planning and Resources Development Act of 1974 (Melhado, 1988).

Traditional health regulation was subjected to increasing attack as ineffective and counterproductive by the 1970s (like regulation in most sectors of the American economy) and is not currently considered a viable policy option at the national level. However, the Eighties saw the rise of what has been termed "the new regulation" (Meyer, 1985). Focused on the problem of controlling costs, these new regulatory measures are based on prospective payment mechanisms implemented by public and private third-party payers. Based on Diagnostic Related Groups (DRGs) that determine the rate of compensation per discharge, the Medicare pricing mechanism established through Public Law 98–21 is the most prominent of the prospective payment systems. Since the passage of PL 98–21 in 1983, other private and public payers have implemented payment mechanisms that are similar to the Medicare system (Hsiao *et al.*, 1986; Russell, 1989).

As stated earlier, the United States has attempted to combine regulatory intervention with the simultaneous movement toward more market competition in order to control costs and provide acceptable access to the health care system. This combination of regulation and competition can be defended intellectually. In practice, however, the dual approach results from the lack of coordination and effective control over the U.S. health care system. Since there is no focal point at which control can be exerted, those attempting to contain costs have little choice other than to pile one measure upon another and hope for the best.

Have these regulatory efforts (prospective payment mechanisms in particular) controlled costs more effectively than the market approach? The record is mixed. There is some research indicating that prospective payment mechanisms have constrained the cost per admission, the cost per day, and the cost per capita for hospital systems (Rosko and Broyles, 1988). On the other hand, prospective payment systems as used in Medicare have encouraged hospitals to control costs by compressing the average length of stay for affected persons (Russell, 1989). All of the above-mentioned cost savings raise the issue of possible risks to the ultimate quality and effectiveness of care delivered (Allman, 1987). Once again there exists the possibility of a shift of the ultimate burden of cost containment, this time to the patient. The shell game of cost-shifting has flourished in the era characterized by prospective payment arrangements. Whatever the actual effects have been on cost containment, the Medicare pricing system has reduced the commitment of the federal government, forcing other payers to take up some of the slack. During the four fiscal years following the implementation of DRGs, the rate of increase in Medicare payments declined from a prior average of 10% per year to 3.4%—significantly less than cost increases for treatment of the elderly during the same period (Guterman and Dobson, 1986; Beebe *et al.*, 1988).

To a substantial extent, the costs that exceed prospective payment rates have been transferred to private health insurers. In response to the higher costs of claims, private insurers have increased their premiums—in 1988 by an industry average of twenty percent (American Management Association, 1988). This in turn has led employers to raise employee contributions and deductibles, restrict benefits or, in many cases particularly in the small business sector, eliminate employee health insurance entirely.

State governments have clearly followed the federal lead in developing payment policies that restrict their obligations and transfer costs to other parties. In 1982 only 14 Medicaid programs operated prospective payment systems. By 1986, 36 states had adopted such measures—ten of them directly based on the Medicare DRGs (Swan, Barrington, and Grant, 1988).

The transfer of financial responsibility from government programs to private insurers and employers is clearly undesirable from the latter's standpoint (Altman, 1987). However, given the pressures to reduce the deficit, it is highly unlikely that the federal government will modify the Medicare pricing mechanism to eliminate cost transfers. Consequently, private insurers have increasingly adopted an "if you can't beat them, join them" logic by implementing prospective payment arrangements that are similar to those adopted by public programs.

The operational changes brought about by cost shifting can be most clearly seen with the Blue Cross system which in recent years has been faced with steady losses in enrollment to other alternative system providers. The number of Blue Cross plans that employed traditional financing mechanisms declined from 31 in 1981 to 19 in 1985 while those using some forms of prospective payment increased from 29 to 41 (Guterman *et al.*, 1988). The increased dependence on prospective payment increases the burden on employees and health care providers who then attempt to shift costs further back to some other institution.

Efforts to transfer costs have engendered a good deal of political conflict in the U.S. As seen in the cases of the "Baby Bell" telephone systems in 1989 and the railroad companies in 1990, health insurance provisions have become more contentious in labor/management negotiations. When the federal government attempted to shift the cost of Medicare catastrophic health insurance to recipients in 1988, a highly-publicized "revolt" by relatively well-educated and affluent seniors (who had seen their Medicare premiums increase sharply) forced congressional repeal of the entire program. This left less affluent seniors who would have benefited from the program vulnerable to financial disaster from major health problems (Cloud, 1989). In health care, some now charge that government policy-makers have become paralyzed by interest group pressure and are unwilling and unable to take the lead in problem-solving (*Ibid.*).

In response to the shell game, physicians and hospitals attempt to impose higher charges on payers who rely on traditional payment mechanisms in order to compensate for deficits emanating from payers that employ prospective payment. Differential prices create disputes between providers and employers and stimulate the adoption of additional prospective payment systems. In turn, the greater reliance on prospective payment further restricts providers who then respond by searching for yet other non-PPS payers and by developing additional services not yet covered by prospective payment. And so it goes, round and round, while costs continue their upward spiral, tens of millions of U.S. citizens are unable to gain effective access to health care, and policy-holders look on in apparent helplessness.

The regulatory approach in health care, as applied, has therefore been no more effective than market competition in containing costs. The national policy of using both approaches in combination has, to date, constituted "much sound and fury, signifying nothing"—or nearly nothing—in really addressing the issue of health care cost inflation (Tokarski, 1990). To get at the root of the cost problems in American health care, policy-makers will have to end the cost shifting that sabotages current containment efforts. And that in turn means altering the basic financial structure of the industry, for that is where the shell game originates.

PRESCRIPTION FOR ENDGAME

The problem of cost containment in health care is something that all post-industrial societies in North America, Western Europe, and Asia have had to face. To date, most have responded more successfully than the United States. According to the National Leadership Commission (1983:3), "[W]e currently spend approximately 11.5% of our GNP on health care, much more per capita than any other nation, and our cost escalation far outstrips that of any other. Despite 15 years of cost containment efforts by government and the private sector, health costs continue to rise rapidly. At present, there seems to be no natural limit to how high health care costs could rise."

It is becoming clear to an increasing number of policy-makers, administrators, and scholars that current efforts to control costs have not worked, will not work, and *cannot* work, given the current system of payment for care. Present-day cost controls have had one undeniable effect, however: they have eroded the ability of millions to gain access to necessary health services as seen most starkly in the impending collapse of emergency medical services in many large urban areas (Gibbs, 1990). When one considers the developing AIDS epidemic and the steady aging of the American population, it becomes obvious that the financial structure of our health care system is facing catastrophe.

The shell game is not only financially wasteful but also threatens to deal a fatal blow to the American ideal of basic health care as a right that should be guaranteed to all citizens. In this area, at least, our financial common sense and our ethics must lead to the same conclusion—we cannot go on this way. Things must change—and they must change in the near future to preserve the basic economy, effectiveness, and ethical underpinnings of our health care system.

Two additional facts are clear, however. One is that prospective payment is here to stay. The U.S. clearly cannot return to the free spending days of cost-plus reimbursement. Even if the nation develops an effective method of cost control, rapid advances in medical technology and the changing demography of the American population ensure that financing health services will remain a problem in the indefinite future (Janeway, 1989).

Health care planners must also take into account a salient *political* fact: the emergence of a health care system that is increasingly oriented toward competitive markets and profit-making. Whatever the normative arguments might be, it is unlikely (barring some unlikely and unforeseeable national ideological upheaval) that the U.S. will develop a governmentally directed and organized national health system resembling those found in either the United Kingdom or Canada. Faith in governmental activism has steadily declined since the Sixties in the United States (Brown, 1983). The spectrum of American political opinion has shifted to the right, particularly on economic matters, in the last decade. The late 1980s and early 1990s have also seen the worldwide decline of socialism as a credible doctrine of governance. Any system designed to control costs must therefore provide for a robust private sector in health services and competition at the level of care provision.

These considerations undeniably complicate cost control but they need not prevent us from ending the shell game. The United States can indeed maintain a health care financing system that is administered by a central agency or a set of coordinated agencies.

A unified administrative infrastructure is a prerequisite to the implementation of a system that is capable of monitoring a single financing mechanism and controlling the rate or level of compensation in both the private and public sectors. The "nonsystem" characterized by fragmented responsibility for controlling costs and ensuring access must, at least financially, become a real system. In the true fashion of American pragmatism, however, it can involve a shared responsibility and authority that includes all major actors involved with health services.

At this time, the most technically efficient and politically acceptable structure for achieving these policy objectives would involve some form of unified prospective payment all-payer system. As suggested by the New Jersey experience, an all-payer system could equitably ration the costs of uncompensated care among third parties and determine the share of these expenses that needs to be financed by each insurer (Broyles and Reilly, 1984). This all-payer system could be largely operated at the state level but would also require a national coordinating and standard-setting entity that would take regional variations and national needs into account.

As market advocates note, all-payer systems do indeed "interrupt the progress now being made toward establishing competition as a force for appropriate spending in the health care sector" (Navighurst, 1985:19). The crucial issue, however, is whether, even in the long run, a competitive marketplace with minimal cost regulation (none of it centrally coordinated) can successfully balance economy and access in providing health services. Although market competition is an important force in health care, it is unlikely that, unaided, the competitive approach will achieve the necessary balance.

Such an all-payer system could also be combined with some variant of the Universal Access (UNAC) program proposed by the National Leadership Commission on Health Care (1989). A majority of American citizens would receive an adequate and guaranteed level of health insurance through their employers. A universal access would also provide coverage to the estimated 37 million Americans (many already employed) who do not have any health insurance. With an all-payer/universal access system, employers would still have the right to choose their own coverage and providers of care but could not escape from the costs of health services by eliminating benefits, or reducing them below a set level, to their employees.

Care givers could establish their own mix of services, market themselves to preferred population subgroups, and compete on the basis of quality or other characteristics of treatment including non-treatment amenities. They could also retain profits but would be required either to provide an acceptable amount of below-cost care or compensate other local or regional facilities for doing so. They would also have to provide the all-payer/universal access system with full compensation for any subsidized resources utilized for private profit-making purposes.

Health care professionals in this system should also be free to market their services as desired, but payments for specific services made under this system ought to be established under a version of the Resource Based Relative Value System (RBRVS) currently being developed. Nothing would prevent physicians or any other health care professionals from selling their services to unsubsidized payers for unregulated market prices. However, health care professionals who receive subsidized training or access to facilities, equipment, support services or patients would be required to provide an acceptable amount of care within the all payer/universal access system or completely repay the system for privately-used resources.

Health care recipients would also have a specified set of rights and responsibilities. They would be guaranteed access to an acceptable level of care and could assume personal financial responsibility for more care or a higher level of care, if desired. In other words, there would be no ceiling regarding unsubsidized individual health care expenditures. Subsidized health services, on the other hand, would ensure that there would be a floor below which no citizen would fall. The overall amount of care provided within this system would be subject to overall limits based upon costs and resource availability—the heart of cost containment. Adjusted for disposable income, recipients might be responsible for deductibles or copayments for subsidized care that they received, a feature that may discourage overutilization and foster cost-consciousness.

The all-payer/universal system briefly outlined above would certainly have a more complex design, requiring a period of trial and error orientation that extends over several years. Policy planning and implementation would involve numerous technical difficulties and potential administrative confusion.

Most fundamentally, a wide range of political conflicts at all levels would also have to be resolved for a nationally-coordinated all-payer/universal access system to work. Given the pluralism, structural decentralization, and ideological fragmentation currently present in our national policy-making system, a move toward an all-payer/universal access system might be impossible. At the very least, it would entail considerable political and economic risk. At this time, the United States is probably not yet sufficiently dissatisfied with the performance of its current health care system to take such chances.

The authors are convinced, however, that the current structure of health services administration and finance also involves considerable risk—more so than the reforms proposed above. They also believe that the costs of staying on the present course will prove unacceptable to the nation within the next decade. Given the current rate of technological development and the demographic and social changes taking place, the present-day U.S. health care system cannot be sustained much longer.

The question is not *whether* major change is coming to the structure of our health care system, but *when*. The ultimate nature of such change is also open to question—and to national choice. Up to the present, the United States has maintained an uneasy balance between economy and access in its provision of health services. That balance is now being destroyed. If specific steps are not taken in the near future to end the shell game, cost containment will most likely come about as the result of unstructured and increasingly stringent rationing of service in an environment of brutal political Darwinism. In such an environment, the United States will be foregoing, perhaps permanently, the ideal of adequate access to health care for all of its citizens.

By such standards the authors believe that the risks and drawbacks to the establishment of an all-payer/universal access system are small indeed. American health policy has reached a major crossroad. If we as people take the future into our own hands, we can create a system that provides for an end to the financial shell game while preserving much of the current system of health services provision. This would be a future in line with historic American ideals and well worth attaining.

Financing Universal Health Insurance: Taxes, Premiums, and the Lessons of Social Insurance

Thomas Bodenheimer and Kevin Grumbach
University of California, San Francisco

Universal health insurance commands strong support from the American population. Over 70 percent favor insurance coverage for the entire population (Blendon and Donelan 1990; Jajich-Toth and Roper 1990), and over 60 percent support government-financed health care (Blendon et al. 1990; Blendon and Donelan 1991).

But when people are asked whether they are willing to pay for universal access, public support drops. In a 1990 survey, only 22 percent were willing to adopt a comprehensive national health insurance (NHI) program if they had to pay more than $200 per year to make it happen (Blendon and Donelan 1990). A 1987 survey reported that while 68 percent of Americans favored a tax-funded national health insurance program, only 10 percent were willing to pay an additional $100 per year (Pokorny 1988). And in a 1978 Gallup poll, although 76 percent favored national health insurance, the support declined 23 percent when respondents were asked if they were willing to pay more taxes to finance it (Goodman and Steiber 1981). Similar findings have been recorded since 1938 (Blendon and Donelan 1990).

Americans perceive themselves as excessively taxed, even though the United States has one of the lowest levels of taxation among industrialized nations (Blendon and Donelan 1990). Partly as a result of politicians' desire to lower rather

Journal of Health Politics, Policy and Law, Vol. 17, No. 3, Fall 1992.

than raise taxes, the federal deficit has grown from about $5 billion in the 1960s to over $200 billion in the 1980s and 1990s, with state and local governments in perennial budgetary crisis (Rosenbaum 1991).

In this deficit-laden society with its strong antitax environment, the passage of any form of universal health insurance is blocked by an impasse over financing. One prominent proposal for universal access, employer-mandated health insurance, attempts to cover most of the uninsured through mandatory private insurance premiums rather than taxes. Does financing by premiums have the capacity to bypass unpopular tax-based funding? In this article, searching for ways to extricate the nation from the health-financing impasse, we explore the dimensions of tax and premium payment for universal health insurance.

We begin by discussing the differences between taxes and insurance premiums, proposing seven parameters for characterizing health financing mechanisms along a tax-like and premium-like continuum. To illustrate these parameters, we use them to describe existing health insurance programs in the U.S. and proposals for insurance reform. We then review some episodes in the political history of American and European social insurance, applying the same seven parameters to our historical exploration. Our conclusion highlights some lessons that different eras and nations may offer for resolving the political impasse over universal health insurance financing.

TAXES OR PREMIUMS?

The standard alternatives offered for financing universal health insurance are to pay more taxes to fund expanded government-run programs or pay more premiums to purchase private insurance for more Americans. "Taxes" and "premiums" are usually regarded as straightforward, dichotomous alternatives for financing health care. *Webster's Dictionary* (1984) defines a tax as "a contribution for the support of a government required of persons, groups, or businesses within the domain of that government." In contrast, *Webster's* definition of a premium is "the amount paid or payable, often in installments, for an insurance policy."

In the complex world of health care financing, however, the definitions of premiums and taxes are less clear. Employer-mandated health insurance, for example, illustrates these indistinct boundaries. Under employer mandates, the government compels employers to purchase health insurance for their employees. One of the political purposes underlying this arrangement is to avoid the imposition of new taxes. Yet economist Uwe Reinhardt (1988) comments that "mandated benefits are taxes in the sense that they coerce fiscal transfers among private entities in the economy. They are, alas, pseudo-taxes that permit the politician to exercise the government's power to tax without having to book these taxes as government revenue and, thus, without assuming accountability for the disposition of the implied tax revenue" (p. 13). Employer mandates are in effect "a payroll tax in disguise" (Reinhardt 1987: 107).

While mandatory premiums paid to private insurers can be considered pseudo-taxes, direct government receipt of health care payments does not necessarily define those payments as taxes. Some governments rely on premiums rather than taxes to fund portions of their public plans. For example, the U.S. Medicare program charges beneficiaries a premium to enroll in Part B, and British Columbia finances a portion of its government-run health system through premiums.

Where, then, do premiums end and taxes begin? To clarify this question, it is helpful to reduce the general terms *taxes* and *premiums* into their component features. This enables us to characterize different financing methods by specific criteria. The following list of questions covers the major defining ingredients in any health care financing scheme: (1) Is payment voluntary or mandatory? (2) Is coverage contingent on making payments? (3) Are payments earmarked exclusively for health care purposes? (4) Do some people who do not benefit pay for the benefits of others, or are all payers also beneficiaries? (5) Are benefits received directly proportional to payments made, or do some groups receive more (or less) benefits in relation to their contributions? (6) What is the source of the payments (taxpayers, employers, or employees)? and (7) What is the destination of the payments (government or private insurance companies)?

Tax-like qualities include mandatory payments, coverage not contingent on making payment, nonearmarked funds, payers not necessarily eligible to receive benefits, benefits not proportional to payments made, payments from taxpayers, and payments to government. Premium-like features are voluntary payments, receipt of benefits contingent upon making payments, funds earmarked for health care, payers always eligible to receive benefits, benefits received proportional to payments made, funds coming from employers/employees/individuals, and payments going to private insurance institutions. Since taxes and premiums represent a continuum of qualities rather than distinct entities, it is essential to view these tax-premium distinctions as tendencies rather than pigeonholes—analogous to the concept of electron clouds with probabilities, as contrasted with discrete clumps of matter. Thus taxes can be earmarked (e.g., gasoline taxes going to highway maintenance) and premiums, as noted above, can be paid to governments.

PROFILES OF EXISTING FINANCING METHODS

Different forms of health insurance in the United States rarely consist of either pure taxes or pure premiums but typically involve a blend of tax-like and premium-like features.

Medicaid is the most tax-like of these examples. The entire population makes mandatory payments into the Medicaid program through income, sales, corporate, and other taxes. These payments arrive as general revenues to federal and state treasuries; they are not identifiably earmarked for health care services at the time of payment. Enrollment in the Medicaid program is not contingent on making these payments; on the contrary, the payments are perceived as particularly odious taxes, because many of those who pay do not benefit from the program.

The next example, payments for Medicare Part A (the U.S. hospital insurance program for the elderly and permanently disabled), has two important features that distinguish these payments from Medicaid's general tax-funding mechanism. First, the Medicare Part A payroll tax contributions paid by employers and employees are earmarked for the Medicare trust fund. In addition, while working Americans make these payments for a program that primarily benefits retired or disabled Americans, workers' payments contribute to their own future insurance coverage. To qualify for Medicare, a person or spouse is required to work and to pay into social security for at least ten years; persons over sixty-five who do not qualify can enroll in Medicare Part A by paying a monthly premium (U.S. Social Security Administration 1991a). These two features—earmarked payments and enrollment contingent upon payment—give Medicare Part A payments something of a premium-like character.

Medicare Part B (providing medical benefits) also has elements that are both tax-like and premium-like. While much of the funding for Medicare Part B derives from general government revenues similar to Medicaid financing, eligible individual must also pay a flat-rate monthly premium to enroll in the program. Although Medicare Part B is a government-operated insurance plan, enrollment and its attendant monthly payments are voluntary.

The last example, drawn from existing insurance programs, is the conventional American private insurance model. In this model, the destination for payments is a private insurance company instead of a public entity, and premium rates are set by experience rating—with payment levels determined by the amount of benefits a group of people is expected to receive—or by across-the-board flat rates. The private insurance model contains two variants—the individual policy, representing 11 percent of all private health insurance policies in the U.S., and the employment-based group policy, representing the remaining 89 percent of private policies (Levit and Cowan 1990). While the former conforms closely to the "pure premium" model, the latter strays rather far from this prototype. Employment-based insurance has an often-overlooked tax subsidy analogous to the government revenues that supplement the premiums for Medicare Part B. Whereas the Medicare subsidy represents explicit tax revenues flowing into the Medicare program, the government subsidy for employment-based insurance is a tax exclusion, worth $50-60 billion per year (Pauley et al. 1991), represented by the tax-exempt status of health insurance premiums paid by employers.

To summarize, Medicaid financing and payments for private, individual insurance policies represent the tax and premium poles, respectively, of health care financing. Lying between these diodes is a spectrum of financing methods with varieties of tax-like and premium-like qualities.

PROFILES OF PROPOSED FINANCING METHODS

Two major types of NHI proposals are now under consideration in the United States. First are the pseudo-tax models of employer-mandated health insurance—proposed, for example, by the Pepper Commission (U.S. Bipartisan Commission on Comprehensive Health Care 1990), the American Medical Association (Todd et al. 1991), and congressional Democrats (Friedan 1991)—and mandatory individual insurance, i.e., the Heritage Foundation plan calling for government to mandate individually paid private health insurance policies (Butler 1991). Second is the unified public insurance proposal, commonly referred to as a "single-payer" or "Canadian-style" system, exemplified in the Physicians for a National Health Program plan (Grumbach et al. 1991), and the Universal Health Care Act of 1991 (H.R. 1300), introduced by Congressman Marty Russo. How do these proposals measure up on the tax-premium axis?

Both the employer mandate and the Heritage Foundation proposals could be seen, respectively, as instituting pseudo-taxes on business or on individuals, thus providing a compulsory feature that further dilutes the premium-like character of private insurance financing. The employer mandate model shares many features of the Medicare Part A mechanism, such as compulsory employment-based payments, although the destinations of payment differ. Both mandate models would require substantial increases in general government revenues to subsidize private insurance premiums for lower-income people or to promote enrollment in a supplementary public plan.

Most single-payer proposals, with all health dollars flowing to a public health care trust fund, rely on a variety of taxes to finance universal coverage. Earmarking the taxes for health care tints them a premium-like hue. The Russo Universal Health Care plan includes an individual premium to help fund long-term care. One state-level single-payer proposal, the Florida Universal Health Access Plan, would finance the majority of its program through a flat-rate individual premium (Vinger 1991). Other state-level single-payer programs have considered the institution of an income-adjusted premium similar to that used in British Columbia, where health care premiums, collected by the provincial government, are graduated to increase with income.

Late twentieth-century America is by no means the first society to confront a health care financing dilemma. For an entire century, the interplay of premium-like and tax-like financing of public programs has occupied policymakers attempting to implement a political program known as "social insurance." Central to the history of social insurance movements in both the United States and other industrialized nations has been the tension between the universal need for income security, including health insurance, and the political difficulty of funding such programs. As Americans come to terms with the inadequacies of health insurance and grapple with proposals for reform, the rich history of social insurance offers many lessons for reconciling the funding dilemma. To this history we now turn.

HISTORICAL LESSONS OF SOCIAL INSURANCE

The very name *social insurance* reveals its dual nature: *social* denotes tax-like properties, while *insurance* embodies premium-like qualities. Social insurance is a compulsory program of payments to insure against (i.e., to provide financial assistance for) interruption or loss of earning power due to retirement, unemployment, disability, or other causes (Lubove 1968). From the beginning, the social insurance movement included payment for medical care in its list of insurable financial hardships.

What is Social Insurance?

Insurance is a mechanism by which people reduce the adverse financial consequences of an event by paying small amounts in advance to an institution, which in turn pays all or part of the costs incurred by the event. Insurance has two major branches, private insurance and social insurance, which have similarities and differences. Both private and social insurance are based on the pooling of risks over a large population. Both involve payment of premiums or contributions, and individuals have a right to benefits only if they have made contributions. The main distinction between private and social insurance lies in the former being voluntary while the latter is compulsory (Booth 1973). The other major contrast is that the insuring institution is a private company in the case of private insurance and generally (but not always) a public agency in the case of social insurance.

Historically, social insurance evolved as a response to the inevitable periods during which wages were interrupted. The financial effects of sickness, involuntary unemployment, death of an essential breadwinner, old age, or industrial accident became disastrous for large numbers of families. During the nineteenth century, voluntary associations (trade-union-or employer-sponsored benefit funds, fraternal societies, and commercial insurance companies) developed in Europe and America, providing voluntary insurance that paid cash benefits to assist people during periods of income interruption (Rubinow 1916). Most workers, however, earned wages insufficient to allow for the purchase of these mutual benefit programs. In the words of American social insurance reformer Abraham Epstein (1933:21):

> So long as the wage-earner is able to hold his job, he somehow manages to subsist; but when through either accident, sickness, invalidity, unemployment or old age he is deprived of work, he frequently becomes helpless and destitute. Try as he may to provide for a rainy day through friendly societies, trade unions, savings and voluntary insurance, he finds that there are altogether too many rainy days.

To effectively cover the "many rainy days" at affordable cost, social insurance developed, with four mechanisms to make the insurance affordable to the great majority of unskilled workers: (1) spreading the risk very broadly throughout the population, an end accomplished by making the insurance mandatory; (2) requiring employers to pay part of the premium cost; (3) administering the insurance through public or quasi-public institutions with no profits and low administrative costs; and (4) designing the program to allow for some income redistribution from higher-to-lower-income families.

LESSONS FROM THE SOCIAL INSURANCE MOVEMENT

It is not the task of each new generation of health insurance reformers to reinvent the wheel. Rather, the wheel should be adapted to the current and unique historical and political terrain. The history of social insurance provides lessons for American policymakers grappling with reform of the health insurance system.

1. Participation in social insurance programs is compulsory for the great majority of the population of most nations, with limited exceptions (e.g., the affluent are not obligated to join the German health insurance program).
2. Contributory (premium-like) social insurance is popular worldwide because people feel they are getting something for their payments.
3. Payments are generally earmarked to guarantee that they are used to pay benefits.
4. Although in principle social insurance and public assistance are entirely different, in practice these types of programs have overlapping qualities. Especially in health care, many nations (e.g., Germany and Britain) integrate programs of social insurance and public assistance. The United States resembles underdeveloped countries more than other industrialized nations in relegating the poor to separate public assistance health programs. Medical care is unlike other social insurance programs because it is a service rather than a cash payment. Differentials in cash payments between social insurance beneficiaries and public assistance recipients are customary in most developed nations, but differentials in health services are often seen as producing unacceptable inequality.
5. Correspondence between the amount of contributions and the amount of benefits is not a strict feature of social insurance. Generally, social insurance represents a compromise between the contributory principle (a premium-like feature) on the one hand and redistribution of income (a tax-like feature) on the other. Most nations (e.g., Germany and the United States) set contributions for social insurance as a percentage of wage earnings, but some countries (e.g., Great Britain) use a flat premium-like rate.
6. Social insurance may be financed by contributory payments from employers and employees and by general taxpayers in varying proportions. Most nations demonstrate a strong contributory component to social insurance; the degree of general revenue supplementation varies from nation to nation. The intermingling of premium-like and tax-like features is common in the financing of social insurance programs.
7. Social insurance programs can be administered through public, private, or quasi-public institutions. Public institutions have the advantage of simplicity, fairness, and lower administrative costs. Although some nations (e.g., Germany's health insurance program) have retained their existing insurance entities to administer social insurance, others (e.g., Britain's health insurance program) have not. Even in nations where funds are directed to nongovernmental enti-

ties, payments tend to redistribute income and are not guided by private insurance underwriting principles.

Back to the Future

The passage of universal health insurance in America faces at least two major hurdles: (1) how to finance such a major social program and win popular support for a specific financing mechanism in the face of strong antitax sentiment, and (2) how to construct a coalition of interest groups sufficiently powerful to enable the passage of such a program. This paper is concerned with the first of these barriers, and does not attempt to tackle the second. Regardless of the interest group obstacles lying ahead, a popular movement for universal health insurance is likely to stumble in its first steps out of the starting gate if it cannot assuage the public's concern about taxation and compulsory health care payments

The social insurance mechanism has the potential for breaking the financing impasse. The broad mass of public opinion in the United States supports social security, in marked contrast to its view of public assistance (Blendon and Donelan 1990; Navarro 1985; Jenkins 1969). With its contributory foundation and earmarked funds, social insurance is far more acceptable to the voting public than is general revenue taxation. A Harris poll found that 66 percent supported the social security tax as a means to finance universal health insurance (Blendon and Donelan 1990). Public assistance recipients could be folded into the social insurance program, with those recipients making a contribution to help pay for the benefits they receive. Historically, inclusion of a certain measure of income redistribution has not politically undermined the contributory principle.

While it is not our intent to propose a specific financing plan here, an example based on a social insurance-type premium-tax hybrid might be instructive. Universal health insurance could be financed by a mandatory increase in social security contributions by employers, employees, and self-employed people, with the funds earmarked for health care. Payments could be proportional to wages and benefits equal for everyone. To account for the fact that some employers already pay for group private insurance premiums while other employers do not, further redistributive efforts might be needed to soften the impact on small and marginal employers and low-wage employees. Contributions made by the employed population could be sufficient to insure dependents and to cover periods of unemployment, temporary and permanent disability, and retirement.

How would public assistance recipients be incorporated into such a system? Current U.S. health care financing appears to divide society into two groupings: (1) those who pay for their own care through social security contributions and employment-related insurance premiums (note that economists consider most employer payments for employee health insurance as a portion of employees' total effective wages or as included in the prices of goods or services sold by the employer [Reinhardt 1987]), and (2) those whose care is supported by taxes or (in the case of uncompensated care) by surpayments on the premiums of people who do pay. Americans do not want to pay more taxes under such a system because the first (majority) group appears to pay twice, once for themselves and another time (through taxes) for the care of others. Employer-mandated private health insurance, which could be labeled a social insurance program because of its compulsory aspect, has the disadvantage of perpetuating a strict separation of social insurance and public assistance programs rather than melding them together as other industrialized nations have done.

To lessen the division between social insurance beneficiaries and public assistance recipients as other nations have done, the latter could be folded into the social security financing program. To maximize the contributory principle, public assistance recipients could be required to make contributions to their health care coverage; perhaps the often-overlooked payments of low-income people—in sales and other taxes—should become more evident, such that no one is viewed as a "free rider," completely supported by the payments of others.

The lessons of social insurance tell us that people are willing to pay for their benefits as long as they receive the benefits. Contributions need not be proportional to benefits received, but everyone should contribute and everyone should benefit. The history of social insurance also affirms that social insurance benefits, including health insurance, should be financed by earmarked funds, such that there is no mistake that contributions pay for designated benefits. Finally, financing of universal health insurance has the greatest chance of commanding strong public support if it ceases to perpetuate the division of society between those who appear to contribute both for their own benefit and for the benefit of others vs. those who benefit without appearing to pay.

While other nations can provide lessons for the United States, the implementation of these lessons must be consistent with U.S. political culture (Morone 1990). The existing American social security program, a compromise between a contributory and a redistributive system, may provide better guidance for the financing of American national health insurance than Canadian and some European approaches that primarily rely on general revenue financing. If Americans feel confident that everyone contributes and everyone benefits, perhaps our nation can overcome the antitax impasse to the passage of universal health insurance.

Privatization in Health and Human Services: A Critique

Steven Rathgeb Smith
Duke University
Michael Lipsky
Massachusetts Institute of Technology

In recent years public discourse in the United States, many of the European democracies, and most of the Socialist bloc nations has been dominated by the belief that the public sector is overextended, inefficient, and destructive of savings and investment initiative and innovation. Some analysts have argued that the welfare state is in crisis because the growth of the public sector was producing a downward spiral of stagnant or declining economic growth, falling tax revenues, and the resultant inability of government to meet its obligations (OECD 1980; Peterson 1987).

Accordingly, a policy frequently advanced to resolve these concerns has been *privatization*, a broad policy impulse which seeks to change the balance between public and private responsibility in public policy (Savas 1981; Donahue 1989). Privatization encompasses two interconnecting themes. We may call them the ''competition'' theme and the ''load-shedding'' theme.

The competition theme emphasizes the efficacy of market dynamics and the desirability of competition. It promotes the notion that wherever possible the private sector should be responsible for the distribution of goods and services. Competition among private organizations is said to have the salutary effect of

Journal of Health Politics, Policy and Law, Vol. 17, No. 2, Summer 1992.

fostering innovation and minimizing production costs. In contrast, monopolistic government bureaucracies are thought to tolerate inefficiency and destroy initiative. Without the spur of competition, it is said, government programs languish with little care for the quality of services or the costs of producing them. Not only is government inherently inefficient, but it is said as well to foster inefficiency in the private sector when government interference with private activity through regulation leads to higher and unnecessary costs. Privatization has been the ideological umbrella under which the United States has pursued deregulation of the airlines, trucking, interstate bus transportation, and other areas of economic activity previously subject to more extensive regulation. And recently, the health economist Regina H. Herzlinger (1991) recommended "healthy competition" as the solution to the escalating crisis in the cost of health care.

"Load shedding" is the practice of allocating to the private sector work previously carried out by public agencies. In the service sector, "load shedders" have been asking whether there are private alternatives to government provision. The federal government and many local governments have indeed adopted policies that seek as much as possible to engage private companies to do work previously carried out by government. Thus federal agencies have already been contracting with private agencies to provide auditing, computing, and other services when there exists a private agency to do the work. The subway system in metropolitan Boston, for example, has increased its payouts to minority workers by contracting with local businesses to clean its stations. At the municipal level, garbage collection has received a good deal of attention as an area in which private companies may outperform public agencies (Savas 1981; Bendick 1984; Donahue 1989; Stein 1990).

Most discussions of privatization focus on fostering competition or load shedding because in the popular mind the private sector is equated with business. To most people, privatization means enhancing private enterprise and decreasing the influence of government in the economy. However, sometimes advocates of privatization have more expansive concerns than the efficacy of the market. Their views are grounded in the belief that government is an inevitably dominant and coercive influence and should play only a minimal role in society. And they are supported by widespread but by no means universal public opinion that governments are not necessarily good at performing many tasks. Herzlinger (1991:81), for example, ends her article recommending increased competition in health care, "Which would you choose to safeguard your health: a federal government bureaucracy or yourself?"

This view of privatization underlies at least four directions established by privatization advocates. One, which goes back at least to the antiflouridation campaigns of the 1950s, advocates the minimization of government involvement in such areas as gun control, mandatory seat belt and motorcycle helmet laws, off-road vehicle regulation, and other areas in which governments seek to restrict individual choice. A second applies the cautions against big government to fears that the "heavy hand" will fall fatally on community organizations and other private initiatives (Meyer 1982; Glazer 1983). A third, championed by Herzlinger and others, urges the development of policies that maximize individual choice. This perspective leads to support for voucher systems and payment schemes to individuals, as in health care and day-care tax subsidies, which allocate public monies in a way that permits individual choice of provider while fostering competition among private service organizations and individuals.

A fourth direction identifies the public sector with institutions such as public welfare bureaucracies, state hospitals, state schools for the developmentally disabled, and training schools for juvenile delinquents. These institutions are believed to oppress the poor, the developmentally disabled, the mentally ill, and disadvantaged. Advocates of this view see nonprofit organizations, with their community roots, voluntarism, and often greater professionalism, as more effective, humane vehicles for caring for individuals in need.

The extraordinary growth of government contracting for services with nonprofit agencies is an outgrowth of these perspectives on privatization. A guiding premise of contracting with nonprofit agencies—a premise that also underlies contracts with for-profits—is that competition for contracts among private providers will lead to greater consumer choice, innovation, more effective service, and cost reductions. And if we mean by *privatization* consigning public sector activities to individuals and organizations that are simply *not part of government*, we immediately see the appeal to analysts and policymakers predisposed to favor nongovernmental policy development of government contracting with private agencies.

The dramatic rise of the nonprofit sector in the United States has of course received some attention. But with few exceptions (Kramer 1981; Demone and Gibelman 1989), commentary on this development only obliquely addresses its implications for American social policy. Some studies are narrowly (if understandably) focused on the utility of the market model as applied to privatization through contracting (Gurin et al. 1980; Schlesinger et al. 1986). Others are broadly focused on the development of the nonprofit sector as such, encompassing organizations with such diverse purposes as hospitals, museums, orchestras, think tanks, charitable foundations, and the like (Hansmann 1980; Rudney 1987).

Both approaches usually fail to address a central question raised by contracting in human service delivery: What are the implications for the society when governments increasingly seek to achieve social welfare objectives through private agents? In other words, does it matter that the individuals and groups charged with carrying out legislative mandates are at best only indirectly accountable to public officials through modern democratic processes? And more broadly: What are the effects on the public and private sectors, now that public business is carried out in distinctly new ways? Does this form of privatization indeed yield the benefits heralded by its advocates? Partly by reviewing the direct evidence and partly by analyzing the relevance of market logic to contracting in health and human services, we are able to reach some broad conclusions concerning the efficacy of this form of privatization in achieving public purposes.

In a perfect market, buyers and sellers might have no interest in each other beyond the exchange itself. However, governments that go to market for services must nurture the nonprofits they pick to provide the services (to ensure quality and quantity of supply). The nonprofits in turn go beyond setting prices for standardized services and lobby governments (thereby affecting the demands of the buyer). Above all, both parties share the expectation that a reasonable performance will be awarded with a renewed contract.

Having recognized that contracting in health and human services has many nonmarket characteristics, we may inquire into the effects of contracting on the functions of government and then consider nongovernmental interests—those of the organizations that enter into agreements with government and of the sector of society of which nonprofits are a part. Throughout, we should be alert to the ways in which developments on one side of the relationship generate responses on the other side.

Given the rapidly escalating costs of health care, substantial interest exists among policymakers and scholars for contracting and other forms of privatization as a way of checking health care costs and improving the quality of care. Advocates of vouchers as a solution to the health care crisis believe that consumers are capable of evaluating the costs and benefits of health services and willing to take their "business" to the most efficient health care provider. Contracting in health and social services presents government officials with a similar choice: Can government administrators, who are often trained professionals, adequately judge the quality of service and, if dissatisfied, move the business elsewhere? We will argue that professionals often find it difficult to evaluate the quality and cost of health care and, in addition, face substantial obstacles to switching service providers. If professionals find the task of service evaluation daunting and troublesome, surely the citizenry would find the task equally if not more problematic.

WHY DOES GOVERNMENT CONTRACT WITH NONPROFIT AGENCIES?

The ideology of privatization intersects with conventional concerns of public officials to produce a complex rationale for the efficacy of contracting. Among the common rationales for government contracting with nonprofit agencies are the following.

First, it may be cheaper. This is one of the paramount reasons that liberals and conservatives initially support this way of achieving public purposes. *If* it is cheaper to contract for services, it may be cheaper for one of several distinct reasons. First, the dynamics of market competition may lead contractors to pare down their costs in order to win or retain contracts. Second, private providers may be able to provide services at lower cost because they operate in a different environment from government. Specifically, labor may be cheaper because private providers are not bound by civil service hiring requirements or public employee pay scales, or government may have an aging work force with a higher average salary than a new agency operating with relatively young and inexperienced workers. Government agencies may be tied into expensive long-term leases, in contrast to agencies such as home health organizations, which rent space in a local community center or small office building.

The second rationale is that contracting may provide greater flexibility. It is often politically and administratively difficult for government agencies to initiate new programs with existing staff, hire new staff, and locate facilities for new programs. Contracting for services places the work of starting up new programs on private providers. Searching for private agencies to undertake new initiatives can put the burden of planning and initiating new programs on private agencies, who may be able to respond with a flexibility that government bureaucracies do not normally exhibit. Among a dozen private providers of substance abuse services, it may be easier to find several able to mount new programs than it would to move a single state agency. If governments are under pressure to mount new services quickly—say, to provide health care for Spanish-speaking families and children—it may be easier to call upon private Hispanic agencies than to hire and train workers within prevailing government procedures.

Government agencies normally strive for a degree of uniformity of service across jurisdictions. Contracting locally for services solves the problem of tailoring a program to fit local conditions: community agencies know their community needs and sentiments and can design programs to suit them.

Quite aside from tailoring programs to local conditions, contracting permits governments to acquire special expertise and talents for which there is insufficient demand for hiring in permanent government positions. A search, for example, for a Vietnamese-speaking translator for a municipal hospital may be more easily accomplished through private contracting than hiring through civil service procedures, particularly when the extent and the duration of the need is uncertain.

The desire to develop flexible options surely commended contracting to those who sponsored and carried out the deinstitutionalization movements of the 1970s. Disestablishing the state training schools and mental institutions could not have been accomplished by remaking enormous state bureaucracies and service staffs into lean, decentralized state facilities. The possibility of contracting with private agencies made deinstitutionalization "thinkable."

An additional aspect of flexibility is the capacity to change direction or cut back quickly if government priorities change. If those employed in new service areas work for private providers, they may be cut back or eliminated when a contract is not renewed. Cutting back public employment is much more difficult, and the consequences are more severe. When Massachusetts communities cut back on public employees in the wake of a state tax limitations referendum in 1980, the public outcry was intense. Public sentiment is rarely so pronounced, if it is given voice at all, when the employees of private agencies are laid off because of reductions in government spending patterns.

A third rationale for contracting is that it appears to limit government growth. Contracting allows government to extend services without generating growth in the government work force. Public officials may welcome contracting because they can extend the reach of government programs without directly employing new workers.

Contracting may also limit the *appearance* of government growth. Public criticism of government growth tends to focus on taxes, expenditures, and, as a surrogate for growth, the number of government employees. Contracting for services insures that the figures for direct government employment will not rise substantially—particularly (as has tended to be the case) if the growth in contracting is not accompanied by growth in the number of government workers employed to monitor contracts.

DOES CONTRACTING SAVE COSTS?

For the production of some public policies there may be a general case for economizing through privatization. However, the problem of providing human services of high quality on a sustained basis is so different from the problem of producing standardized products at a fixed price (such as automobiles) that it calls into question the simple proposition that government could increase its general effectiveness by stimulating competition by purchasing services. Purchase of services in the long run may turn out to be a positive development. But if this proves to be so, it will not be because of the greater efficiency of the private sector or because contracting spurred competition among private providers.

Consider the assertion that purchased services are cheaper. In straightforward service areas such as garbage collection, car towing, and grounds maintenance, there is evidence that it may pay cities to contract for such services rather than perform them with public employees (Savas 1979; Donahue 1989). But the model does not apply to human services. For one thing, unlike service activities for which there already exists demand, such as private security and word processing, private sector human services providers may not already exist in large numbers. When government in the recent past sought to contract for services to AIDS victims, crack addicts, or chronic mental patients, there were few if any private agencies providing the required services, still fewer with enough administrative capacity to allow prudent contract offices to have confidence in prospective contractors. Every city may have one or several traditional multiservice charitable agencies, but they are hardly numerous and in any event do not necessarily already provide the services government is seeking. Many established agencies either are reluctant or refuse to serve the developmentally disabled and the chronic mentally ill—two groups for which government desperately needs community services because of deinstitutionalization. But if there are few potential bidders, the logic of achieving innovation and cost savings through market dynamics falls apart.

Competition is reduced by the cost of entry into the field. Examples of social welfare programs with particularly high entry costs are residential treatment programs. Community residences for people who are different and despised, such as those who are mentally ill, addicted to drugs, or in trouble with the law, must acquire occupancy licensing and run the gauntlet of community opposition before they can be certified. Thus competition in the health and human services field is often restricted to those few agencies that are already running specialized programs. True, the higher the price government is willing to pay for services, the more potential suppliers there are likely to bid for contracts. In reality, however, cost restrictions limit this logic as a guide to government action.

Another reality of health and human services intrudes to reduce the chances of salutary competition. Some services, particularly those involving residential placement or long-term therapeutic relationships, depend upon continuity of care. In these areas it is important to the service to be delivered that clients are able to depend upon their relationships with providers. In these service areas, responsible state officials must temper their interest in generating competition and cost savings with concerns for client-provider relationships. For example, AIDS patients come to depend upon their home health workers; government officials may be understandably reluctant to switch a contract to another agency if disruption caused by a contract change would cause hardship and suffering.

Still another reason to question the logic of market competition in contracting for service concerns the intimate involvement in policy and practice of nonprofit contractors and their contracting agencies. A public agency responsible for providing services to drug abusers or the chronic mentally ill is charged with very sensitive, delicate, and urgent tasks. Public officials experience excruciating pressures to make sound judgments to treat severe problems, protect the public, and support families and relatives, while in the background lurks the threat of exposure in the press when one out of thousands of decisions inevitably proves faulty and a drug addict dies in a detoxification center. When a public agency contracts this work to a private treatment agency, it becomes dependent upon the agency in the most fundamental way. Close ties develop and public officials find themselves deeply involved in the affairs of their contractors as the nonprofit becomes in a sense part of government in the discharge of these obligations. Nonprofit executives, in turn, involve themselves directly in legislative and government affairs in order to influence payment rates, service standards, and other aspects of policy. The effectiveness of their activities is enhanced by the increasing number of exchanges of top personnel between public and private sectors that comes as a result of contracting. Such relationships of mutual dependence are hardly the arm's-length transactions envisioned by market theorists.

In summary, the efficacy of competition is severely dampened if there are few bidders, entry into the market is restricted, buyers have a stake in relationships with previous sellers, and sellers actively participate in structuring market demand. If one takes a closer look at the claims made in services where cost savings do seem to be realized through privatization, it appears that the most substantial reason is that private firms pay workers less. Private firms do not have to pay government-scale wages, conform to civil service job definitions, retain another and therefore higher-paid workforce, or offer full-time employment for work which is episodic, seasonal, or, like the rush hour, involves predictable, significant variations in daily demand. Thus the weightiest reason for superior cost/benefit ratios of private providers is not so much their leaner organizational structure, acquired in a competitive market, as the relief they offer from public laws and prevailing government practices, which cannot be, or at least in the present political environment have not been, repealed. No wonder public employee unions regard privatization as an anathema.

This is not to deny that privatization may result in lower costs. It is to say that a substantial portion of the savings where they are realized seems to be associated with avoidance of public employee wage levels and civil service practices and has little to do with the theory of competition touted by advocates of privatization. In theory, governments could achieve the same savings if they had more flexibility in establishing wages and terms of work.[1]

When we turn to claims of cost saving in health and social services specifically, we find additional reasons to doubt that privatization ultimately will be cost-effective. Private agencies may pay workers less than public agencies, but they can do so only so long as working for a private agency itself constitutes a psychic benefit or provides compensating advantages that induce workers to accept wages below public wage scales. (Consider the lower salaries of private school teachers, who presumably prefer to work in the more refined, sheltered private school environment).

Three developments may conspire to render lower private agency salaries obsolete. First, if the attractiveness of working in private agencies changes as they become more regulated and lose their original quasi-voluntary character, the willingness of skilled professionals to work in the nonprofit sector will diminish, forcing wages up or the quality of services down. Second, when tight job markets develop, it will be hard for private agencies to attract and hold workers if they can make significantly more money elsewhere. Third, a vigorous nonprofit sector is likely to organize to reduce wage disparities.

These three propositions summarize the Massachusetts experience of the 1980s. Wages in nonprofit agencies in the state were so low compared to wages for comparable public sector jobs that nonprofit providers could not attract or retain staff, experienced destructively high turnover, and often allowed jobs to go unfilled for long periods. Many nonprofit organizations were forced to turn to temporary help agencies at a high cost to fill essential staff vacancies.

After tolerating these growing disparities for a decade the Massachusetts Council of Human Service Providers gained support for state budgetary redress to achieve wage parity. Many public officials conceded that the state could not continue to provide reliable human services to citizens and save money at the expense of workers in private agencies. Lower private sector wages also result in higher turnover rates and longer time periods in which jobs go unfilled, resulting

---

1. In a personal comment to one of the authors, Burton Weisbrod points out that government could also save costs if it used volunteers. Theoretically, there is nothing to prevent the public sector from tapping volunteers on a large scale.

in loss of continuity in care. Agencies forced to turn to temporary help had to bring on workers who were completely unfamiliar with the individual needs of particular clients. They incurred higher recruitment costs as well. Faced with a tight human service labor market, some Massachusetts mental health providers went looking for prospective employees in Pennsylvania and Great Britain.

The decade of the 1990s opened with a severe fiscal crisis in Massachusetts and many other state governments, for a time obviating concern over the balance of public and private wage rates. However, the experience of the 1980s suggests that savings from privatization arise from the conditions that structure wages in the public and private sectors, not from market-driven logics. In the long run, lower wages paid by private agencies may be seen as a temporary and transient feature of privatization. The dynamics of privatization contain within them pressures that may eventually surface to end wage disparities.

HOW FLEXIBLE IS CONTRACTING IN PRACTICE?

Some human service policy areas change slowly, primarily in response to changing conceptions of professional responsibilities. There are not likely to be swift changes in facilities for profoundly retarded people, for example.

Some service areas, on the other hand, may change rapidly. Shifts in the ethnic background of urban newcomers, for example, generate quite rapidly changing perceptions of needs in health and social policy. Thus the arrival of Southeast Asian, Cuban, Haitian, and other immigrants in recent years has strained existing services, which also have to cope with the requirements of older urban populations. Shifts in perceptions of needs also generate demands for scarce resources. In recent years, AIDS, alcohol and drug abuse, respite care, and infant mortality have gained high places on the policy agenda. To provide new services public agencies may receive new appropriations. But it is just as likely that they will be expected to juggle existing funds to cover new priorities. Shifts in the relative responsibilities of federal, state, and local governments have placed new pressures on state and local governments, even when general social policy concerns are stable.

Contracting for services provides government with flexibility in programming. In every budget cycle government agencies can assert new priorities by amending or fully changing their program profiles. A state department of public health can change priorities from alcohol and drug abuse prevention, to AIDS education, to rape prevention and counseling in successive budget cycles without batting an eye. The same non-profit agency can provide the services or different agencies can accommodate changing policy priorities. Contracting out permits public agencies to change directions without firing staff or deploying inappropriate staff members in new assignments. The tendency has long been observed that organizations may fail to adapt to new circumstances because they are comfortable with what they currently do and the costs of change (in firings, learning new skills, and so forth) are too high. In a way, contracting out frees public agencies from these familiar restraints.

However, in practice, the flexibility gained by contracting is sometimes compromised by one or other consideration and loses its clear advantage.

The dependence of public agencies on private providers, for example, limits the extent to which government officials are willing to move funds around. If the local neighborhood health center depends upon state contracts for half its revenue, public officials will be reluctant to jeopardize the fiscal health of the agency if they are dependent upon the health center for some of its services. If the center is one of the only providers in a small city, officials will be very cautious about taking actions that might jeopardize the existence of one of the few organizations with the capacity to deliver private services. The need to retain a capacity to treat certain classes of clients creates an incentive to continue contracting with important providers rather than seeing each contract period as a fresh opportunity to buy this year's bundle of service requirements. In considering defunding the center, public officials also must confront the political pressures, particularly from powerful community supporters, that will be brought to bear to insure that the center has a reasonably stable funding stream.

Like many other complex government decisions, therefore, contract times are approached by public agencies as periods of incremental adjustment. Most contracts are renewed if indeed providers seek renewals. A few are adjusted upward to reward good performance or as expressions of changing public priorities. Some are marginally reduced to sanction inadequate performance. Major shocks to the provider networks tend to be avoided, and this is more the case the more government depends on particular providers for service delivery.

THE DIFFICULTIES OF PERFORMANCE ASSESSMENT

The model of market competition cannot be used as a means to improve government effectiveness through contracting because in health and social services it is particularly difficult to measure performance (Hasenfeld and English 1974; Lipsky 1980; Demone and Gibelman 1989). Many contracts for service essentially provide for the purchase of the discretionary judgments and actions of workers who interact with citizens by selecting them, assessing them, and carrying out one or another individualized intervention—this is obviously so in home health services (assessing family strengths and client health and risk), mental health services (diagnosis and treatment), and other areas involving education, therapies, and treatment. Whereas one can hold a service worker accountable for making a visit to a mentally ill person's family, following up with phone calls, and performing other appropriate tasks, one cannot know if her judgment was sound and her intervention ultimately effective. This is why mental health agencies seem so vulnerable to criticism when, tragically, a client commits suicide or violence against someone else; it is very difficult to demonstrate that the routine practice of the agency is effective.

Admittedly, the state often contracts with nonprofit providers whose work may be assessed simply by recording the production of service units. For example, state government may fund a homeless shelter solely for the purpose of shelter and not for the improvement of a client's abilities to cope or integrate into society. If the state is also indifferent to which homeless families receive shelter, then a shelter's contract performance can be straightforwardly assessed by taking a nightly census. A similar situation may exist for immunization campaigns when government wants as many people vaccinated as possible.

Rarely, but increasingly, client outcomes can be assessed validly, and in these instances, the performance measures govern contract appraisals. In recent years, many states have implemented performance-based contracting with community mental health centers by rewarding them for good performance on key indicators such as the number of hospital days prevented (Miller and Wilson 1981; Gaynor 1990). Success in such programs is readily operationalized and verifiable, although government may rely excessively on agency reporting rather than spend money on independent auditing of the agency's claims. Performance-based contracts in health care, mental health, and other health and social policy areas are currently the object of intense interest among policymakers.

Performance-based contracting is often opposed by providers who fear that the measures to be employed are unrealistic or not reflective of effective practice. They also worry that they will be held to performance standards without being given the resources to achieve their quotas. They are concerned as well that performance standards will require them to accept clients who are inappropriate for their agency. Thus, it is not entirely surprising that private agencies are often reluctant to leave the cozy shelter of mutual dependence on the state for the cold world of performance assessment.

But most services cannot be judged on the basis of decisive client outcomes. They cannot be standardized in their treatment approaches, nor can auditors effectively intrude into the interactions between workers and clients to determine whether decisions were made appropriately and consistently with existing policy. Thus in many cases it is impossible for government to know whether it is getting effective selection, diagnosis, and intervention. What happens to contracting when one party cannot know whether it is getting the value for which it pays?

Even if the public agency could know what it wanted it would be defeated in monitoring the providers. While government contracting for services has vastly increased in volume the program-auditing capacity of the public sector has not kept up. Contractors typically file reams of reports which, except for basic fiscal information, are ignored. There is little independent auditing of the accuracy of program numbers submitted, and hardly any capacity to assess the effectiveness of contractors' programs. As a result, the public sector may not know what it is purchasing even when it can define what it wants.[2]

Public officials seeking to obtain services which cannot be tested against performance criteria still need to fall back on some reason to support their choice of one or another contractor. Let us accept that public officials seeking to purchase

2. The problem of monitoring provider performance is usefully addressed by Pratt and Zeckhauser (1985).

services experience severe difficulties in measuring performance. Let us say further that they are motivated not only by a desire to obtain high-quality service (as they define it) but also by a need to justify their choice of contractors and maintain a stable provider environment in future. Then five observations on contracting appear to follow.

First, public agencies accept process measures as surrogates for performance. The number of beds, places, seats, and slots filled by clients are accepted as instances of treatment or policy delivery, without extensive inquiry into how they were filled or what happened to clients.

Second, government officials try to control the inputs into the agency. For example, governments have established procedures and regulations which give them effective control over the placement of clients in the contract agencies, including programs serving AIDS patients (Kennedy School of Government 1989a: 9–10) and deinstitutionalized mental patients (Taube and Goldman 1989). Thus the service provider does not have the authority to turn down clients it deems incompatible with its mission or staffing capabilities.

Third, official service standards are accepted as standing for quality. Perhaps the state cannot determine whether AIDS victims, mental patients, or drug abusers are getting good advice and counseling. It can, however, require that an AIDS service agency maintain "continuous nursing services, provided by either a registered nurse or licensed practical nurse" (Kennedy School of Government 1989b: 17). Adherence even to minimal process requirements can come to stand for quality in the absence of a better alternative.

Fourth, orderly administrative processes may be taken as significant in justifying contracting relationships. If public officials cannot truly know how effective their contractors are, they may give weight to the agency's ability to relate to its contract office. The timely and orderly submission of documents, ingratiating relations with agency officials, and swift return of telephone calls all contribute to the agency's standing in the eyes of public officials. These impressions are supplemented by information gained through site visits and anecdotal evidence of successful client outcomes. And they certainly are affected by any negative publicity generated by the agency.

Fifth, the reputation of the agency in the specialized communities in which it works becomes important, as public officials look to contract with "good" agencies and nurture the long-term capacity of the community to provide services.

Consider a contract bidding process in which evaluators award "points" to proposals to lend the evaluation a degree of apparent rigor. Weight is typically given, as it should be, to what is actually being proposed. But consideration will also be given to feasibility of the plan, organizational capacity, and previous performance, all of which relate simply to the agency's reputation.

The futility of looking at health and human services contracting through the prism of saving costs by competitive bidding is most apparent when "sellers" of contract services are limited or nonexistent. To insure service continuity, for example, governments sometimes negotiate the renewal of existing contracts without opening up the process to new bidders. And under some circumstances, such as providing services for emergency needs, contracts can be let without any competition at all. The Massachusetts Department of Public Welfare created an unprecedented homeless shelter network not through a process of soliciting competitive proposals but, as an emergency matter, by working with as many community groups as possible to develop acceptable proposals and get them funded. Likewise, many neighborhood health centers, community mental health centers, AIDS service agencies, and home health agencies were created without competitive bidding procedures by government officials in concert with interested community leaders, lay activists, and professionals.

In the end, despite the lack of objective measures of performance quality, public officials tend to have surprisingly firm and, in their minds, accurate views of contractors' performance. They tend to agree on which programs are "outstanding," "so-so," and "in trouble." But these beliefs in contractors' performance are largely the opinions of craft (Schon 1983). Public officials know programs are good because they have run well-regarded programs themselves, or have considerable experience in comparing impressions of similar programs over a long period of time.

To be sure, the public benefits from canny and experienced administrators. The problem with relying on craft knowledge, however, is that it is unevenly distributed. Effective program evaluation depends upon the individual talents of the program evaluators.

Nonetheless, efforts to develop more objective program assessments should not be rushed if the result would be to denigrate this intuitive approach. What is clear is that there are major inconsistencies in the belief that contracting in human service can take substantial advantage of the discipline offered by market dynamics.

THE IRONY OF PRIVATIZATION THROUGH CONTRACTING

A significant appeal of contracting with nonprofit organzations for public officials, particularly those with a conservative ideological bent, is the ability to accomplish public purposes without increasing the size of government. The public work force need not increase. Government intrusion into society can be minimized, because private agencies will do the work. This form of privatization appears to combine the pragmatic objectives of keeping costs down and maintaining flexibility in policy options with the ideological objective of minimizing government's role in society while turning to charities and other community agencies to play their traditional role.

However, only in the limited sense that the public work force has not expanded greatly can it be said that the government role has been curtailed or expansion restricted by this version of privatization (see Smith and Stone 1988). And, it should be noted, government has at times been severely criticized for its unwillingness to expand in order to manage its new responsibilities. The failure of governments to increase their oversight capacity while they increase contracting has subjected them to criticism from a variety of groups concerned with government accountability and oversight (Tanzer 1980).

In two other respects privatization through contracting has resulted in *increases* in government roles. First, governmental expenditures in human services have expanded enormously, as we already indicated. Contracting for services may actually be credited with facilitating a larger growth in public services than might otherwise occur. Contracting has permitted the expansion of a service sector unconstrained by the difficulties public agencies would experience in hiring a huge number of new workers for new tasks. It has also permitted an expansion unconstrained by the popular opposition that might be mobilized against a rapid increase in the public work force. Politicians are regularly criticized if the number of pubic employees has increased while they have been in office. They are virtually never criticized if the number of employees working for agencies under contract to the state has increased dramatically.

Contracting, up to a point, thus hides the growth of government from public scrutiny. It does so because the press and government critics are not accustomed to making contract employees an issue. And it does so, in part, because contract employees often work for private agencies that receive funds from many sources. In private agencies supported by endowment, fees, and charitable contributions as well as government funds, the total work force is not the equivalent of the number working under contract. Thus statistics on employment increases attributable to contracts are hard to obtain.

Second, privatization has led to government penetration of the private sector through the regulations, obligations, and restrictions that accompany contracts. It has created rules and regulations for private agencies that otherwise would not be subject to government control. Thus, a home health agency that seeks to help the elderly or AIDS victims finds that it must do so according to government standards. Privatization has also led to the creation in the private sector of whole agencies that accept government restrictions and standards from the beginning. Some of these agencies, such as halfway houses, day treatment programs for the mentally ill, or home health agencies, have never had another source of support. These are prepenetrated private organizations. Moreover, the proliferation of these organizations in the last twenty-five years has increased the pressure on other nonprofit organizations to adopt government norms and standards as well.

This is the irony of privatization through contracting. Supported by some as a development to reduce the size and influence of government, privatization as contracting instead has resulted in unprecedented growth and involvement of government in the affairs of private organizations.

HEALTH CARE SERVICES AND THE MARKET

Advocates of market competition in health care often propose that vouchers for health care insurance be given to everyone. Consumers would then use these vouchers to purchase health care insurance and stimulate competition among private providers. In this case, consumers would be in a similar position to government contract administrators, since they would have to evaluate the quality and effectiveness of health care: How much drug therapy is enough? When should I try an aggressive, expensive therapy instead of a low-cost option? What do I do when there is only one health care provider in a particular town willing to help me? Am I willing to break my long-term relationship with my provider (the doctor or hospital) for simply the possibility of better care from a different provider?

The experience of contracting for social services should raise serious questions for policymakers that a voucher system would actually stimulate anything approaching market competition. The voucher model is flawed because it is based on faulty assumptions, first, about the way individuals and organizations behave in the real world and, second, about the problems of evaluation in the health care and social services field. Individual consumers, like government contract administrators, do not exist in isolation from one another. Instead they are subject to peer and community pressure, the marketing efforts of provider organizations, and the desire to build a relationship with their service provider.

Consumers, like contract administrators, face significant transaction costs. Monitoring and evaluating a service provider entails significant time and energy. Moving from one provider to another is very costly, both in terms of resources and the disruption to the care and treatment offered by service providers. Then, there is the problem of defining quality, effectivness, and efficiency. Contract administrators have tended to address this problem by focusing on process measures such as the number of professionals and the timeliness of reporting. There is no reason to expect that consumers would be any different. Thus, consumers are likely to be attracted to hospitals and providers with well-educated professionals with good reputations. This is entirely reasonable. However, the effect on over-all health care costs could well be perverse, because hospitals and other health care providers would have an incentive to attract professionals with good reputations and a stable client base with high salaries, benefits, and concessions.

In a voucher scheme, service providers are likely to exhibit the same types of defensive behavior characteristic of contract agencies. The agencies have an incentive to limit the risk and intrusiveness of the contract official trying to monitor their performance. In a voucher system, service providers would strive to minimize their risk of unforeseen costs by limiting access for individuals with the likelihood of serious disease or insufficient insurance. Providers would also make it difficult for patients to evaluate service quality.

Maldistribution of services presents another problem. Contract officers are constantly faced with the problem that organizations do not exist in the desired location. Government administrators may want to develop an early intervention program for low-income Hispanic children but find that no nonprofit agency exists in the targeted neighborhood to provide the contracted service. With vouchers, consumers will find that the urologist they would like to consult does not practice in their town or that they will have to travel long distances if they want to switch service providers because of dissatisfaction.

Contracting, in contrast to vouchers, may still be a good idea in some circumstances, but the reasons for contracting should be based on the needs of programs rather than on the elusive benefits of market competition. Thus, government should recognize that private contract agencies are extensions of the state and make the investment and commitment necessary for them to provide quality services. Private agencies should be allowed to invest a reasonable surplus earned from a contract in the organization. Government should assist agencies with capital needs, including access to low-interest loans. Government should also improve its monitoring capacity, although it should encourage efforts by nonprofit agencies to develop methods of self-evaluation that could ease the monitoring and evaluation burden of public authorities. And finally, government should retain its own service capacity, especially for difficult-to-serve clients, such as individuals who combine mental illness and substance abuse. Retaining a service capability provides two overall benefits: it gives government leverage in its relations with contract agencies, and it offers a way to serve clients whose treatment is most difficult for government to evaluate and for private agencies to provide.

Many of these suggested reforms in the contracted service system will have to await an improvement in state and local economies. In the meantime, we should be under no illusion that contracting for services approximates the classic model of free-market competition. Indeed, the mistaken belief that market competition is occurring and should be encouraged further is having destructive consequences on the existing service system and preventing the implementation of needed changes in public policy that would help contract agencies provide improved services.

Symbols, Rationality, and Justice: Rationing Health Care

Daniel Callahan

One of the most important domestic tasks before the United States is to put in place a just and universal health care plan. Most people seem to believe, however, that such a plan would obviate the need for rationing health care, indeed that it is an alternative to rationing. This Article argues that universal health care is neither feasible nor plausible without health care rationing. This contention is based not on some theory of just health care but on the the experience of other countries that have some form of universal health insurance already in place. Each provides a decent level of health care. None provide all the health care that people might want, nor necessarily provide it in the way in which they would most like to have it.[1]

Why do these countries set such limits? Because early on they came to recognize what might be called the economic iron law of universal health care plans: to be affordable they must be limited. If you want universal coverage, then be prepared to ration. If you are not prepared to ration, abandon all hopes of an affordable plan of universal coverage. To these general propositions, good for all countries and times, must be added a specifically American point: if we ever hope to persuade American politicians to enact a plan of universal coverage, then we

---

American Journal of Law & Medicine, V. 18, n. 1 & 2.
Director and Co-founder, The Hastings Center, Briarcliff Manor, New York; Ph.D., 1965, Harvard University.
1. *See* Mark Pauly et al., *A Plan for "Responsible National Health Insurance"*, HEALTH AFF., Spring 1991, at 5, 20–21 (comparing experiences of the United States, the United Kingdom and Canada).

must show them in advance how such a plan will control costs and how it will have built into it the ingredients to keep it from breaking the bank.

It is hard to say such things in the United States. Any discussion of the possibility of rationing health care in this country begins under a cloud. Symbolically, the very idea seems to offend a nicely tinted picture of ourselves as a rich, powerful nation, one that can afford to do whatever it takes to do whatever we want.[2] A nation that can put a man on the moon, that can afford Desert Storm and that can afford the S & L bailout is a nation that does not have to stint on health care. Especially for liberals, for whom the idea of universal health care has long been a high goal, any embrace of rationing seems a great betrayal. Since the main motive of the push for national health insurance has been coverage for the poor, the prospect of rationing care for that same group seems particularly offensive. It would seem to build into a program for the poor precisely those features that have so long burdened them: limits on what they can receive, while the more affluent can buy whatever care they want. As a symbol, then, rationing has nothing at all going for it. It seems, in fact, the perfect negative symbol of a weak and unjust society.

A strong and generous society must, however, be realistic if it is to do what needs doing. In case anyone addicted to symbols has not noticed, we have yet to enact universal health insurance in this country, and that failure comes at the end of at least forty years of trying. It is at best naive, at worst obstructionist, to continue invoking some idealized picture of ourselves to justify a failure to do what can be done, in a way it can be done, and to put in place something better than we now have. We can have universal health care in this country, but only if we can convince legislators and the American public that it is sensible and affordable. The only way to make such a case is to build an acceptance of rationing into it. What is now a negative symbol must be turned into one that is powerful and forthright: we can get what we need if we are prepared, in the process, to restrain ourselves. Rationing should be understood as a symbol of reasoning and restraint.[3] So understood, it can have great power, showing that we are concerned enough about the poor to pursue reasonable policies. However wonderfully symbolic, an anti-rationing policy is not reasonable.

There are other, more literal objections to rationing. It has often been taken for granted that health care rationing would positively harm the poor,[4] and that it would also represent a precipitate abandonment of efforts to control costs and

---

2. *See, e.g.*, Robert J. Blendon, *The Public's View of the Future of Health Care*, 259 JAMA 3587 (1988); Cindy Jajich-Toth & Burns W. Roper, *Americans' Views on Health Care: A Study in Contradictions*, HEALTH AFF., Winter 1990, at 149.

3. *Cf.* David C. Hadorn, *Emerging Parallels in the American Health Care and Legal-Judicial Systems*, 18 AM. J.L. & MED. 73, 85 ("The problem of rationing merely is another instance of the need to balance individual welfare and public good.").

4. *See, e.g.*, Joan Beck, *Oregon Health Plan Faces the Reality of Care Rationing*, CHI. TRIB., Mar. 2, 1992, at C15; Spencer Rich, *Advocates for the Poor Hit Oregon Health Plan: Governor Vows to Prevent Inadequate Care*, WASH. POST, Sept. 17, 1991, at A3.

eliminate waste.[5] It need not do any of those things. On the contrary, rationing is likely the only way in which we can improve care for the poor and manage our health care system in a more efficient manner. This Article's argument, therefore, is strong and direct. Both as a symbol, and as a way of organizing the health care system, rationing represents the most promising route available to us. Or, put somewhat differently, so long as it builds a method of rationing into it, the United States can have, and can afford a solid, decent and just health care system.

In this Article, "rationing" means an action undertaken when there is: (a) a recognition that resources are limited, and (b) when faced with scarcity, a method that must be devised to allocate fairly and reasonably those resources. Rationing is the effort to distribute equitably scarce resources. This definition is consistent with much common usage.[6]

Rationing may be understood in a hard and a soft sense. The hard sense is that of the lifeboat at sea, where a limited amount of fresh water must be shared. In that case a method of distribution must be devised that accepts the fact that there will be no more water. The limits are absolute.

The soft sense of rationing is the kind that we confront with health care, and just about everything else, in the United States. The limits to resources are not absolute. We could, if we chose to do so, spend far more on health care. We could go from 12% of our GNP[7] to 20%. We could, for that matter, declare superb health care to be the main goal of American society, and the delivery of health care our main industry.

That is not likely to happen, and for a good reason. There are practical political constraints on how much money can be spent on health care. Limits are imposed by an unwillingness to pay higher taxes, to increase the burden of employers to provide health care, or to pay personally out of our own pockets. Public opinion polls time and again show that Americans, however, high their aspirations for good care, are not willing to pay an unlimited amount to have it or to put up with the restrictions that it might entail.[8] There are, as politicians know all too well, limits to a public willingness to tolerate tax increases, both across-the-board and for health care. For their part, employers cannot afford to jeopardize the overall fiscal soundness of their businesses by readily tolerating

---

5. *See, e.g.*, David Lauter & Edwin Chen, *Health Care For All: Three Plans Compete*, L.A. Times, Nov. 11, 1991, at A1.

6. *See* Kai N. Lee, *Salmon, Science and the Law in the Columbia Basin*, 21 Envtl. L. 745, 776–77 (1991) ("[In] rationing lifesaving medical care . . . societies must attempt to make allocations in ways that preserve the moral foundations of social collaboration."); Pascal Fletcher, *Feeding Family Food Basket is Frustrating Chore in Cuba,* Reuter Libr. Rep., Sept. 30, 1991, BC cycle ("The authorities say the rationing system is the only way to ensure a fair distribution of scarce resources.").

7. *See* George J. Annas et al., American Health Law 121 (1990) (11.1% of GNP in 1987); Robert D. Ray, *Health Tax Credits? A Sickly Idea: Here's A Plan That Won't Do Anything to Make the System Work,* Wash. Post, Jan. 26, 1992, at C5 (13% of GNP in 1991).

8. Robert J. Blendon, *supra* note 2, at 3588–90; Cindy Jajich-Toth & Burns W. Roper, *supra* note 2 at 153.

constant cost escalations. The Hastings Center[9] has had to put up with average increases of 25% per year for the past three years, and that is not atypical. Neither the Hastings Center nor more affluent organizations can afford to continue that pattern.

Limits are further imposed by common sense. We ought not to spend excessively on health care. We do so spend only at the cost of other important recipients of limited resources. We need a good educational system, good parks and roads, good welfare and poverty programs, good industrial research and development policies. Health is not the only human good. Despite the great hand-wringing about the state of our health care system, for the most part American citizens already have a high and adequate level of general health. No special national gain adheres in increasing average life expectancy, or in trying to conquer each and every human disease. It would be nice, but it is not an imperative goal for the overall well-being of the country. Only a nation that over-values health could think we need more of it.

This Article speaks primarily about the health status of middleclass white people, those who can expect, on average, to live a long life, well into old age. But what is true of this group is not true of everyone. The most immediate pressing problem is whether we can bring to the poor and deprived the same benefits now available to the rest of us.

This Article proposes the following ideal for the American health care system. Every American should be guaranteed a decently adequate, affordable level of health care. The poor, in particular, should be provided such care. The goal would be universal access to decent care. The achievement of that goal will require significant government expenditures; the government should provide the base guarantee for the poor. Beyond that, a combination of employer and personal contributions can provide the remainder of the needed money for everyone else.[10]

Such a system would not make economic sense without some form of rationing, at least in its public government programs and its private employer programs. Why rationing? Because the government would be foolish to promise an unlimited system of health care, one devised independently of the costs of that system. No country on earth, including one with the most generous system, has done that. The government cannot say, in effect, that it will pay whatever it costs to give you the most advanced health care. It cannot promise to pay for every technological advance, however efficacious and however expensive. It cannot promise to help all of us live as long as we choose, regardless of what private hopes we might have. It cannot promise to jeopardize other important societal needs in the pursuit of improved health. It cannot promise to conduct an unending struggle against mortality.

The American Congress has a long memory. It can recall how it was assured, in 1972, that the kidney dialysis program would cost no more than $250 million

9. Daniel Callahan, Director.
10. This Article does not address the details of that kind of system.

per year in its fourth year of operation or thereafter.[11] It now costs over $3 billion per year.[12] Congress can recall when it put Medicare in place in 1965,[13] assured that the costs would be manageable. Those costs now are expected to bankrupt the Medicare Trust Fund within the next decade.[14] In neither case were any methods conceived or developed to keep the costs under control; they were not thought to be needed. With memories of this kind, Congress cannot be expected to initiate major new entitlement programs that do not show, in advance, how the costs are to be managed. Blank checks will not be issued. The estimate of the Pepper Commission in 1990, the major bipartisan congressional effort to formulate a response to the problem of indigent and long-term care, was a cost of an additional $69.6 billion per year for decent coverage.[15] That estimate was for the first year. Nothing was said about the second year; the Commission knew better than to do that.

In short, both because no nation on earth, not even the United States, can promise unbounded health care regardless of the cost, and because Congress will not pay for such health care, some system of limits must be put in place. I call such a system a "rationing." It is rationing in the worst sense if it is capricious and discriminatory, as is our present method of using ability-to-pay as a way of limiting costs. But it can be rationing in the best sense of the term if, in response to the need for limits, a fair and reasonable way is developed to set and maintain these limits.

But of course, for symbolic and practical reasons, every possible rationale, every conceivable evasion, is being developed to avoid the need for rationing. If we could just organize our present system better, it is said, we could have all the necessary health care we want.[16] If we could simply wring the waste, inefficiency and excess bureaucratic and malpractice costs out of the system, we would not even have to think about rationing.[17] The basis for this faith in efficiency is not groundless. We know that our administrative costs are high, approximately 20% of all costs (in comparison with approximately 10% in Canada).[18] We know that

---

11. 118 CONG. REC. 33,004 (daily ed. Sept. 30, 1972) (statement of Senator Hartke in sponsoring the end-stage renal disease section of the Social Security Amendments of 1972).
12. *See* GEORGE J. ANNAS ET AL., *supra* note 7, at 890.
13. Health Insurance for the Aged Act, Pub. L. No. 89–97, 79 Stat. 290 (1965) (codified as amended at 42 U.S.C. A. §§ 401–426 (West 1991)).
14. John Holahan & John L. Palmer, *Medicare's Fiscal Problems: An Imperative for Reform,* 13 J. HEALTH POL., POL'Y & L. 53, 77 (1988).
15. THE PEPPER COMM'N: UNITED STATES BIPARTISAN COMM. ON COMPREHENSIVE HEALTH CARE, 101ST CONG., 2D SESS., A CALL FOR ACTION 17 (S. Print 1990).
16. *See Administration Health Care Proposals: Hearings Before the House Ways and Means Comm.*, 102d Cong., 2d Sess. (1992) (statement of Dr. Louis Sullivan, Secretary of Health and Human Services) ("Indeed, one of our principles is to increase the efficiencies in our system because of my belief that we already have enough dollars in the system, but we're not spending them wisely."), *reprinted in* FED. NEWS SERV., Feb. 20, 1992.
17. *See* Amitai Etzioni, *Health Care Rationing: A Critical Evaluation,* HEALTH AFF., Summer 1991, at 88–95.
18. Steffie Woolhandler & David U. Himmelstein, *The Deteriorating Administrative Efficiency of the U.S. Health Care System*, 324 NEW ENG. J. MED. 1253, 1255 (1991).

a huge amount of money is spent in response to malpractice problems and on our present system of tort compensation.[19] These costs are not incurred in other countries.[20] We know that we waste billions of dollars on untested or misused technologies.[21] We know that most other developed countries can show as good or better mortality and morbidity outcomes for considerably less money per capita[22] and for a smaller percentage of their GNP.[23] It is not, in a word, hard to show that we could get much better value for the money that we do spend and probably even could get as good or better an outcome for less money.

Nonetheless, we are profoundly mistaken in believing that we should not move to open and conscious rationing *until* we have wrung all of that waste out of the system. This is a version of what this Article calls the "best of all possible worlds fallacy": if we could just organize ourselves more efficiently, we could have all the necessary and affordable health care we want.

Why am I skeptical, and why do I call that a fallacy? Mainly because I have heard the same refrain again and again, for well over a decade now. Yet during that time, and despite a variety of highly touted cost containment programs, nothing has worked to any substantial degree to control costs or to bring much greater efficiency into the system. We have tried DRGs,[24] managed care,[25] HMOs[26] and competition.[27] No attempt has had any striking success, although some evidence shows that Medicare cost increases are being controlled.[28] The most that we can say is that costs might have been higher without these alternative health care plans. Overall health care costs continue to increase at two to three times the rate of inflation in general, and have risen even more sharply over the

---

19. *See* Leonard S. Weiss, *Finding the Remedies for Ills in Health Care: They Don't Come Easy, but They Do Exist,* NEWSDAY, Mar. 5, 1992, at 97 (defensive medicine adds more than $18 billion to healthcare costs).

20. *Cf.* Frank A. Sloan & Randall R. Bobvjerg, *in Medical Malpractice: Crises, Response and Effects,* HEALTH INS. ASS'N OF AMERICA, RESEARCH BULLETIN 43 (1989) ("Price rises for liability coverage and heightened fears of litigation with its many uninsured costs have surely affected the climate of American medical practice.").

21. INSTITUTE OF MEDICINE, ASSESSING MEDICAL TECHNOLOGIES 211–27 (1985).

22. *See* George J. Schieber & Jean-Pierre Poullier, *International Health Spending: Issues and Trends,* HEALTH AFF. Spring 1991, at 106, 114 exhibit 6.

23. *Id.* at 110 exhibit 2.

24. Diagnosis-related group, which is a Medicaid payment plan under which hospitals receive a lump sum payment on the basis of discharge diagnosis, without regard to actual treatment provided. *See* GEORGE J. ANNAS ET AL., *supra* note 7, at 215–16, 234–48.

25. Under a managed care system, the patient chooses, or is assigned to, a primary care provider who then controls the patient's access to hospitals and specialists. Under most plans, the provider's income decreases if the provider approves expensive specialists or hospital care. *Id.* at 784.

26. Under a health maintenance organization system, the patient pays a fixed sum and the organization promises to provide a defined package of inpatient and outpatient services. Doctors may be paid as salaried employees or on a fee-for-service basis. *Id.* at 774–75.

27. *See* DANIEL CALLAHAN, WHAT KIND OF LIFE: THE LIMITS OF MEDICAL PROGRESS 76 (1990).

28. *Id.* at 76–77. *See also* Sandra Christensen, *Did 1980s Legislation Slow Medicare Spending,* HEALTH AFF., Summer 1991, at 135.

past three years.[29] Why should we expect some great shift in the historical pattern? Why, if we have failed for years in controlling costs, should we expect a transformation—the equivalent of a religious conversion experience—of the national character and of the present system?

It is a fallacy to conclude that because there is room for great savings, which there is, it therefore follows that we will have, and can get, those savings. On the contrary, one can conclude only that the surest prescription to maintain the unfair and costly status quo is to continue talking about all the money that we can save simply by eliminating waste, malpractice excess and bureaucracy. This is a method that surely has worked well toward that end so far. Nothing changes and there is no prospect of any immediate change.

Why? We do not know how to eliminate waste in behavioral practice (even if we do in economic theory). In fact, we make things all the harder to change by posing the elimination of waste as an alternative to rationing. On the contrary, we will eliminate waste only by rationing. Only if we understand that we must live within restraints, and take the steps consistent with that recognition, can we contain costs. To be undertaken seriously, cost containment must be understood as another form of rationing. Responsible cost containment means saying "no" to some things that physicians, patients and administrators want. Serious cost containment means establishing practice guidelines and making them stick. Serious cost containment means the setting of priorities.

The issue before us is not a matter of cost containment *or* rationing. Both are necessary. They should be thought of as two sides of the same coin, not as alternatives. The experience of the European countries should sober those who think cost containment will make unlimited beneficial care available. Those countries—which have already in place most of the reforms that are desired in the United States—are beginning to feel the strain.[30] They have managed to control costs, but at the price of limiting services and requiring long waiting times for many procedures.[31] With the same demographic forces at work in those countries as here (that is, with an aging population), with an increase in high technology medicine, and with rising patient demands, these countries will be forced, as will we, into even more rationing in the future. They are quietly beginning their own rationing discussion—and are immensely curious to see how ours progresses.

The main concern about rationing in the United States is that the burden will fall upon the poor.[32] That is a serious problem. How can it be avoided? The overriding requirement is that this country have national health insurance and, with it, an adequate baseline of care. Inevitably, this baseline will have to be set

29. *See* Stuart M. Butler, *Coming to Terms on Health Care*, N.Y.Times, Jan. 28, 1990, at C13; Robert Pear, *Social Security Benefits to Go Up 3.7%*, N.Y. Times, Oct. 18, 1991, at A10.
30. *See Yesterday's Mirage: Why Britain's NHS Needs Competition*, The Economist, Apr. 28, 1984, at 26 [hereinafter *Yesterday's Mirage*]; *see also* Daniel Callahan, *supra* note 27, at 88–89.
31. *See Yesterday's Mirage*, *supra* note 30, at 26–30.
32. *See* George J. Annas et al., *supra* note 7, at 70–74, 104–06.

at a level lower than the richest people can set their baseline. Rich people can hire limousines to get to their medical treatment, and helicopters to take them from their resort villas to daily psychoanalysis. Rich Americans can fly to Switzerland to use experimental treatments not available here. Rich people can seek out the very best specialists in the country and use them rather than their local doctors. No conceivable government program could offer benefits of this kind to everyone. No private employee benefit program could offer them either.

Why should that matter anyway? What does matter is not whether the rich do better than the poor, but how well the poor do. The crucial issue is whether the baseline of care for the poor is set high enough to eliminate the most serious disparities between rich and poor. It could not eliminate all of them. It would take a totalitarian state to keep the rich and powerful from the health care that they want. The communist countries of Eastern Europe, as well as the Soviet Union, had the pretense of a single-tier, egalitarian system. The reality was that powerful party members got care not available to others, and that ordinary citizens had to bribe their way through the system to get good care. A democratic society would not even attempt to impose a single-tier system. It would invite corruption and evasion. But a democratic society would try to make certain that the poor have decent health care.

Yet if decent care is not the same as maximal care, how can the former be determined? It will, by definition, be rationed care. A fair system of rationing will have to set some priorities. If not everything can be made available to everyone, what is comparatively more or less important? The Oregon initiative is of great national importance. Using a combination of technical and economic considerations, and tempering them with expressed public values, that state has set up a system of priorities.[33] The Oregon legislators determined that it is better to provide health care coverage to everyone falling below the federal poverty line than to eliminate some people altogether in order to give virtually unlimited care to those who qualify. To make the new system possible, Oregon plans to limit services by means of its priority list.[34] The plan will also mandate that small businesses provide health insurance or pay into a pool that would make that insurance available to all employed persons.[35] The long-term goal is a system of universal health care in Oregon.

As the Oregon planners recognized, any process of rationing health care will have to find a way to balance medical judgment, economic possibilities, and public values. Yet it took some years to gain that insight. When the Medicaid program was established by Congress in 1965 to provide health care for the

33. *See* Charles J. Dougherty, *Setting Health Care Priorities: Oregon's Next Steps.* HASTINGS CENTER REP., May–June 1991, at special supp. 1–16; Sara Rosenbaum, *Mothers and Children Last: The Oregon Medicaid Experiment,* 18 AM. J.L. & MED. 97 (1992).

34. Sara Rosenbaum, *supra* note 33, at 104.

35. Act effective July 1, 1989, ch. 836, 1989 OR. LAWS 836 (codified as amended in scattered subsections of OR. REV. STAT. § 414 (1989)).

poor,[36] it specified that the indigent were to receive care that was "medically necessary."[37] Congress did not, unfortunately (but perhaps deliberately) specify what that term meant or what means would be appropriate to make such a determination. It may have presumed that a purely medical standard of medical necessity could be determined.

If that is what Congress believed, it was wrong. As the intervening years have demonstrated well, it has turned out to be impossible to specify a purely scientific standard of medical "need," the basic concept that lies behind the idea of that which is "medically necessary." The problem is that "need" admits of no precise definition, ranging as it does over mental and physical needs, life-saving and life-enhancing needs. It is a notion, moreover, that is subject to different interpretations, open to the changed possibilities provided by technological developments, and subject to different valuative interpretations. Thus although "medically necessary" and meeting health care "needs" have about them the ring of objectivity, then turn out to be flexible and malleable concepts. They combine both a descriptive and a normative content. They are at once scientific and moral concepts. This was not so obvious in 1965.

As time has gone on, it has been possible to trace a steady enrichment of our understanding of the ingredients necessary to specify a decent minimum of adequate health care.[38] Such care must include, in some plausible way, first, some reference to medical need; it must be rooted in commonly accepted notions of what people characteristically look for in health care. Yet, for all the above-mentioned reasons, it cannot use such a standard exclusively. Inevitably, many questions about the extent of those needs and the various evaluations required to deal with the borderline cases[39] will arise. Second, therefore, a decent minimum of average health care must include judgments about the efficacy of available treatments to meet those needs; that is, what works and what does not work? A consideration of efficacy will, however, force a third set of considerations—that of the relative costs and benefits of different treatments. What will it cost to provide different benefits and is there a good return on the money spent?

Next a decision will have to be made. If not everything can be afforded, what treatments and benefits are relatively more or less important? At this point, it should be abundantly clear that this question and those that preceded it require a central political component to be properly answered. Because these questions address fact and value, and the weighing of costs and benefits, they transcend a technical level. The questions call for collective judgment, judgment of a kind

36. Pub. L. No. 89-97, § 1901, 79 Stat. 343 (1965) (codified as amended at 42 U.S.C.A. §§ 1396a–1396u (West 1992)).

37. *Id.*

38. CHARLES J. DOUGHERTY, *supra* note 33, at special supp. 3–4. *See also* Daniel Callahan, *Medical Futility, Medical Necessity: The Problem Without A Name,* HASTINGS CENTER REP. July–Aug. 1991, at 30.

39. For example, coronary artery bypass surgery for an elderly person, or resuscitation efforts with a very low birthweight baby.

that will combine both expert and lay opinion. Thus, the fourth consideration is that a political process will have to be devised.

Since the political process almost certainly will encounter resource limitations, a question will then be raised: what is relatively more or less important in the provision of health care? The setting of priorities, then, will be a fifth consideration. How might that best be done? The state of Oregon has devised one method to do this,[40] and perhaps one could imagine others. Whatever other possible ways they might use to set priorities, however, other states would be wise in following the lead of Oregon in organizing community discussion of health care policy prior to the more formal political process of priority setting. Thus, the sixth consideration is the importance in giving the public not only a chance to express its opinions and preferences on priorities, but also a chance to become educated on the issues.

In a sharp attack on the Oregon approach to rationing and priority-setting, one of our most astute health care analysts, Lawrence D. Brown, wrote that "rationing has been elevated to the panethon of fashionable solutions—competition, managed care, prudent purchasing, and more—that policymakers intermittently embrace as all-American answers to uncontrollable health care costs."[41] He then goes on to say that

> [v]iewed in cross-national context, Oregon's contribution is mainly to show that, at least today in the United States, rationing is not a profound but a spurious issue. . . . The United States should worry less about rationing and more about constructing a rational policy framework whose watchwords are budgeting, planning, regulation, and negotiation. If the polity has declined to make those hard choices, rationing cannot save it from itself. American policymakers have not earned the right to ration health care, and the very policies that would earn it would eliminate much of the need to exercise it.[42]

Dr. Brown is wrong. First, rationing has not been proposed as one more solution to be put alongside competition or managed care, but as a strikingly different kind of proposal. The other approaches were all designed to control costs within the present system of health care, not to change the system altogether. For many, in fact, they were meant as ways of avoiding rationing, as rationing is a generically different kind of approach. Second, what Dr. Brown proposes is perfectly sensible, but it *also* is fashionable. For what has been more common of late than to call for "a rational policy framework," and the national health insurance that would embody it? It is the best solution, and even those of us who support rationing would prefer such a framework as our starting point in an ideal world. But Dr. Brown neglects to mention that there has been no national progress of any significance toward that goal. There has been neither the political will for

---

40. OR. REV. STAT. § 414.720 (1991).

41. Lawrence D. Brown, *The National Politics of Oregon's Rationing Plan*, HEALTH AFF., Summer 1991, at 46–47.

42. *Id.* at 50.

such a framework nor, in the face of budget deficits, any serious, politically potent constituency for it.

Third, the real genius of the Oregon initiative is that it shares with a recognition of limits as the first step toward a comprehensive health care system.[43] Its organizers say that in the present American political climate, the best way to get to Dr. Brown's goal of "budget, planning, and negotiation" is to concede at the very outset that rationing is necessary, and that the setting of priorities is the most sensible way of effecting it.[44] It is striking that none of the major national universal health care plans that have been proposed make any serious provision for controlling their costs. The Oregon plan takes limitations at its *point of departure* and then works from there.[45]

In effect, the Oregon plan stands Dr. Brown's approach on its head. Dr. Brown says that "American policymakers have not earned the right to ration health care, and the very policies that would earn it would eliminate much of the need to exercise it."[46] The organizers of Oregon's plan, by contrast, say that only by a willingness to embrace rationing—the orderly, equitable allocation of scarce resources—can we make progress toward universal health care, not the other way around.[47] They also say, moreover, that it is high time we stop talking about how a better, more rational system would obviate the need for rationing.[48] No universal health care system could avoid some degree of rationing. In any case, we are still far from significant national reforms, and the need now is to find a good starting point. In the absence of the will, leadership and public support necessary for national health insurance, Oregon is actually taking some real steps in that direction. The other states and the federal government are just talking.

The animus against rationing in the United States, symbolically and literally, expresses in one sense some of our most admirable values. Those are our touching faith in the power of efficiency, our commitment to egalitarianism, and our reluctance officially to pick upon the poor to test our social schemes. Rationing is thought to offend all of those values and thus is rejected.

We deceive ourselves. Serious efficiency would require the equivalent of rationing, and that is why we have not achieved it. Our egalitarianism is more rhetorical than it is real. We tolerate a radically inegalitarian health care system

43. *See* Daniel Callhan, *Ethics and Priority Setting in Oregon,* HEALTH AFF., Summer 1991, at 78–87.

44. *See Oregon Medicaid Rationing Experiment: Hearings Before the Subcomm. on Health and the Environment of the House Comm. on Energy and Commerce*, 102d Cong., 1st Sess. 19 (1991) [hereinafter *Hearings on Oregon Rationing*] (statement of Jean I. Thorne, Director, Medical Assistance Programs, Dep't of Human Resources); *id.* at 83 (testimony of Tina Castanares, Oregon Health Servs. Comm.).

45. *See id.* at 65 (testimony of Rep. Les AuCoin) ("Oregon's health plan is a program of expansion, not of limits.").

46. Lawrence D. Brown, *supra* note 41, at 50.

47. *See Hearings on Oregon Rationing, supra* note 44, at 157, 160 (statement of Sisters of Providence in Oregon).

48. *See id.* at 151 (statement of Peter O. Kohler, M.D., President, Oregon Health Sciences University); *id.* at 157 (statement of Sisters of Providence of Oregon).

as a day-to-day affair but then rail against anyone—in the name of perfection—who would accept some degree of inequality as the first step on the way to a genuinely fair system. Although we carry out social experiments with the poor all of the time, including the crazy mess that is our Medicaid system, we rail at efforts to bring some sensible priorities and planning into that system, as Oregon is trying to do.

The usual approach to American problems is to say that since we are such a powerful and rich nation, we can afford nothing less than the best: the most lavish health care system and, with reform, the fairest and most efficient as well. So we reject any notion of limits, boundaries or self-restrictions. We live with our dreams. We should give them up and put realism and sobriety in their place. An acceptance of rationing would be a good place to begin. In fact, if we want national health insurance, it is likely to be the only feasible place to begin.

Seeking Social Justice

As long as resources are allocated by socioeconomic status and not medical need or scarcity, ethical problems arise.

Ron J. Anderson, MD

Until the relatively recent groundswell of support for national health-policy reform, discussions about universal health insurance had stalled on zero for nearly half a century. Efforts to legislate reform began with President Harry S. Truman and the Democratic party in 1948, when they proposed national compulsory health insurance. In doing so, they helped forward the concept that health care is a right every American should enjoy.

Unfortunately, the notion of guaranteeing a baseline of medicine benefits to every citizen didn't get very far.

Today, an estimated 16 percent—approximately 40 million—of Americans have no health insurance, and at least 50 million others have insurance inadequate to cover serious illness. Many of these men, women and particularly children suffer preventable illnesses; the direct result of a status quo that tolerates lack of

---

Health Management Quarterly, Second Quarter 1992.
Ron J. Anderson, M.D., is president and chief executive officer of Parkland Memorial Hospital in Dallas, chairman of the Texas Board of Health, and chairman of the National Association of Public Hospitals.

health care for certain groups at the same time it spends staggering sums on high-tech and boutique medicine.

This is the sorry legacy of a trend in this country to allocate health care on the basis of socioeconomic class. This ugly habit was formally endorsed in 1965 with the creation of Medicaid—a joint federal-state health-care program where eligibility is unrelated to medical need. Like welfare, Medicaid allows state-by-state latitude in the amount, duration and scope of services. Consequently, costly last-minute, "resurrection" medicine is usually favored over early intervention and preventive services.

Most of the current proposals for reform continue to build on these fundamental flaws, and few would significantly alter the plight of today's uninsured and underinsured. Many are just cost-shifting schemes based on the "price rationing" that Uwe E. Reinhardt calls "integral" to free-enterprise medicine: the withholding of truly needed health care from those unable to pay.[1]

As long as resources are allocated by socioeconomic status and not medical need or scarcity, ethical problems arise. Ethically skewed proposals seek to preserve existing rationing, which occurs when health care is regarded as a private obligation and public programs contain eligibility criteria unrelated to health status. Implicit rationing occurs everyday through inconvenience and long queues in public hospitals and health clinics because no one else will care for the poor.

This undeclared rationing is more egregious than Oregon's proposal to openly limit care among Medicaid beneficiaries, but neither is ethical in the midst of today's abundance. For rationing to be ethical, a scarcity must exist. Indeed, rationing assumes scarcity. The fundamental definition of rationing is the equitable allocation of scarce resources—hardly the case in a country whose annual health-care expenditures were more than $700 billion, higher per capita than any other nation.

As much as a third of the total cost may comprise waste, fraud and ineffective care.[1] Administering our bureaucratic system, which comprises more than 1,500 insurers,[2] costs up to 24 percent of total spending.[3,4] Providers, insurers, lawyers and bureaucrats obviously are benefiting more than patients, employers or taxpayers who pay for health care.

Waste of such magnitude allows the invisible business of price rationing to refuse otherwise deserving women a technology as beneficial as mammography. The United States is saturated with four times as many mammography machines as usage warrants[1], and the resulting low utilization rate must be subsi-

1. U. E. Reinhardt, "On the Economics and Ethics of Rationing Health Care," *Decisions in Imaging Economics 5* (April 1992): 10–16.
2. D. U. Himmelstein and S. Woolhandler, "A National Health Program for the United States," *New England Journal of Medicine* 320 (January 12, 1989): 102–108.
3. A. S. Relman, "The Health Care Industry: Where Is It Taking Us?" *New England Journal of Medicine* 325 (September 19, 1991): 854–859.
4. S. Woolhandler and D. U. Himmelstein, "The Deteriorating Administrative Efficiency of the U.S. Health Care System," *New England Journal of Medicine* 324 (May 2, 1991): 1253–1257.

dized through unnecessarily high fees of $100 or more—usually not covered by insurance. Similarly, the 1990 measles epidemic could have been averted if all insurers covered immunizations. Instead, this easily preventable disease killed 68 children in a raging nationwide epidemic of 26,500 reported cases.

Meanwhile, the debate about rationing continues, with each side arguing over whom to exclude; but as Daniel Wikler so aptly describes the ethics of rationing care, "one loses some debates simply by joining them."[5] Only when health care is every American's right can the debate at last be elevated to an ethical plane.

Certain principles are not debatable; and from an ethics perspective, equal access to a socially defined level of health care should be a right, not a privilege. It is a need-fulfillment right that is a prerequisite for the full expression of many of our constitutional rights. The right to vote and freedom of expression are difficult to exercise when you are debilitated by hunger or compromised by pain.

For many years, the state of Hawaii has been virtually alone in attempting to correct such wrongs by making health care more equitable among its residents. Hawaii's State Health Insurance Plan is a near-universal program that has been in place since 1974, and its Canadian-like access is responsible for increasing the percentage of insured residents to 98 percent of Hawaiians. (More recently, Florida, Minnesota and Vermont have also announced plans to provide universal access.)

In stark contrast, Oregon's Health Plan proposal completely sidesteps the rights issue and reallocates existing resources in a manner that doesn't affect the wealthy or insured. Only certain Medicaid patients are affected—the aged and disabled are exempt. The plan's stated goal is to contain costs by providing a baseline of health care to each of Oregon's estimated 400,000 uninsured residents and reducing the overall number of health-care measures now open to a smaller Medicaid population. The plan makes more money available to provide the reduced services to all Oregonians living in poverty, or so the argument goes.

Clearly, the plan is being funded on the backs of the poor.

By basing the provision of care on nonmedical criteria, we are continuing the dubious American trait of blaming victims for their diseases and socioeconomic class. This is a silent and cruel discrimination tool that helps perpetuate inequity, particularly among the races. The majority of minorities are low-income Americans and therefore have limited access to health care.

The United States and the Republic of South Africa are the only industrialized nations that consider health care a privilege, and the parallels of the two nations are shamefully evident. Blacks in both countries suffer higher rates of infant mortality, and there is a greater prevalence in blacks of diseases such as tuberculosis, pneumonia and measles, which have been nearly eliminated among whites in both countries.

5. D. Wikler, "Ethics and Rationing: 'Whether,' 'How,' or 'How Much?' " *Journal of the American Geriatrics Society* 40 (April 1992): 398–403.

As long as we tolerate inadequate health care for any of our citizens, each of us is vulnerable to a similar plight. Increasing numbers of us are being eliminated from health care, as exemplified by the current disintegration of the health-insurance market for small businesses—employers of half this country's uninsured workers. Insurers increasingly are adopting practices that limit the ability of small groups to obtain sufficient insurance, including dropping a firm from coverage if just one of its employees uses high-cost treatment, such as chemotherapy.

True reform cannot occur as long as health care is a commodity and defined by piles of pills or procedures to be parceled out. It is not a static snapshot of someone's life. It's a fluid motion picture drawn by many social influences and should be viewed as such.

Health care cannot be addressed separately from the collateral social ills of illiteracy, unemployment and underemployment, crime and unfit housing. As Reed Tuckson, M.D., so eloquently stated in a recent interview, "health is the place where all the social forces converge to express themselves with the greatest clarity."[6] The absence of health is personified in babies who don't get enough to eat and children shot as they lay sleeping in their beds or playing outdoors. It's no longer unusual to read about toddlers gunned down, the innocent victims of crazed gunmen or hostile gangs.

What difference is there between killing our children with the stray bullets of drive-by shootings or the miserable public health neglect that kills with measles?

We should hold ourselves to a higher standard and begin acknowledging the value of every citizen—implicit in guaranteeing basic health services to everyone.

Fundamental to reforming our health-care system should be the equitable, managed health-care concepts of outcome, utilization review and continuous quality improvement. Through rational reforms that rid the system of defensive medicine, excessive bureaucracy and other waste, price rationing won't be necessary.

But in doing so, we also will have to reform our thinking, viewing the poor through a new pair of glasses that permit us to see them as an opportunity, not a social burden. By acknowledging the value of each citizen's humanity, we will rise above the "us and them" mentality that now permits us to step over homeless people sleeping on the sidewalk. When we begin to do something to reduce the physical suffering of others, true reform of our health-care system can occur. Perhaps that's where the Canadians have risen above us. They seem to value people more than we do.

---

6. R. Tuckson, "A Question of Survival: An Interview with Reed Tuckson," *Second Opinion* 17 (April 1992): 48–63.

Comparing Health Care Systems: What Nations Can Learn from One Another

William C. Hsiao

How should a nation structure its health care system? Varied forces around the world cause many countries to search for answers to this question. In the United States and the Netherlands, rapidly escalating health care expenditures and the lack of universal health insurance coverage drive the desire for reform. Further east, a shift from centrally managed to free market economies has caused Russia and other eastern European countries to restructure their social protection programs, including their health care. In newly industrialized nations such as Singapore, Taiwan, and South Korea, a swelling middle-class population demands better health care service at an affordable cost. Meanwhile, in many developing countries, the process of macroeconomic structural adjustment compels governments to reform their health care sectors. In China, as well, reform of both collective farming the state enterprises forces policymakers to redesign its health system.

Developing an optimal structure for a health care system has been an elusive task, however, for three reasons. First, a health system is a means to an end. In the abstract, most countries embrace three goals for their health care system: universal and equal access to reasonable health care, control of health care costs at an affordable level, and effective use of resources. When trying to develop the specifics of a health system, however, many nations find that they have not reached a consensus on the relative importance of these goals. It is only when

Journal of Health Politics, Policy and Law, Vol. 17, No. 4, Winter 1992. Duke University.

socioeconomic and political objectives have been clarified that a nation can begin to build an effective health care system to achieve its objectives.

A second obstacle to developing a health care system is the ideological debate between those who favor free enterprise and those who believe in the merits of government planning as a means of structuring an efficient economy. This long-running debate has spilled into the health sector and has impaired rational discussions on the best approach to structuring a health care system. In redefining the economic doctrine in the health care context, the debate is between the demand-side and the supply-side approaches.

The final obstacle is inadequate knowledge and insufficient empirical information. We still know little about the performance of various types of health systems and the key dynamic forces that influence outcomes.

By confronting theory with empirical evidence, we can move beyond this ideological gridlock. A comparison of the performance of health systems based on demand-side theory with those based on a supply-side approach can provide useful information about various outcomes of the different systems.

While many experts engaged in comparative research believe useful lessons can be learned from other countries, others warn of the difficulties of transferring a specific approach across national boundaries (Stone 1980–81). The goal, however, is not to duplicate another country's system, but to understand better the key factors that affect one's own health care system.

THREE FUNDAMENTAL POLICY QUESTIONS

Every society must formulate policies to address three fundamental questions. First, a nation must face the question of what proportion of its total resources are to be spent on health care. Rapid development of both expensive medical technology and new drugs has pushed health care costs beyond what even the most affluent of nations can afford. Aging of populations and newly emerging diseases such as AIDS also strain resources. Consequently, in order to stem spiraling costs, a nation needs to impose an effective fiscal constraint on total health expenditures. Otherwise, health care costs will be driven out of control by the desire to have the newest fancy technology, particularly when this technology will boost the reputation of hospitals and fascinate the specialists. There also needs to be a budget constraint so that patients, physicians, and hospitals have to take costs into account when making difficult decisions regarding the desirability of a certain test or procedure and resuscitation of terminally ill patients.

Second, a nation must decide how and by whom scarce health resources are to be allocated among programs, diseases, and regions. The resources can be allocated by market forces or by a planning agency, which bases its decisions on criteria that take into consideration equity, need, and cost-benefit analysis, as well as the political implications of each decision. In addition, resources will ultimately be used by individuals. Societies must choose whether to allocate services among these individuals by price—according to the consumer's ability and willingness to pay— or by some other means, so that at the point of delivery the health services can be free.

Third, nations must endeavor to obtain maximum efficiency in the production of health services, or, as the British put it, "value for your money." Two factors affect the productive efficiency of health services: the nature of ownership, organization and management of health facilities; and the incentive structure, comprised of the compensation method and compensation level of health care providers. This incentive structure influences the type of health services supplied and the way in which they are produced, as well as the number of physicians and their specialty choices. Furthermore, the compensation level determines the amount of wealth transferred between patients and health professionals. As Uwe Reinhardt (1990) noted, a heath care system can be viewed as a bazaar. Physicians, nurses, technicians, etc., possess real resources—their labor, skill, and knowledge. They sell these real resources in exchange for money. Patients transfer their wealth to these providers for those resources. Each nation must determine how much wealth should be transferred in exchange for labor and who should make that decision in order to assure that the health sector is as efficient as possible.

THEORETICAL FRAMEWORK: SUPPLY-SIDE VERSUS DEMAND-SIDE

Each nation must choose macropolicies that address the three questions discussed above. Such policy choices reflect a nation's historical antecedents, culture, social values, and the balance of political power among the stakeholders in health affairs. A nation that lacks a clearly defined policy and lets natural forces take their own course chooses a laissez-faire free enterprise system by default.

Two basic economic theories exist to guide the formation of health policy: on the one hand the demand-side theory, and on the other the supply-side.

Demand-Side Approach

The demand-side school argues that health care is like other goods: consumers can exercise control over what services to buy and at what price. Purchasers and providers are evenly matched. Providers have little ability to induce patients' demand or market power to set prices. Thus, a health system maximizes welfare by atomizing economic power in the hands of each consumer. Competition for consumer dollars forces providers to produce services efficiently. In the long run, production occurs at the lowest possible average cost. The level of total resources devoted to health care is of little concern to the demand-side school, because it assumes that expenditure decisions are the direct result of consumer utility maximization (i.e., they want to spend that much for health care). Fundamental aspects of the demand-side approach include the allocation of resources according to consumers' willingness to pay and the privatization of organizations that provide health services.

Singapore and South Korea are examples of nations that rely on the demand-side approach to constrain the system and to allocate health services. Wanting to assure universal equal access, Singapore mandates an individual savings plan (Medisave) for every worker, which is dedicated to covering health care expenses (Phau 1991). When a worker is in need of services, she spends funds from her own Medisave account. South Korea takes a somewhat different approach. Its universal health insurance plan imposes high coinsurance rates on patients—55 percent for general hospital outpatient services and 20 percent for inpatient services—trying to constrain demand for health services (Yang 1990).

Supply-Side Approach

The supply-side school argues, on the other hand, that health care has many distinctive features. Since health services are necessities for maintaining life and relieving suffering, everyone is entitled to reasonable access to health care, regardless of his or her ability to pay. In addition, serious market failures arise in the health care sector, due to three major factors: (1) the presence of insurance, which reduces both the consumers' and the providers' sensitivity to price; (2) the propensity of high-risk individuals to buy insurance (adverse selection) and the selection of favorable risks by insurers, both of which impair competition in insurance markets; and (3) a disparity between the amount of information that a physician has and what patients have (information asymmetry), which leads to physicians' strong professional dominance over medical decisions and enables physicians and hospitals to induce demand and set prices. To remedy these market failures, supply-siders advocate the placement of fiscal power in public or quasi-public agencies, which use a political or bargaining process rather than the flawed market to determine a total budget constraint for health care. Under this approach, government plays an important role both in allocating resources to regions and programs and in setting payment rates for providers.

Differing Approaches Taken by Five Nations

Unlike Singapore, with its pure demand-side approach, or the former Soviet Union, with its pure supply-side approach, none of the five nations reviewed in the articles that follow—Japan, Germany, the United Kingdom, Canada, or the United States—has followed either theory to its extreme. Instead, they differ in the degree to which they rely on market forces and regulation to constrain health care expenditures and to allocate resources.

At one end of the spectrum is the U.S., which, as Robert Evans puts it, is distinct from all other major industrialized nations because of its extensive reliance on consumer demand and market competition. Rather than use a pure demand-side approach, the U.S. uses a mixture of strategies. Uwe Reinhardt's paper describes how, since the late 1970s, the U.S. followed a procompetition strategy by shifting health care costs toward the individual consumer through increased coinsurance rates and increased premium payments by consumers. Alain Enthoven (1977; Enthoven and Kronick 1989) fathered a second strategy. He argues that consumer sovereignty and simple market competition will not result in efficient production and allocation of health care resources, because of information asymmetry and professional dominance. To remedy these market failures, he has advocated a managed competition strategy. Under this strategy, the consumer chooses an insurance plan or a health maintenance organization basing this choice on price, benefit coverage, and perceived quality of service. In order to compete, insurers must act as informed group purchasers and attempt to contract hospitals, clinics, and physicians for the highest quality services at the lowest possible price. Under either strategy, the U.S. depends on consumer demand to provide the fiscal constraint.

In contrast, the U.K., Canada, Japan, and Germany[1] use supply-side approaches to constrain total health expenditures. Culyer and Meads's paper describes how the U.K. uses the central government's budgetary process to limit total health expenditures, by forcing health care expenditures to compete with other conflicting claims on total tax revenues.

Evans describes Canada's similar adoption of a supply-side policy to control health care expenditures. However, rather than use its central government as the locus of power, Canada allows provincial governments to make financing decisions under a set of strict federal guidelines. In contrast to the U.S., the Canadian federal government explicitly discourages the use of consumer demand (i.e., price and income elasticity) as a means of establishing budget constraint and rationing health services.

Schulenburg's paper analyzes the supply-side policy under which Germany imposes a budget constraint on health care expenditures. Instead of using a budgetary process, the federal government creates a national council composed of representatives from all major stackholders in the health sector. This council creates policy guidelines which the states follow. In each state, a global budget for health care is decided upon as a result of negotiations between providers and payers.

According to Ikegami, Japan also relies on a supply-side approach to control health expenditures. Instead of developing an explicit global budget, Japan uses its pricing structure to control health care costs. Prices are set with a global budget in mind. Administrative measures and peer pressure are subsequently used to limit the volume of tests ordered and drugs prescribed.

RESULTING STRUCTURAL DIFFERENCES

Demand- and supply-side principles both influence the specific structural form of a nation's health care system. While many authors have conducted comparative analyses, few have defined or developed an overall classification scheme for health care systems. Milton Roemer (1985) gave a comprehensive and broad definition of a health care system that incorporated cultural, historical, political, social, and economic aspects; however, this characterization is too broad to be

1. The data for Germany are for the former West Germany only.

useful in examining how a system affects health outcomes. We view different health systems in a narrower context, concentrating mainly on their economic aspects. For comparative purposes, we define the operational structure of a health system by its financing, its organization, and its incentives.

Financing and Fiscal Constraint

Financing and fiscal control of health care systems are inextricably linked. The financing mechanism decides which stakeholders have the fiscal power to determine both the budget constraint for the health care system and the allocation of resources within that system. In this section, I compare how the five nations discussed in these papers finance their health services and evaluate their ability to achieve universal coverage, the degree of equity in their financing, and the cost of their administration.

Nations may use either the public or the private sector to finance health care. The demand-side approach manifests itself in pluralistic methods of financing. Consumers decide whether to buy insurance or to pay directly at the point of delivery. Principles of consumer soveriegnty preclude the government's mandating insurance and regulating benefit design and premium rates. Instead, many insurance plans compete in the marketplace and select the risks they want to insure. The U.S. follows this approach; consequently, its system has neither mandated coverage nor a minimum benefit standard. U.S. health services are rationed by price, according to a patient's ability and willingness to pay.

The combination of adverse selection by consumers and selection of good risks by insurance companies caused failures in the health insurance market. Moreover, some people cannot afford or do not choose to buy health insurance. After recognizing that there were gaps in insurance coverage, the U.S. enacted compulsory social insurance for the elderly and disabled and extended a welfare program to finance health services for the poor. However, despite these efforts, 15 percent of Americans remain uninsured.

In contrast to this demand-side approach, supply-side has developed four different financing structures. All four provide universal coverage. With the first, the central or provincial government finances health care and determines the amount to be spent by weighing the benefits of health expenditures against the merits of other claims on total tax revenues. Subsequently, the government either provides health services directly through the public sector (as in the U.K.) or facilitates private sector provision of services (as in Canada). Under the second financing structure, paying for health care is the responsibility of the local government, which must balance health expenditures with expenditures for other local services (as in Sweden). The third financing structure uses a separate tax, like the Social Security payroll tax, to fund health care. In this case, expenditures do not have to compete directly against other claims on general tax revenues. Finally, under the fourth structure, health care is paid for by health insurance, which is provided through a mixture of private and public plans. Under this scenario, the government uses extensive regulation to control health insurance. Such regulatory measures include mandating universal coverage, regulating risk selection, and specifying a minimum benefit standard. Moreover, under this structure, representatives of payers and providers negotiate a total budget with a single channel for paying providers. This budget limits total health expenditures for the following year. The single channel of payment allows the insurers to identify which providers abuse the system for higher revenues.

The supply-side approach would plan the quantity and location of hospital beds and expensive equipment. Some nations extend their regional planning to physician training and placement.

Other than the U.S., all major industrialized nations have either a national health service or compulsory health insurance coverage. These nations have found that they cannot rely on voluntary action in the marketplace to assure universal coverage.

The U.K. promotes equal access to health care and makes health services available to its population, through the public provision of services that are financed with general revenues. Canada, Japan, and Germany have chosen the compulsory health insurance route and use different sources of financing. Canada funds its national health insurance through a revenue-sharing program between the federal and provincial governments. The federal government gives each province a fixed amount of revenue for health care, which, on the average, finances 40 percent of the province's health care costs. Any additional amount comes from the province's tax revenues. In contrast Japan and Germany finance their national health insurance through a combination of public and private nonprofit health insurance plans called sickness funds.

The key criteria in evaluating a system's financing structure include the extent of universal coverage provided, the equitable distribution of financial burden according to an individual's ability to pay, and the administrative efficiency of the financing scheme. A financing mechanism funded through general revenues, such as that used by the U.K. and Canada, is the most equitable, since general revenues are derived largely from progressive income taxes, while the Japanese and German methods of pooling risks and assessing premiums by occupation or by industry are more regressive, because health conditions and costs vary systematically by occupation and by industry. Schulenburg's paper points out, for example, that the payroll tax varies from 8 percent to 16 percent among sickness funds in Germany. The U.S. has the most regressive form of health care insurance, because it is employment-based, and insurance companies pool risks by individual employer. Firms that pay their workers higher wages pay a smaller portion of the wage bill for insurance premiums. Companies that employ young, healthy, white-collar workers pay lower premiums than companies with older or less healthy workers. Thus, risks of the healthy and the sick are pooled less, and insurance costs are shared less between the wealthy and the poor.

As for administrative costs, public financing and direct provision (as in the U.K.) undoubtedly involve the least amount of individual transactions and paperwork and thus the least administrative cost. On the other hand, the free-choice competitive approach of the U.S. prompted insurers to spend a large amount on marketing and sales commissions to attract customers. In order to differentiate products, each insurer has its own distinct claim form, designs its own computerized system to review and pay claims, and employs an army of health professionals, whose jobs are to second-guess the providers' decisions, contributing to the ''hassle factor'' in American medicine today. This complex administrative apparatus may help to reduce unemployment in the U.S., but it increases health care costs.

With regard to capital planning, the governments of the U.K., Canada, and Japan regulate investment in hospital beds and expensive equipment in order to distribute the resources more evenly, to control the diffusion of technology, and to minimize duplication and excess capacity. Germany does not regulate capital investments; rather, resources are allocated within each state according to patients' demand. The U.S., meanwhile, delegates the authority to regulate regional investment to the states, which often take a laissez-faire approach. Overall, we lack adequate empirical evidence about the extent to which regional planning has produced a more even distribution of facilities across communities and how much capital planning has increased efficiency by reducing duplication.

Organization

Demand- and supply-side approaches to the organization of health services differ in two critical areas. The first is in the patients' choice of providers. Under the demand-side approach, patients are given a free choice of doctors, hospitals, and pharmacies; the supply-side approach may restrict options. While Canada, Japan, and Germany rely on a supply-side approach to finance health care and control expenditure inflation, they allow free choice of physicians and hospitals, as does the U.S. In the U.K., although people select their own family physician, they have little choice of specialists or hospitals. Their options were, however, expanded somewhat under the 1989 reform, when family physicians who are budget holders were given greater freedom to select the hospitals and specialists for their patients.

The second area where approaches differ is in the public or private ownership and management of hospitals. Ownership rights affect how a hospital or clinic is organized and managed. In turn, organization and management affect both the availability and quality of services provided and the productive efficiency of institutions. The demand-side school relies on profit motives and market competition and encourages for-profit organizations to provide health services. According to economic theory, profits motivate firms to minimize costs and to respond to consumer demand. Inefficient firms are driven out of the market, as free entry of new firms maintains competitive pressure. Thus, it is argued, privatization yields the most efficient production of health services. On the other hand, the supply-side school argues that public interest motivates workers better than profit and believes that publicly owned facilities produce services more efficiently than do private facilities.

In the U.K., hospitals are owned and managed by district health authorities. There is some evidence that publicly owned hospitals under pressure from hospital-based physicians organize their services more for the convenience of medical staff than for patients (Day and Klein 1991). A mixture of public and private hospitals prevails in Canada, Japan, Germany, and the U.S., with nonprofit community organizations owning many hospitals. In the U.S., recent evidence shows that private nonprofit hospitals are more efficient than public hospitals (Burgess 1992). However, there is conflicting evidence concerning the relative efficiency of nonprofit and for-profit ownership (Herzlinger and Krasker 1987). If for-profit hospitals are more efficient, cost savings may still be retained as profits rather than passed on to consumers in the form of lower prices. Also, for-profit hospitals have been accused of treating only the most healthy patients or those with proven ability to pay; thus, productive efficiency may; not be the sole consideration when defining effective hospital management.

In addition to differences based on ownership, the relative efficiency of public and private institutions depends on the extent to which services are integrated and coordinated. Often, outpatient services can be substituted for inpatient services, and medical treatment can be substituted for surgical treatment. Moreover, the services of primary care physicians and specialists and those of community and tertiary hospitals all need to be coordinated. The demand-side school believes that market forces will push providers to integrate services in the most efficient manner, while supply-siders assert that rapid change in technology and the hierarchy of medical personnel require government intervention to bring about an efficiently integrated system.

Under the German system, ambulatory and hospital services are totally separated from each other. This separation has led to duplication, inefficiency, and higher costs, according to Schulenburg. In contrast, the U.K. has a more integrated system, while systems in Canada, Japan, and the U.S. are fragmented. We currently lack comprehensive studies designed to ascertain empirically how fragmentation of services impacts health care cost and quality.

Another test of efficiency is a nation's ability to balance supply and demand. When demand exceeds supply, the supply-side approach may use nonmonetary means, such as waiting times for nonemergency procedures to ration services. The U.K., for instance, suffers from an inadequate supply of elective surgical services. When shortages exist, waiting lines are used to allocate nonemergency surgeries and explicit rules are established to restrict eligibility for services (Aaron and Schwartz 1984). For example, patients over the age of sixty-five are not eligible to receive kidney transplants funded by the National Health Service. However, in the U.K., patients can usually see their primary care physicians within a day or two, while there are often considerably longer waits in the U.S.

By and large, demand and supply are in balance in Canada. In several isolated instances when demand exceeds supply for several elective surgical procedures, the available supply is allocated on the basis of a professional judgment of the patients' needs and waiting times. Up to the time of reunification, western Germany seemed to be able to match supply and demand reasonably well. There also does not seem to be any serious imbalance between supply and demand in Japan.

Reinhardt shows that the supply of hospital beds in the U.S. currently exceeds the demand, with occupancy rates of 60 to 65 percent. For other services, supply and demand seem to be in balance, but it is not clear how much of the demand is consumer-initiated and how much is induced by providers. The evidence seems to show that the supply-side approach can balance supply and demand reasonably well, and although the U.K. may have over-restricted the supply, it has restrained its expenditures on health care to about 35 percent of the U.S. costs—in 1990, the U.K. spent only $909 per capita on health care, while the U.S. spent $2,566.

Incentives

The performance of health care systems depends heavily on the roles and behavior of patients, physicians, nurses, and pharmacists. The behavior of these actors, though, is motivated by incentives.

While demand-siders let providers set prices according to market conditions, a supply-side approach adjusts provider compensation, which in turn affects medical and prescriptive practices. Payment methods and rates are set by specialty, by type of service, and by region.

All payment methods produce some undesirable responses. The question is, which one is the least objectionable? A demand-side approach most often results in a fee-for-service system, which encourages practitioners to render a greater number of services. With a supply-side approach, practitioners are often salaried, which induces them to reduce their workload by lengthening the time of each visit, decreasing the number of patients to be seen, and restricting work hours. Another method of payment is capitation, but it gives practitioners the incentive to spend as little time as possible with each patient during each visit.

Primary care physicians in all the nations represented, other than the U.K., are compensated on a fee-for-service basis, which encourages them to render increased quantities of services. The U.K., on the other hand, compensates its family physicians with a combination of a small fixed salary, a capitation rate, special fees for preventive services, and a fixed sum for practice expenses. As for hospital-based specialists (other than chiefs of service), the U.K. and Germany pay them a fixed salary. Japanese physicians based in public hospitals are also paid a salary, but many surgeons and specialists receive side payments from patients.

Canada, Germany, and the U.K. use the same process to set hospital payments. In this process the governments or insurance plans negotiate a global budget with each hospital for the next year. The budget is based on anticipated utilization of hospital services, measured by the total number of patient days.

Consequently, there is an incentive for hospitals to lengthen the average length of stay for patients. Japan, on the other hand, sets a packaged fee to be paid to hospitals for each diagnosis. A portion of this payment is for the compensation of salaried physicians.

Under the U.S.'s pluralistic system, hospitals are paid at different rates for the same service. The Medicare program makes prospective payments according to diagnosis-related groups (DRGs) of treatment. This payment method has encouraged hospitals to increase admissions, to reduce the length of stay, and to shift services to unregulated settings—outpatient clinics and freestanding surgical centers. Meanwhile, some private insurance plans negotiate a price with the hospital, while other plans pay the charges set by hospitals. Uninsured patients are often billed higher hospital fees than those charged to insurance companies.

Japan consciously uses its payment rates to influence medical decisions. Fees favor primary care and outpatient services and penalize surgical procedures and inpatient hospital services. Meanwhile, because of market imperfections or for political reasons, the German fee schedule benefits providers of diagnostic tests, and U.S. fees favor provision of surgical procedures. On 1 January 1992, Medicare reformed its physician payments by establishing a national fee schedule based on the resource cost of each service (the resource-based relative value scale, or RBRVS system). Twenty-two Blue Cross/Blue Shield plans say they intend to follow suit. Differences between nations in the quantity of services utilized per capita seem to be correlated with the incentives inherent in their fee schedules.

A COMPARATIVE ANALYSIS OF PERFORMANCE AND OUTCOMES

The test of either approach, demand-side or supply-side, should include a measure of how much each spends on health care and what the outcomes are. Health expenditures are one reasonably reliable indicator of resource utilization; the health status of the population is another, but appropriate outcome measures of health status are less easy to find. Health care is both an investment in human capital and a consumption good. Whereas health status largely reflects the investment aspect, we also need to assess its value as a product for consumption. Measures of public satisfaction with the quality of care are sometimes used to indicate this outcome. Another outcome that needs assessing is the accessibility of health care, since most nations want equal access for all their people.

Expenditures

One performance measure of a health care system is how much of a nation's resources are spent on health care. The U.S. spent the most and the U.K. spent the least. In 1990 the U.S. spent $2,566 per capita, 43 percent more than the second highest nation, Canada, which spent $1,795. The U.K. spent only $909. Japan and Germany spent $1,113 and $1,287 respectively. If we measure health expenditure as a percentage of GNP, the results are the same. The U.S. ranked highest (11.5 percent) and Japan the lowest (6.7 percent). Intrinsically, we cannot say whether a nation spent too much or too little for health care. The "right" amount to be spent is revealed either through a competitive market or in the political arena. The American people certainly feel their expenditures has reached an unreasonable level, as demonstrated by the fact that controlling health expenditure was a top political issue in the 1992 presidential election.

Health Outcomes

Turning to health outcome measures, we have only primitive measurements of a population's health status. The common indices of health status are infant morality and life expectancy, but they are crude measurements indeed. Health care is only one among many factors that determine infant mortality and life expectancy. Nutrition, sanitation, housing, and personal habits may have greater impact on these health status indices. The marginal contribution of health care to these health status indicators is very difficult to isolate. Nonetheless, in the absence of better indices, we used infant mortality and life expectancy as health outcome measurements.

Infant mortality is used first as a health indicator because it may also reflect how equitably a nation's basic health services are distributed across regions, income classes, and races. Among the five nations, infant mortality ranged from a low of 4.6 per thousand (Japan) to a high of 9.7 in the U.S. The U.K. has the second highest infant mortality rate of 9.0, while Canada and Germany are 7.2 and 7.5 respectively. In other words, the U.S. performed the worst.

We also compared life expectancy among the five countries and again, the U.S. had the worst outcome of 75.6 years, and Japan and Canada had the best performances of 79.2 years. The U.K. ranked second worst with 76.3, and Germany fell in the middle.

Public Satisfaction

Consumers derive satisfaction from both tangible and intangible benefits of health services. Besides health benefits, consumers may also value free choice of providers, easy access to health services, and quality of services received. The Canadian system produced the greatest public satisfaction with regard to their personal health care; 94 percent of Canadians are satisfied, while only 88 percent of Americans are satisfied. The British are only slightly behind the U.S., with 87 percent satisfied, in spite of the much lower expenditure per capita and the explicit rationing mechanisms used. The Japanese were reportedly the least satisfied: only 60 percent of Japanese are happy with their own health care.

A health care system consists of many complex parts. Satisfaction with personal health care is only one dimension of it. As consumers we are also concerned about how much we have to pay for the services, through taxes, insurance, and at the point of delivery; about how much paperwork we have to do; how well our neighbors and relatives have been treated, etc. One measure of this wider concern is how satisfied people are with their own nation's health care system. Surveys found, again, that Canada comes out best, with 56 percent of its people satisfied with its health care system. Meanwhile, Americans are the least satisfied: only 10 percent of Americans reported satisfaction with the U.S. health system. The British (27 percent), Japanese (29 percent), and Germans (41 percent) all did better than the Americans.

Access

Health services are not only used to prolong life. A great many health services are rendered for the relief of pain and anxiety and to provide comfort and assurance for patients. Thus, we must consider access to health care to be a value in itself. To examine this factor, we used utilization rates as a measure of a system's performance. The number of patient visits per capita as well as hospital admission rates were compared. We found that Americans have the fewest contacts with their physicians, while Germans and Japanese have the highest number. However, the number of patient visits does not reflect the amount of time or quality of care rendered during the visit. For example, while the average time for a routine visit in the U.S. is about fifteen to twenty minutes, in Japan it is five to eight minutes. Nonetheless, the data show that the populations of the other four countries have greater and more frequent access to their physicians than in the U.S. As for hospital admission, it ranges from a low of 8.1 percent in Japan to a high of 21.5 percent in Germany. Japan has a much lower surgical rate and hospital admission due to its culture, epidemiology, payment systems, and other factors. Germany has the highest hospital admission rates, partly due to strict separation of primary care physicians and hospital-based services.

These outcome data on utilization seem to show that countries that rely on the supply-side approach give their people much greater access to physician services and have lower health expenditures. This indicates that the transfer of wealth from patients to physicians is lower in those countries than in the U.S.

Overall, other than having middle ranking in public satisfaction with personal health care, all other outcome measures indicate that the U.S. system produces the poorest health outcomes and satisfaction while spending the most. A closer look at the apparently more effective health systems of the other four nations may provide insight into areas for U.S. improvement.

WHAT OTHER NATIONS CAN LEARN

Nations choose different economic bases to formulate their macropolicies for health care. These macropolicies result in different health care systems in terms of financing, organization, and payment. The outcome and performance of these systems also differ. By going beyond ideological debate and examining the evidence, valuable lessons can be learned from the experiences of various nations. In a comparison of the five advanced industrialized nations, the U.S. stands out as the only nation that has chosen the demand-side approach, while

Canada, Japan, Germany, and U.K. have chosen supply-side approaches. Canada, Germany, and the U.K. see universal and equal access to health care as an integral part of building national solidarity. They design their systems to achieve this social goal.

The first lesson we learned was that the U.S.'s demand-side approach cannot produce universal health insurance for a population. Market failures are so severe that even with government intervention to provide insurance to the elderly, permanently disabled, and very poor people, the U.S. still has 15 percent of its population uncovered. Therefore, one clear lesson is that the government must intervene if equal access to reasonable health care is a goal of the nation.

Secondly, the four nations that use the supply-side approach found they could establish effective fiscal constraints on health care expenditure inflation. Using the demand-side approach, the U.S. spent much more than the other four nations and found its expenditure inflation rose faster as a percentage of GNP, reaching a level unacceptable to the public. Yet paradoxically, nations that spent less found their people to be more satisfied with the performance of their health care systems, measured in various ways.

How can we explain the higher cost and worse outcomes in the U.S.? There are several explanations. Studies have found that surgical rates in the U.S. are higher than in other nations (McPherson 1989). Other studies have discovered that approximately 15 to 25 percent of the most frequently performed surgeries and diagnostic tests in the U.S. were unnecessary. The appropriateness of an additional 20 percent of these surgeries and tests was highly questionable (Chassin et al. 1987; Greenspan et al. 1988; Winslow et al. 1988). American doctors seem to have a greater zeal for invasive procedures and tests, while physicians of other nations have more restrained practice patterns. These inappropriate services not only consume resources, but, more importantly, they cause suffering and sometimes harm patients. Another explanation lies in higher costs of administration due to the reliance on competition, which results in pluralistic financing, multichannel payments, and complex methods of scrutinizing physicians. Finally, the U.S. suffers from duplication of expensive high-technology equipment and an excess of hospital beds. These additional costs arose from the way in which the U.S. chose to structure its health care system. It would take a concerted political commitment to alter it.

Without harming patients or restricting access to reasonable care, the U.S. could lessen its health care expenditures by at least 20 percent. First, invasive procedures and tests could be reduced by 15 to 20 percent without significant health consequences. A more conservative approach could also be taken in the use of heroic efforts in extending the lives of terminally ill patients. These reforms in medical practice could easily reduce expenditures by 10 percent. The U.S. could save an additional 5 percent by reducing administrative costs through the reorganization of its financing and payment systems. Finally, elimination of excess capacity and duplication could also result in a 5 percent expenditure reduction.

International experiences teach us that neither an extreme demand- or supply-side approach yields the best outcomes. The structure of the U.K. system produces social equity and low-cost health care, but suffers from rigidity, over-centralization, and inadequate responses to patient demands (Enthoven 1991). On the other hand, the structure of the U.S. system produces innovations and high-quality services for those who can pay, but suffers from high costs and social inequity. There must be a middle ground where we can combine the best of demand- and supply-side approaches. The U.K. is trying the internal market. Perhaps the U.S. is not far behind, in adopting the supple-side macropolicy to constrain the health system yet preserve choice and some competition within it. How to do this practically remains to be worked out. There are other lessons to be learned from comparing health systems. How did the nations that effectively limit the resources that they devote to health care still produce such a high degree of patient satisfaction? The answer must lie in the doctor-patient relationship. It seems that, within reasonable limits, doctors have considerable discretion in giving patients effective medical care and leaving them satisfied. How it is done is a mystery that remains to be solved.

Desperately Seeking Solutions

Though we can learn valuable lessons from other nations, Americans still must make painful decisions for themselves.

John K. Iglehart

The American health-policy community, wracked by uncertainty over how best to curtail the uncontrolled growth of spending for medical care, has become fascinated with how other industrialized nations provide their citizens with these services, usually on a universal basis and for considerably less money. The findings have been enlightening, but they do not provide any real American-style answer to the essential question that haunts all advanced industrialized nations: How should finite health-care resources be allocated when the very human instinct to relieve the burdens of illness, disability and death is without limit?

Over the last decade, I have examined how other industrialized nations (Canada, Germany, Japan and the United Kingdom) have organized their health-care systems and have addressed this eternal resource-allocation question. Along the way, I was asked innumerable times why *The New England Journal of Medicine* would send its national correspondent to other nations to examine their health-care systems when, as conventional wisdom holds, America has "the best

---

Health Management Quarterly, Third Quarter 1992
John K. Iglehart is editor of *Health Affairs* and national correspondent for *The New England Journal of Medicine*.

system in the world.'' I readily recognized the pitfalls of such cursory examinations and, for the most part, avoided direct systemic comparisons, given the countless variables that make them suspect, if not totally misguided. I settled on a rationale that was best summed up by Canadian economist Robert G. Evans, who wrote:

> ''Nations do not borrow other nation's institutions. The Canadian system may be 'better' than the American. I believe it is, though that is a very complex question, and as I have just pointed out, my views, like yours, are contaminated by my origins. Even if it is better, I am not trying to sell it to you. You cannot have it. It would not 'fit' because you do not see the world, or the individual, or the state, as we do. . . . The point is that by examining others' experience you can extend your range of perceptions of what is possible.''[1]

Whatever the experience of a country in formulating its health-care policies, an ever-present reality punctuates the dialogue. It is represented by the ideologic pendulum that swings between individual accountability and social responsibility. This dynamic, which is constantly in motion, is particularly important in the new environment of freedom that has provided the countries of Eastern Europe the opportunity to chart reforms that redress imbalances that favored centralized decisionmaking over individual freedom. It applies as well to the industrialized democracies that are driven by capitalism because governments and individuals live in a constant state of tension on questions of resource allocation.

To elaborate, the peoples of Czechoslovakia, Hungary, Poland and former East Germany yearn for systems that reflect meaningful private-public collaboration in the provision of medical care, rather than systems run by government fiat, to which they were long subjected. Thus, health-care system reforms in these newly free nations are moving in that direction.

In Western Europe, where mature health-insurance schemes feature universal coverage financed through taxation or employer-employee contributions, there is pressure to mix some market-oriented features with government regulation in an effort to give individuals a greater voice in decisionmaking and to encourage providers to become more efficient. The Netherlands and the United Kingdom have embraced reforms that reflect these priorities without changing their basic systems. These reforms reflect the influence of the thinking of economist Alain Enthoven of Stanford University, whose proposed ''managed competition'' model has been embraced by key Washington policymakers as well.

Lastly, in the United States, the world's bastion of individual freedom and unfettered capitalism, there are pressures for government to adopt more compulsory policies that would guarantee universal coverage, mandate ''play-or-pay'' financing schemes and not allow physician billing of patients beyond health-insurance reimbursement limits. These proposals represent swings of the political pendulum. While they are strong and growing as a consequence of the millions

---

1. R. Evans, ''The Spurious Dilemma: Reconciling Medical Progress and Cost Control,'' *Health Matrix* 1 (1986): 25–34.

of Americans who lack health insurance, they are as yet no match for our steadfast beliefs in low taxation and limited government. Nevertheless, even the most conservative reform approaches, including the one advocated by the Bush administration, call for an unprecedented degree of government intervention in the American health-care system.

As the United States moves ahead, in the halting fashion that has become a trademark of its paralyzed processes of health policymaking, what might we take from other industrialized nations that would be meaningful to our debate? I believe three essential lessons can be derived from studying the health-care systems of the other major industrialized democracies. Overriding all three is the fundamental reality that all nations approach their problems differently, based on their cultural beliefs, political priorities, medical imperatives and economic standings. In this respect, it is important to recognize that the United States is distinguished by its sheer physical size and diverse population. The subpopulations of the United States are no less diverse in many respects than are the Greeks and the Swedes, or the Dutch and the Italians.

Lesson One: All major democracies have placed government in a more prominent position in relation to their health-care systems than has the United States. Not only do more of the monies flow directly through governments via taxation or indirectly through quasi-government structures that collect employer-employee contributions, but other governments also chart policies that affect entire systems, regardless of the financing mechanism. The principal government mandate in all of the other major democracies is to guarantee access to medical care for all citizens.

This has been a priority in other nations since World War II. One way to illustrate it is to point to Canada's experience. Although the flow of people, commerce and culture—including television programming, sports teams and a wide variety of other exchanges—have long marked the dynamic relationship between Canada and the United States, the health-care systems of these two neighboring powers have diverged sharply in the last three decades. In 1960, the systems of both nations were dominated by solo, fee-for-service practitioners and nonprofit community hospitals. Medical care was financed through a multiplicity of private insurance plans, out-of-pocket payments and minimal government support. And millions of citizens in both countries lacked adequate coverage.

Underscoring its binding belief in equality, many of Canada's 10 provinces, led by Saskatchewan's initial step in 1947 to create a health-insurance plan for its people, developed schemes that eventually forced the national government to bring the programs into conformity. By 1971, all the provinces had adopted insurance programs that met the basic conditions set out by Parliament to qualify for federal funds covering 50 percent of the programs' costs. In the process, Canada made illegal the sale of private health-insurance benefits that were offered by the provincially based plans.

This action, an impossible step for American policymakers to seriously contemplate given the domination of the U.S. system by private interests, arose from "deep-rooted suspicion of class-based systems of any kind," Evans wrote recently. Private schools are only a small part of Canada's educational system before college, private universities do not exist, and in public transportation only a single class of travel is usually available, except in some air and train travel. As Evans put it, "equality before the health-care system" in Canada is a political principle similar to equality before the law.[2]

The health-care systems of other major democracies better reflect the value that Americans attach to private-public collaboration than does Canada's system, but they also place government in a far more commanding position. For example, as the General Accounting Office pointed out in its study[3] of the systems of France, Germany and Japan, they resemble the U.S. system in four important ways: They provide health insurance using multiple quasi-public insurers, or payers. People typically get health insurance for themselves and their dependents at their place of employment, and they have free choice of doctors, who charge on a fee-for-service basis. Both private and public hospitals deliver inpatient care. But a key differentiating characteristic is that the French, German and Japanese systems are extensively regulated by government. Among the consequences of this regulation: All citizens are guaranteed access to health insurance; insurers' payments to physicians and hospitals are standardized, thus avoiding cost-shifting between payers; and all three countries use price controls that place ceilings on physician fees or daily hospital charges.

Lesson Two: The profit motive is far less pervasive in the health-care systems of other countries than it is in the United States. Though the private companies—indeed, many are multi-national, American-based companies—that manufacture pharmaceutical products and medical devices are operated on the same for-profit basis in other countries as they are in the United States, the insuring function in other countries is performed for the most part by nonprofit organizations with a more social orientation than is the case with commercial health insurers and many Blue Cross and Blue Shield plans in the United States.

The values Americans attach to profits, wealth and business acumen are also influencing their health-care system. Arnold S. Relman, M.D., whose 1980 essay[4] on the medical-industrial complex underscored the growing importance of these trends, acknowledged 11 years later that his earlier paper painted an incomplete picture. He wrote: "What I had not fully appreciated in 1980 was that the pressures on our voluntary hospitals would lead many of them to behave just like their investor-owned competitors. . . . We are witnessing a pervasive change in the

---

2. R. Evans, "We'll Take Care of It For You, Health Care in the Canadian Community," *Daedalus* 117 (1988): 155–89.
3. U.S. General Accounting Office, *Health Care Spending Control: The Experience of France, Germany, and Japan,* GAO/HRD 92-9 (Washington, D.C.: Government Printing Office, 1991).
4. A. S. Relman, "The New Medical-Industrial Complex," *New England Journal of Medicine* 303 (October 23, 1980): 963–970.

ethos of the voluntary hospital system in America from that of a social service to that of a business.''[5]

I am struck by the different nature of the health-insurance organizations that operate in other major Western countries. Most of these organizations are either heavily regulated private carriers or are quasi-public insurers with more socially oriented objectives than is the case with their U.S. counterparts. U.S. commercial health insurers offer no excuses for their reluctance to protect medically risky people who are employed in marginal industries; they are in business to make a profit. But a number of nonprofit Blue Cross and Blue Shield plans, launched as part of a social movement in the 1930s to help people pay their hospital bills, now are difficult to differentiate from their commercial competitors in terms of their restrictive medical underwriting practices, their reluctance to insure people in need of financial protection and their entrepreneurial instincts.

Lesson Three: The health-care systems of other nations maintain a better balance of medical generalists and specialists than does the United States. Other systems, through a variety of mechanisms, assume that primary-care doctors will act as gatekeepers to specialist care. This places the primary-care doctor in charge of the patient and generally provides for a more efficient allocation of resources. In some countries, governments regulate the number of training positions in given specialities and do not rely on the marketplace to sort out this ratio, as is the case in the United States.

There is no precise ratio of generalists to specialists that all countries strive to achieve, but the accepted standard is about 50–50. Canada has been able to maintain such a balance over a long period of time. If Canada has a problem in this regard, it is a surplus of primary-care doctors. In the United States, the opposite is true. Medical training programs in family medicine and internal medicine are experiencing difficulty in filling their positions, although such doctors are in great demand, particularly as managed-care enrollments rise.

In conclusion, American health policymakers have identified a number of important differences between the systems of other industrialized nations and the United States. The differences have shown that other systems have a more social orientation and that their overriding emphasis is on providing all citizens with access to medical care. On the other hand, these exercises have not uncovered a magic pill that is going to spare the United States the painful decisions that lie ahead in its debate over reforming the American system. To paraphrase the advertisement of a Wall Street brokerage firm, American policymakers are going to have to address a range of very difficult issues ''the old-fashion way,'' by debating the pros and cons and then actually making decisions, painful though they may be.

In the absence of such decisions, the United States remains an outlier in the

5. A. S. Relman, ''The Health Care Industry: Where Is It Taking Us?'' *New England Journal of Medicine* 325 (September 19, 1991): 854–859.

advanced industrialized world. It does not provide universal health-insurance coverage to all its citizens, and that which is provided is the most costly in the world. Americans seem prepared to accept paying a premium for quality medical care, but the system's inequity of coverage may be a shortcoming that will ultimately determine whether we are indeed "our brother's keeper."

Health Care Reform Now

Robert B. Smith

Health care is a salient political issue for well-known reasons: costs of health care and medical insurance have skyrocketed; the number of Americans under sixty-five who lack health insurance has increased from 33.6 million to 35.7 from 1988 through 1990; and, during the recent recession, insecurely employed and newly unemployed citizens are living in fear of losing their insurance and not being able to pay their medical expenses. More than forty bills are before Congress addressing these problems. Many offer specific provisions for reform of the small business insurance market. Full-time workers in small businesses and their dependents often lack insurance coverage because many small businesses cannot afford employee benefits. Under the present laws, which do not require community rating of risks, commercial insurers may determine the premium they charge a small business only on the basis of that business's experience. Its risk pool may be so small, however, that one expensive episode of health care may radically increase the premium. To avoid higher costs, the insurer may drop the company or refuse to cover a high-risk person, and the employer might fire the high-risk person or shift to an insurance company that offers lower rates by excluding that person from coverage.

The lack of community rating of risks is consistent with the public's individualism. When asked if it was unfair to require the majority of the people, who are healthy, to pay for most of the treatment cost for those who are sick and are heavy

Society, March/April 1993.

users of hospitals and doctors, 47 percent of Americans polled by Humphrey Taylor and Uwe Reinhardt agreed (thereby supporting experience rating of risk) and 49 percent disagreed (thereby supporting community rating). Among Canadians, 27 percent agreed with the statement and 70 percent disagreed—about 21 percent more supported the communitarian alternative.

HEALTH POLICY ALTERNATIVES

Many prominent plans for insuring the uninsured can be classified by three dichotomous taxonomic attributes. The first category of each dichotomy is represented by an "x" and the second by a "y", with no value judgment implied. The first attribute is economic, assessing whether the plan is based on private insurance (x) or requires some new public insurance (y). Then, within the above two categories, plans can be distinguished politically, according to the relative degree of systemic change that is required—either incremental reforms (x) designed to ameliorate market failure, or more comprehensive restructuring (y). Finally, plans are distinguished socially, according to the extent of consumer choice of health plans that they allow—either somewhat limited (x) or broad (y) choice of health plan.

To simplify this exposition, I have grouped these diverse plans into three strategic types: 1) private sector strategy composed of mandated employer-provided insurance, small business market reform, and managed competition among health care plans; 2) strategies requiring private and public funds—the Republican plan for comprehensive health care reform and the Pepper Commission's employer and public insurance "play-or-pay" plans supported by Democrats; 3) national health insurance with or without managed competition—that is, with or without some private sector participation.

PRIVATE SECTOR STRATEGY

If implemented as an integrated system, the following three types of plans could solve the problem of insuring the uninsured without recourse to new public insurance—private sector funds would be used to provide private health insurance. The package would mandate employers to provide insurance (marginal small businesses and those who are self-employed would receive a means-tested government subsidy), reform the small business market, and offer consumer choice of competing government-approved indemnity and managed care health plans.

Some policymakers advocate the Hawaiian plan, which provides universal health care coverage through state-mandated employer-provided insurance. They believe that near universal coverage can be obtained without creating new government bureaucracies if the federal government structures the conditions of the insurance market for small and medium-size business and mandates that employers provide insurance for their employees and dependents. About 85 percent of the working uninsured are employees of businesses with 100 or fewer employees. Only those not covered by the universal employer mandate would receive public insurance.

The state of Hawaii requires all employers, regardless of the size of their business, to provide comprehensive health insurance for all employees who work twenty or more hours per week after thirty days of employment. Two plans provide almost all insurance: Blue Cross/Blue Shield is the dominant payer with 80 percent of the market and Kaiser Permanente, a Health Maintenance Organization (hereafter, HMO) has most of the remainder. Because only two major insurers are available, consumer choice of health plan is restricted, but the fee-for-service plan along with the HMO allows choice of physicians for those desiring it. The dominant payer limits increases in costs by streamlining administration, preventing excessive proliferation of expensive high technology diagnostic tools, and encouraging a strong emphasis on primary care and preventive medicine. Besides enjoying savings engendered by these limitations, small business would be able to afford health insurance because costs will have been reduced by the following regulations: 1) all employers with one hundred or fewer employees are placed in one risk pool; 2) community rating is used for that risk pool; and 3) individual employees are not denied coverage for any pre-existing medical conditions. Those not covered by their employers are enrolled in the State Health Insurance Program (SHIP), which is supported by general tax revenues. Blue Cross/Blue Shield and Kaiser Permanente provide the coverage under contract to the state, so no new public insurance is needed. Liberal Medicaid eligibility covers the unemployed and those on welfare.

To recommend legislation that would ensure that all Americans have adequate health and long-term care coverage, Congress created the U.S. Bipartisan Commission on Comprehensive Health Care—renamed the Pepper Commission in memory of its founder, the late Claude Pepper, a Democrat from Florida. Jay Rockefeller, a Democratic senator from West Virginia, the commission's chairman, and a strong majority on the commission would encourage small businesses to provide private insurance, thereby reducing the pool of the uninsured. To facilitate this coverage, the commission would reform the small business market, guarantee access for high risk people, subsidize the cost of insurance, and replace many state-mandated benefits with new federal standards. Uniformity of standards would lower costs.

Lloyd Bentsen introduced a bill—"Better Access to Affordable Health Care Act of 1991," S.1872—and Eugene Rostenkowski introduced a similar, though not identical, bill—"Health Insurance Reform and Cost Control Act of 1991" (H.R. 3626)—in the House that would facilitate implementation. Both bills aim to reform the insurance market for businesses with up to fifty employees. At present, about 77 percent of the working uninsured are employees or dependents in small businesses so defined. Most probably, numerous insurers and HMOs would compete in the reformed small business market; therefore passage of these bills would provide the consumer with a broad choice of health plans.

Both bills define a universal core benefits package and enforce the requirement of guaranteed issue. This contrasts with the present law, which allows commercial insurers to screen employees of small companies. Under the proposed laws an insurer of small businesses could not exclude from coverage any eligible employee (or dependent), deny coverage on the basis of health status, or require an excessive waiting time for coverage for preexisting conditions. Furthermore, insurers providing insurance to one small business in a geographic area would be required to offer insurance to all small businesses in that area. An insurer who offers a managed-care plan to larger employers in a state, must offer the same plan to small employers. The insurer could not terminate coverage for one small business unless it terminates coverage to all small businesses. Otherwise the insurer would not be allowed to insure small businesses in the state for five years. Small businesses would be community rated (the minimum community size is a standard metropolitan statistical area) with adjustments for the age and sex distributions of covered individuals in a small business. Variation in premium rates between sets of policyholders could not exceed 20 percent.

The Bentsen bill would establish federal requirements for certification of utilization review programs and managed-care plans; Rostenkowski's bill would establish a health care cost commission to study administrative costs and to formulate standards for managed care. Both bills would ease Medicare eligibility for diagnostic procedures, increase the medical insurance tax deduction for the self-employed, and require research on rating practices. Neither bill mandates that employers provide insurance for their employees.

A third type of plan is ''managed competition,'' which was first formulated by Alain Enthoven, developed by the Jackson Hole Group of health policy notables, and transformed into legislation by the Conservative Democratic Forum. By organizing all consumers into state- or city-wide Health Plan Purchasing Cooperatives, known as HPPCs, this bill addresses the problem of market failure that occurs when risks are spread over a small number of people. HPPCs would create competition among accountable health plans as accountable, define the basic benefits package, guarantee the provision of insurance regardless of health risk, subsidize the insurance of low income and Medicaid enrollees, and report on the effectiveness and quality of the health plans. Employees of small businesses and the poor would be enrolled in HPPCs and would select their coverage from a portfolio of open health plans. An occupational group or a large employer, one with at least 1,001 employees' contributions from their paychecks, but it neither mandates nor prohibits employer contributions for health insurance. In theory, costs would be contained because individuals choosing a richer plan would pay more and the competition among the plans would lower costs and assure high quality care.

By aggregating the uninsured into HPPCs, this plan leverages the group's purchasing power and provides its members with choice. Because organizational units, not the individual, negotiate the insurance coverage and purchase the health plans, this plan would mitigate any informational and bargaining asymmetries between the individual and the insurance organization. It thus differs from the Republican plan, which would ask individuals—many of whom are financially strapped—to make informed choices about complex health insurance policies.

The managed competition plan could be financed through a change in the tax treatment of employee health benefits or through a play-or-pay mechanism. Contributions of employers to their employees' health insurance are at present fully deductible from pre-tax profits as a cost of doing business; employees' benefits are not counted as income and are tax free. Under the Cooper Boren bill the employer's exclusion would be limited to the cost of the basic plan and contributions over this amount would be taxed at 34 percent. Employees could deduct their payments for the basic plan, but would pay taxes on employer-provided benefits above this minimum. The Jackson Hole Group would also tax employees but would continue to allow employers to deduct their contributions as business costs. They would finance this insurance by mandating employers to pay 80 percent of the premium and a payroll tax on the earnings of their part-time workers they do not insure—which tax would provide the funds for the HPPC-sponsored plans.

The managed competition plan has not been installed at a large test site in the United States. Consequently, there is little empirical information about whether such a plan would provide the promised benefits of consumer choice and competition among providers that would enhance quality and constrain cost. However, the Federal Employees Health Benefits program (FEHB) does share many features of managed competition and, with a few changes in the law, could provide a nation-wide test of the plan.

A yearly open enrollment period in the present FEHB plan allows federal employees to choose their health plan from a portfolio that includes Blue Cross/Blue Shield for indemnity insurance and more than three hundred managed-care organizations. The plans vary in coverage and price, with the government paying about 60 percent of the premium, giving employees an incentive to choose a more expensive, richer plan. As a result, many retirees who are not eligible for Medicare choose the richer plan and the plan's risk pool becomes unfavorable. The insurer then must raise the premium, which in turn will motivate people with low health risks to leave the plan. Even so, the FEHB cost increases (about 8 percent in recent years) have been no higher, and may be lower, than those of most other plans.

If FEHB were to be used as a test of managed competition, the following changes would have to be made first: 1) the plans must have a uniform minimum of core benefits, but each individual plan could include richer benefits than those in the core plan; 2) the government must pay a fixed dollar amount rather than a fixed percentage of the premium; and 3) plans with benefits richer than those in the core plan must be allowed to charge more. These changes would create an incentive to choose less expensive core plans and discourage overuse of medical care.

To test whether managed competition can solve the problem of insuring the uninsured, the latter and those on Medicaid should be given access to FEHB in several large urban areas and in some rural areas. They could be enrolled in new groups or allowed to join existing plans. Vouchers or tax credits would enable them to purchase insurance through the FEHB portfolio. All three types of reforms would cost relatively little to implement and they hold the promise of core benefits without recourse to new public insurance. Employer-mandated insurance would lower the number of working uninsured, small business market reforms would lower the cost of the insurance, and the competition among health plans would give consumers a choice and would reduce costs. To comply with the insurance mandate, some small businesses would receive a means-tested governmental subsidy.

PRIVATE AND PUBLIC FUNDS

The Republicans would use private and public funds for private health insurance only. Some Democrats would use private and public funds for new public insurance in addition to employer-provided private insurance. The Republican Comprehensive Health Reform Program, which was first announced by the Bush administration in February 1992, would enable the self-employed, poor, and nearly poor—regardless of pre-existing conditions—to use tax credit certificates (vouchers) and tax deductions to join managed-care networks—HMOs and Preferred Provider Organizations (hereafter PPOs). It would also enable small businesses to purchase private health insurance from a reformed small business insurance market.

This plan would provide income tax incentives of up to $3,750 for low income families to buy their own private insurance, create incentives to steer people toward less costly prepaid managed-care health systems, and reform the private insurance market so that people who change jobs or have high health risks could purchase core health insurance. In the area of reform of the small business market, the Republican legislation would be similar, but not identical, to the Bentsen and Rostenkowski bills. However, none of these bills and plans require employers to provide insurance. Cuts in Medicare and Medicaid would make available some of the funds needed, as would hypothetical savings from administrative streamlining, the use of the managed-care plans, and changes in liability laws that now encourage physicians to practice defensive medicine.

Unlike the Bentsen and Rostenkowski bills the Republican plan implicitly discourages employers from insuring their employees because the promised tax credits and deductions are reduced by the amount employers contribute to their employees' health insurance. The plan clearly states: "Applicable credit and deduction amounts will be reduced by the amount of any contribution made by the employer to the employee's health plan. Individuals with employer contributions exceeding the applicable credit or deduction will receive neither the credit nor the deduction." Some employers may desire to reduce the financial burden of their employees' benefits and would therefore eliminate these benefits altogether or significantly increase employee contributions.

The Republican plan would allow such reductions to be replaced in part by larger federal contributions, enabling these businesses to shift some of their benefit costs to the government. A similar cost shifting already occurs for certain employee disability payments. Rather than paying these benefits, employers can shift costs to the Social Security system for payment, and they do. The cost-shift provision would also weaken the effectiveness of the proposed Health Insurance Networks, groupings of small businesses that would band together to obtain insurance for their employees. Economies of scale and the leveraging of purchasing power would reduce the cost of insurance for these companies. Rather than providing health insurance, however, such businesses might find it more profitable to shift their costs to the government by encouraging their employees to take advantage of the full tax credit and deduction amounts.

The instability created by such a disincentive to employers to insure their employees would reduce the value of the proposed core medical plans and increase the cost to the individual for more extensive coverage than that in the core plans. The Republicans propose that each state define a core benefit package equal in value to the maximum value of the health tax credit. Thus, there could be at least 100 different core benefit plans (two insurers per state multiplied by fifty states) rather than the one plan the Bentsen and Rostenkowski bills stipulate. Such a proliferation of core plans would make it difficult for large, national carriers to provide the insurance.

States with expensive medical care (New York) would not be able to offer much coverage for the fixed dollar amount, whereas states with less expensive care (Hawaii) would be able to offer more extensive coverage. This state-to-state variation would increase the administrative costs of such plans and this would, holding constant cash value, reduce the extent of the coverage. In effect, the Republican plan would create diverse state-mandated benefits—variations it aims to eliminate. The weakening of employer-based health insurance would tend to shift the coverage from group to individual insurance policies, which are more expensive than group-based plans. The Health Insurance Association of America (hereafter, HIAA) has critiqued individually purchased plans on three grounds:

1) inefficiency—the marketing and administrative costs would be higher than in the present employee benefits system;

2) adverse selection—insurers would compete by trying to attract health individuals, whereas high risk individuals would have to pay much more;

3) erosion of financing—without the present strong tax incentives many employers would not pay for employee health benefits. The Republican plan is susceptible to all three of these weaknesses and, given projected rates of medical inflation, will not provide affordable insurance for the poor. Its dual promise of wide consumer choice and efficiencies achieved through competition are probably illusory.

Some of the ideological sources of the Republican plan and related legislation come from The Heritage Foundation, perhaps following the ideas of Milton Friedman. The Heritage Foundation advocates a family-based free market system in which individuals or the head of the household—not the employer— would be responsible for purchasing health insurance. Friedman would like to see the end of all government insurance and the end of the employee tax exemption for employer-provided health insurance. The Heritage Foundation would require employers to compensate their employees in cash with the amounts they now pay for health insurance. This money would be taxable income. The individual family, aided by tax reductions and government subsidies if poor, would be required to use this money for the purchase of health insurance, the cost of which could be deducted from their income tax. The family would be able to shop around and choose a health insurance policy or a managed-care plan from a private sector company, which would have to compete for business. In theory, health costs would be controlled because individual consumers would be more cost-conscious in purchasing health insurance than they are now, and they would resist any medically unnecessary treatments that would increase their premiums.

Drawing upon these ideas, the Republicans proposed transferable tax credit certificates that would enable poor families to purchase private health insurance. But unlike The Heritage Foundation proposal, this plan would not require employers to transfer health care insurance funds to their employees. The lack of a mandate, coupled with the inverse relationship between employer and government contributions, would encourage employers to shift some of their benefit costs to the government.

The HIAA recommends incremental reforms of small business insurance markets that would expand private coverage through the workplace. The HIAA also recommends public coverage for the poor and near-poor. The Republican plan proposes an alternative. The poor would purchase private insurance using tax credit certificates. Many full-time workers in small businesses and their dependents lack insurance coverage because under the present law insurers can screen small companies to assess which employees they are willing to insure. The HIAA aims to reform the small group market so small employers will have continuous, private coverage and high-risk employees cannot be denied insurance. Both HIAA and the Republican plans favor requiring "guaranteed issue" (as do Bentsen and Rostenkowski), under which all employees must receive health insurance if one employee gets it.

Under the HIAA plan small businesses would continue to receive a tax incentive for the purchase of private insurance with coverage for full or limited care for their employees. Employers would not be mandated to provide insurance, but there would also be no government-provided disincentive to insure employees, as there would be under the Republican plan. Small group market reforms would enable private insurers to spread losses for high-risk groups and individuals across the market without recourse to community rating. It would also reduce costs of the insurance, which now may be prohibitively high. Cost containment strategies and managed-care networks would be applied in the private and public sectors to control costs. The HIAA plan would also expand Medicaid income eligibility to the poverty level in all states.

Congresswoman Barbara Kennelly, Democrat from Connecticut, has introduced legislation ("Health Access and Affordability Today Act of 1991," H.R. 3410) for incremental reforms similar to those of the HIAA among other changes.

To improve access to care, this bill would expand Medicaid eligibility for individuals with incomes below 133 percent of a state-adjusted poverty level, levy new excise taxes on those providers who fail to treat Medicare and Medicaid patients, levy new taxes on employers with discriminatory health benefits plans, develop community and migrant health centers for under-served areas, and encourage college and university health plans for students who have graduated. Kennelly's bill would also pre-empt state regulations concerning the inclusiveness of health insurance coverage and the number, type, and compensation of providers in managed-care networks. It would allow the self-employed to full deduct their health insurance costs from their income tax. It would also fund research on fraud in the health care industry and establish a national health outcomes research data base.

Finally, to guarantee access to coverage regardless of the health risk of a group or individual, it would require the states to implement small group market reforms. These reforms would provide access to coverage, guarantee the issue and continuity of insurance to all employees of a small business, and set up a reinsurance mechanism (community rating is not stipulated) to distribute the risks across the market.

Although in its final recommendations it presented a compromise between those who desired either less or more government responsibility for the provision of health care, the bipartisan Pepper Commission was closely divided on key issues. The tally was eight in favor and seven opposed on the recommendations concerning health care access and financing for those under age sixty-five. The commission's chairman cast the deciding votes. The weak consensus engendered numerous bills, some favoring direct implementation of the commission's recommendations and others expressing the objections and opposing views of the dissenters. With respect to long-term health care, eleven members favored the commission's recommendations and four opposed it.

PLAY-OR-PAY PLANS

The essence of the commission's health care plan, which is less comprehensive than national health insurance, is a pragmatic private and public sector "play-or-pay" system. Employer-provided insurance would be supplemented with new public insurance for the uninsured. The federal government would mandate employers either to provide health insurance for their employees and their dependents, that is, "to play," or to contribute to a public insurance fund by paying an 8 percent payroll tax on the salaries of employees they do not insure, that is, "to pay."

The reforms of the small business market would enable many businesses to play rather than pay for public insurance. The new public insurance could be administered in conjunction with, or as part of, Medicare. Any business subject to the insurance mandate would have the choice of purchasing private insurance or coverage from a public plan that would limit consumer choice. Congressional

Democrats—Kennedy and Mitchell (S. 1227), Rockefeller (S. 1177), Waxman (H.R. 25350), Rostenkowski (H.R. 3205), and Roybal (H.R. 3535), and former presidents Ford and Carter (through the National Leadership Coalition on Health Care Reform) support a mixed private and public strategy. A key difference among their various bills—all of which would retain private insurance through qualified employer health plans—is the structure of the public insurance plan.

The original Pepper Commission bill, jointly introduced by Jay Rockefeller (S. 1177) and Waxman (H.R. 2535), would have created a new public program administered by the federal government and funded in part by state contributions similar to their expenditures for Medicaid. Although Waxman voted with the majority of the Pepper Commission, he felt the states should be free from responsibility of financing the new public program. He believed that flexibility in funding at the state-level led to asymmetries in the administration of Medicaid—many states have been unwilling or unable to fund Medicaid adequately and have restricted eligibility, scope of benefits, and reimbursements to save money.

Congressman Roybal's United States Health bill would, in addition to providing benefits for long-term care, expand Medicare to cover the poor, the self-employed, those not covered by employers, those presently covered by Medicaid, as well as workers whose employers find the public plan more affordable. Utilization review and Medicare's prospective payment methods—DRGs (Diagnosis Related Groups) for hospitals and RBRVSs (Resource Based Relative Value Scales) for physicians—would be applied to control costs. A United States Health Board would establish overall spending targets.

To limit the numbers in the public plan, the drafters of the play-or-pay legislation aim to set the payroll tax at a level that would maximize private coverage for the working population. Even so, some of the commission members and some policy analysts affiliated with The Heritage Foundation who oppose national health insurance believe that many employers would find it easier and cheaper not to enroll their employees in private insurance and simply to pay the tax. The Urban Institute, under contract from the Labor Department, has explored this problem by developing computer simulation predictions of the total number of non-elderly people (workers, dependents, and non-workers) who would be enrolled in the public plan under two different payroll taxes set at 7 percent and 9 percent. The original model predicted that under the lower tax 52 percent of non-elderly Americans would be in the public plan; under the higher tax, 40 percent.

Because the model did not take into account the income tax benefits employers gain by insuring their employees, the simulations probably overestimated the expected numbers in the public plan. In fact, an expanded version of the original model now considers variations in employer behavior and predicts a much lower percentage in the public plan. For example, if the payroll tax were set at 7 percent and workers lobbied to stay in the private plan, then the predicted number of persons covered by the public plan would drop from 112 million to 71.8 million, a decline of 36 percent.

A recent survey of 196 employers corroborates the lower expected number in the public plan. About 58 percent of the companies surveyed were very unlikely to terminate their private health plans and instead pay a 7 percent to 10 percent payroll tax; an additional 21 percent were somewhat unlikely to change (for a total of 79 percent who would retain private insurance). Contrariwise, about 8 percent were very likely and 13 percent were somewhat likely to drop their private plans (for a total of 21 percent who would shift to public plans). To further control the number in the public plan, the legislation would stipulate that only the employees of small businesses with less than a certain number of employees could be enrolled. This change would reduce opposition from those who wish to limit the growth of public health insurance programs.

THE MITCHELL REVISION

Senator George Mitchell's bill, "Healthamerica: Affordable Health Care for all Americans," S. 1227, would have states (or regional groupings of states) administer the new public program following federal guidelines for minimum benefits. Mitchell's bill would retain Medicare for the elderly but would replace Medicaid (except for long-term care) with a new program—AmeriCare—that would enroll the poor, the near-poor, uninsured, and employees of businesses choosing the public plan. It would reform the small group insurance market and would provide incentives to small businesses to purchase private insurance. It would control costs of streamlining administration and establishing a Federal Health Expenditure Board that would recommend budgets and payment rates.

Rostenkowski's parallel bill (H.R. 3205) differs from Mitchell's in that the cost control board would be given greater power to set rates, the payroll tax percentage would be fixed at 9 percent, and the administration of the public plan would be more centralized. Mitchell's bill would allow the public plan at the state level to be converted easily to one of managed competition. States, at their option, could implement the public plan through private-sector insurers and managed-care health plans, which would provide public plan enrollees with a choice of health care options. The bill offers new public insurance to replace Medicaid.

Capsule summaries of Mitchell's bill have stressed its play-or-pay aspect and not its flexibility with respect to managed competition. Such oversimplifications may have weakened the political consensus in support of the plan and for the benefits the marginally employed and poor would receive from the bill's passage. This bill, at least potentially, is a managed-competition plan that allows private-sector participation and ought to be referred to as such.

Mitchell plan is similar to the private sector strategy and includes: 1) employer-mandated insurance (or to pay a tax); 2) small business market reform, core benefits, and guaranteed issue; and 3) managed competition at the state-level. The AmeriCare program would compete with private insurance and could eventually lead to national health insurance.

NATIONAL SOCIAL INSURANCE

Canada's joint federal-provincial social insurance system, which provides universal coverage, has served as a model for several American plans. To control costs, the Canadian federal government—the single payer—sets a yearly budget for total health care expenditures, restricts doctors' fees, and limits the availability of providers, some services, and high technology medical equipment. Each province gets a share of the total budget and is responsible for administering the program in its geographic area.

The American public has supported such a plan. An HIAA survey asked, "Do you prefer the Canadian System or the system we have here [in the United States]?" Fifty-nine percent responded they preferred the Canadian system, 26 percent said they preferred the present system, and 15 percent said they did not know. Robert Blendon summarized ten national and statewide surveys conducted since 1989 and found that between 60 percent and 72 percent of the public say they support a national health insurance plan financed through taxes. The favorable percentage drops when arguments pro and con are presented and when the plan is linked to tax increases.

Current legislation in the United States concerning national health insurance systems includes two single-payer plans, one directly modeled on the Canadian system, and the other an expansion of Medicare to cover everybody. A single governmental payer would eliminate the choice of insurer, but both plans would give free choice of physicians.

Congressman Martin Russo, along with sixty-five co-sponsors, has introduced a bill called the "Universal Health Care Act of 1991," H.R. 1300. By replacing all private and public health insurance coverage, this legislation would create a single-payer national health insurance system similar to Canada's. The federal government would set a global health care budget, thereby limiting total health care expenditures. Each individual would be issued a national health insurance identification card for processing of claims. In each state an agency would administer the national program and enroll everyone. By law, no co-payments, deductibles, or alternative insurance for covered services would be allowed. Each hospital would negotiate for and receive an annual payment to cover all operating expenses.

None of these funds could be used for capital purchases of equipment, expansion, or profit. The three payment options for physicians would be fee-for-service, salaries in institutions receiving global budgets, and salaries in group practices and HMOs receiving per capita payments. A National Health Trust Fund would fund the program by consolidating monies from Medicare and Medicaid (these programs would be dropped), state and local government health care expenditures, employer contributions, private insurance revenues, and general tax revenues.

Congressman Fortney (Pete) Stark, a dissenting member of the Pepper Commission, believes that the commission's play-or-pay system is a patchwork approach that would not adequately provide insurance for transiently employed people, divorced spouses and their children, the elderly, and employees of small businesses; nor would it control the spiraling costs of health care. Stark advocates a single national plan, operated by the federal government, that would achieve universal coverage and control costs by using the prospective payment methods of Medicare. Stark introduced a bill (''The Mediplan Health Care Act of 1991,'' H.R. 650) that would expand Medicare to provide coverage for all Americans.

Robert Kerrey's ''Health USA Act,'' S. 1466, which is similar to Mary Rose Oaker's ''Claude Pepper Comprehensive Health Care Act,'' H.R. 8, would further control costs and widen consumer choice by adding several cost containment mechanisms to Russo's national health insurance: deductibles, co-payments, and managed competition at the state level. In effect, the state agency would become a HPPC that would approve a portfolio of private and public health plans—fee-for-service and per capita—that meet minimum federal standards.

The HPPC would negotiate fee schedules with doctors, hospitals, and HMOs, which would be paid a risk-adjusted fixed amount for each person enrolled. All private and public insurance plans would have to cover doctors services, hospital care, preventive care, diagnostic tests, prescription drugs, and nursing home care. No family would have to pay more than $2,000 a year for medical care. The HPPC would receive 87 percent of the needed funds from the Federal government, financed by a 5 percent payroll tax, a 2 percent tax on non-wage income, and increased income taxes on the wealthy.

PUBLIC OPINION AND POLICY OPTIONS

Democratic and Republican congressional leaders all support some form of health care reform but advocate diverse weightings of private and public sector solutions and different degrees of consumer choice of insurance and of physicians. The health policy alternatives are numerous and complex and opinion polls, as guides to health policy, are only of limited use. No survey has covered all plans discussed, and changes in the wording of questions and in context change the percentages for or against a particular alternative. Even so, poll data may provide some insight into the public's preferences, which in turn may help guide the legislative agenda.

Public opinion pollsters presented these three mutually exclusive choices: 1) leaving things the way they are (status quo), 2) requiring businesses to provide coverage for all employees or to contribute to a federal fund (play-or-pay), or 3) creating a national health care plan run by the government (all government). In response, only 22 percent favored the status quo and 74 percent favored change, then defined as requiring some public insurance. Thirty-four percent favored play-or-pay and 40 percent favored an all government plan.

The public's attitude toward three health policy alternatives with different mixes of public and private insurance was assessed in an HIAA survey. The respondents were first informed about the problem of the uninsured, including the unemployed, some employees of small business, and those who are uninsurable because of prior illness. The interviewers then asked whether the respondents favored or opposed any of these proposed plans:

- Incremental Change—making private insurance more available and affordable and providing tax subsidies so low-income workers and small employers can afford it (87 percent favor, 52 percent strongly favor).
- Mandated Employer-Provided Benefits—requiring business to either provide health insurance for all their employees or pay into a fund to cover uninsured Americans (67 percent in favor, 40 percent strongly in favor).
- National Health Insurance—adopting a nationalized health insurance plan that would be run by the government, financed through new taxes, and would cover all Americans (54 percent favor, 32 percent strongly favor).

The response pattern of the HIAA survey (January 13, 1992) suggests that choices may be ordered hierarchically, from plans that are mainly private and incremental to public and more comprehensive plans: 87 percent of the respondents favored market reform. Of these many respondents (67 percent of the total sample) also favored mandated employer-provided benefits, and some (56 percent of the total) also favored national health insurance. Thirty-six percent favored all three options. A national survey (January 10, 1992) found 59 percent favored private sector reform and at least 36 percent (down from the 56 percent above) favored some governmental involvement (with 9 percent favoring mandated employer-provided benefits through play-or-pay and 27 percent favoring a Canadian-style plan).

The public's support for national health care is volatile. In an election night survey of voters (Fredericks/Schneider, November 3, 1992), 48 percent of those polled responded that federal operation of the health care system would be better than the present system; 44 percent said worse. When given a choice between a combination of public and private insurance or an all-government system, 70 percent favored the former and 26 percent the latter. Clinton and Perot voters (31 percent and 33 percent respectively) were more likely than Bush voters (17 percent) to support a national single-payer plan.

Each of the health plans discussed contains a core benefit plan that would pay for a minimum of decent health care. The Republicans would allow the states to define their own plans; the Democrats would legislate universal standards that states could supplement. The core plan should include coverage for inpatient and outpatient hospital and physician care, mental health services, prenatal and well-baby care, and diagnostic tests including Pap smears, mammograms, and colorectal screening. A plan with a universal core would be easier to administer than widely disparate ones, and minimal state-to-state differences would inhibit people from moving from parsimonious to generous states for health care benefits.

It is clear that the public desires change and will at least support bills that aim to reduce the number of uninsured by reforming the small business market through inexpensive federal initiatives. If such reforms are not implemented soon, the number of uninsured employees of small businesses will increase—over the next few years cost increases will force about 30 percent of small businesses currently providing insurance to drop their coverage.

To end the legislative gridlock on health care reform, at a minimum bills such as those sponsored by Bentsen and Rostenkowski or those that build on the HIAA recommendations, such as those by Congresswoman Kennelly's bills, should be passed. All plans, except those based on national health insurance, which may economically or politically not be feasible now—require reform of the small business insurance market. The reforms should guarantee the issue of affordable, continuous insurance without discrimination by health status or by preexisting conditions. Some plans would apply community rating, as is now required in New York and Vermont, and others would apply experience rating and reinsurance of high risks, as is now done in Connecticut. To facilitate a consensus about the relative effectiveness of community and experience rating, these initiatives should be objectively assessed.

To assure that only medically necessary care is provided, the approved plans should utilize cost-management techniques, including certification of care, utilization review, and managed care. The federal government should support cost containment efforts and formulate universal criteria for utilization review and managed care organizations. State-to-State variations in standards for utilization review organizations and managed care plans may make the provision of these services difficult. If such services are in fact useful, as research seems to indicate, then these services should be facilitated. Federal standards would have this effect.

The above reforms will reduce the number of uninsured, but they will not make all small businesses to insure their employees. A recent survey of 501 knowledgeable executive of small businesses concluded that even with a reduction in cost as large as 50 percent, only half of all small businesses that now do not insure their workers would voluntarily provide insurance. Whether mandating employers to provide coverage, changing the tax treatment for employee benefits, implementing a play-or-pay rule, subsidizing marginal employers, using vouchers, providing government insurance, or some combination of these funding mechanisms, reform is necessary to insure all uninsured.

Because the partisan debate about health care reform has led to diverse estimates of the costs and benefits of the various plans, collective action has been stymied. However, reforms can be made on the basis of the credible research done thus far. The consequences of the reforms on access to care, choice of provider, quality of care, and cost should be evaluated.

The protagonists in the health policy debate have diverse values, interests, and power—some consider health care an individual right; others, a privilege. The issues are complex, and as Senator Bentsen has concluded, "Reforming our health care system will be neither simple nor easily achieved."

How Drug Companies Operate on the Body Politic

Pharmaceutical firms have friends in high places.

Viveca Novak

The scene was right out of middle America's worst nightmare about what goes on under the Capitol dome. Special interest lobbyists prowled the halls buttonholing lawmakers. Debating in the chamber, senators parroted industry-supplied talking points and attacked the legislation at hand as a threat to the American way of life. Senators trotted out charts and graphs, the snazziest of them provided by industry.

At the end of the wearying eight-hour debate last March, Sen. David Pryor's (D–Ark.) amendment to restrict a tax break enjoyed by U.S. pharmaceutical makers with factories in Puerto Rico went down by a margin of almost two to one.

Chalk up another one for the drug industry, a lobby that ranks among the most muscular in Washington, D.C., adept at deploying plenty of both political action committee (PAC) money and lobbyists—many of them former congressional aides—to make its arguments and usually carry the day.

"I believe that the drug industry is more feared than respected by Congress," says Pryor, a perpetual foe.

A look at how this industry operates in Washington gives a glimpse of how tough it will be to enact any meaningful national health-care reform. At even the

Business and Society Review, Winter 1993

hint that Congress might curb the skyrocketing price of prescription drugs, the drug lobby enters with guns blazing:

- When Congress tried to control drug prices for the Medicaid program, the industry persuaded minority leaders to warn of "second-class medicine" for the poor.
- When lawmakers were debating a landmark Medicare bill to cover catastrophic illness, the drug industry helped whip up senior citizens, ultimately bringing the law crashing down—because it included a prescription drug benefit that might have led to cost controls.
- When legislators sought to limit profits on drugs for rare diseases, the industry divided the disease victims' advocacy community.
- When Pryor and others tried to cut the industry's Puerto Rico tax subsidy, the industry wailed about the threat to the free market system—even though the subsidy is a basic government giveaway.

Pharmaceutical firms, in short, want it both ways—to preserve their freedom to charge what they want for drugs and still hold on to various government blessings such as tax breaks and generous patent protection. Unlike physicians and hospitals, drugmakers have so far fended off virtually all government attempts to control prices.

CAPTIVE MARKET

It's the public that pays, through inflated healthcare costs and medications that are often priced beyond the reach of many who need them. In 1990, Americans spent more than $67 billion for prescription drugs. While drugs are less than one-tenth of the nation's health-care budget, their prices shot up at three times the rate of inflation in the 1980s—a startling 152 percent, far outpacing even the rise in other health-care costs. Pharmaceutical companies are the darlings of Wall Street. The recession scarcely bothers an industry that is the most profitable in the country and has a relatively captive market.

As the population ages, the industry's future can only get rosier. More than one-half of all Americans over age 45 regularly take prescription drugs. Among those 65 and older, the rate is 76 percent. Surveys show that prescription drugs are the largest out-of-pocket expense for three out of four seniors. Sixty-four-year-old Mary Mitchell of Atlantic Beach, North Carolina, for example spends more than $100 per month—from a Society Security income of $398—on four medications to treat a skin condition, high blood pressure, and asthma. "I think the drug industry is going overboard," Mitchell says.

Or consider the growing populations of AIDS patients, who on average spend $4,000 a year on medications—with some spending more than $10,000 a month.

Since 1981, twenty-nine drug industry PACs have handed out more than

$8.5 million in contributions to House and Senate candidates, including more than $1.7 million in the 1992 elections. Drug company PAC spending is on the rise—up 25 percent in the most recent election cycle over the same period in 1989–1990. Top recipients Sens. Dan Coats (R.-Ind.) and Orrin Hatch (R–Utah), both conservatives, can be counted on to make the industry's arguments in Congress. Sen. Bill Bradley (D–N.J.) is a more complicated case. More liberal and often a consumers' advocate, Bradley also represents a state that is home to many drug companies. He ranks fourth in drug industry PAC receipts and argued against Pryor's recent amendment.

Money isn't everything, of course; there are other ways to get close to lawmakers. Last spring, a group called the Alliance for Aging Research threw a filet mignon-and-salmon dinner to hand out awards to Health and Human Services Secretary Louis Sullivan and Sens. Pete Domenici (R–N.M.) and Jay Rockefeller (D–W.Va.). More than one-half the event's organizing committee were drug industry lobbyists, and fourteen big drug firms helped fund it. The industry sponsored parties and were a big presence at the 1992 Democratic and Republican presidential conventions.

"From my experience, the pharmaceutical manufacturers are one of the best lobbies out there," says a Senate staffer.

But the sheer chutzpah of the drug industry is starting to stir public and congressional resentment. Sensitive to this, the Pharmaceutical Manufacturers Association (PMA), which represents name-brand drugmakers, launched a $7 million advertising campaign that portrays the industry as vibrant, visionary, and even thrifty. Drugs are expensive, they say, because research and development (R&D) is costly—and besides, drugs often help prevent even higher-priced treatment like surgery.

Critics on and off Capitol Hill counter with compelling arguments of their own. Of course drugmakers spend a lot on R&D, they argue—new drugs bring lucrative patent protections and unlimited pricing freedom. Besides, they say, the industry spends at least as much on marketing as on research. And while drugs may be cheaper than other choices, they add, that's little comfort if people can't afford to buy them.

Pryor's longtime efforts to get a handle on drug prices took a new turn last year when he proposed cutting a tax break for manufacturers with factories in Puerto Rico. His bill stalled, but he offered virtually the same measure—slicing the tax break by 20 percent for each percentage point over inflation that a drug company raised its prices—as an amendment to the pending tax bill last spring.

Section 936 of the tax code, designed to create jobs in Puerto Rico, is no small write-off. Drug companies save an average of $70,000 in taxes for every Puerto Rican worker they employ, according to the General Accounting Office (GAO). From 1980 through 1990, the industry's tax savings topped $10 billion.

Internal industry memos show that PMA and its members responded quickly with a coordinated state and national campaign—an effort "tied closely to the industry's direct lobbying, media outreach, and suggested company grass-roots activity on the issue,'' one memo says. PMA simultaneously began a campaign of ads in major newspapers and magazines that tackled the cost issue head on. ''Why does one little pill cost so much?'' began one, answering with the industry's boilerplate arguments.

Last March saw Senate offices flooded with letters and lobbyists from the drugmakers—Glaxo, Bristol-Myers Squibb, SmithKline Beecham, Pfizer, Warner-Lambert and others. They and PMA developed talking points for sympathetic senators to use: The proposal unfairly singled out drugmakers; it was ''back-door price control''; it would hurt R&D investment and the industry's strong balance of trade. They even invoked the Cold War: ''At a time when state-run economies are crumbling around the world,'' read a PMA letter sent to Hill offices, Pryor's measure ''would move the United States in the opposite direction, toward government command and control of one of America's brightest business and scientific success stories.''

Though the amendment was supported by a few heavyweights of its own—the AFL–CIO, the American Association of Retired Persons (AARP) and others—the lobbying was distinctly lopsided. Pryor tried to pin down his colleagues in the crucial final hours of debate, even sacrificing several provisions in a bid to save the rest of the measure.

The next day, March 11, drug industry lobbyists met at 7 A.M. in PMA's boardroom for a final council of war. Then they blanketed the Capitol.

For eight hours, the debate dragged on. Arguments against the measure came from top recipients of industry contributions—notably Hatch and Coats. Among Democrats, Bradley and Sen. Chris Dodd (D–Conn.), another drug PAC favorite, were vocal opponents.

Two of the drug lobby's main points—that it costs an average of $231 million to develop a new drug, and that industry has increased R&D spending to nearly $11 billion in 1992—were repeated over and over, sometimes nearly verbatim from the industry's talking points. Other lawmakers, avoiding the substance, argued against cluttering the tax bill with amendments.

At the end of the day, Pryor lost sixty-one to thirty-six. One ally of the drug industry in that dispute was Sen. John McCain (R–Ariz.), who in a floor speech praised Pfizer, Abbott Laboratories, and a few other firms for holding down prices. Days later, Pfizer, Abbott, and the PMA were among those who threw him a $1,000-a-plate fundraiser. According to the *Arizona Republic*, the invitation said McCain had been central in several health-care measures, ''including drug pricing.''

The day after the vote, PMA President Gerald Mossinghoff wrote his members' Washington lobbyists. Their coordinated effort ''showed in sharp relief what this industry can accomplish when we are united in our objectives,'' he said. But PMA didn't drop its guard. A few days later, it assembled a follow-up task force with the assumption the tax issue would rise again.

GOUGING CONSUMERS

Industry's critics say it bought its own bad image by boosting drug prices to an extreme. Particularly hard-to-swallow examples aren't hard to find. ABC's *Prime Time Live* recently reported that Johnson & Johnson markets identical drugs for sheep, at a cost of $0.06 a pill, and for humans, at $6 a pill. (A company spokesperson denied the preparations are the same.) The price of the controversial tranquilizer Halcion, made by Upjohn, went up more than 75 percent between 1986 and 1991. Even Orrin Hatch has warned drug companies against gouging consumers.

It doesn't have to be like this. In Europe, where most countries regulate drug costs, consumers pay 54 percent less for pharmaceuticals than Americans. In Canada, a review panel can shorten a drug's patent period if drug prices are too far out of whack with the inflation rate.

Drug firms defend high prices, saying that it takes hundreds of millions of dollars to bring a new drug to market and that drugmakers lead all domestic industries in R&D investment. The business also entails costly risks—Abbott recent had to pull its new antibiotic, Omniflox, from the market after several deaths and other adverse reactions.

But critics point to weaknesses in the industry's claims. For one, it may or may not cost an average $231 million—the figure repeated ad nauseam in debate over Pryor's tax measure—to develop new drugs. A draft study last year by the Office of Technology Assessment called the figure "an arbitrary number with no intrinsic meaning."

Also, drug firms' R&D budgets are often equaled or exceeded by what they spend on pushing their products. Drug companies are famous for spending lavishly to wine and dine doctors and send them on conference junkets. Some firms plan to invest millions in a venture by Whittle Communications to bring doctors a daily broadcast of medical news laced with drug ads.

The drugmakers' refrain of heavy costs is further undercut by the fact that some of their work is done—for free—by federal scientists. Taxol, for instance, a promising new treatment for ovarian cancer derived by the bark of the Pacific Yew tree, was developed through research by the National Cancer Institute. Last year, the government agreed to give its research exclusively to Bristol-Myers, which will bring taxol to market—and get the profits.

AZT, the AIDS drug, also was developed in large part by the government. Burroughs-Wellcome initially priced AZT at $10,000 for a year's supply. Pressure from AIDS activists helped bring the price down, but it still costs about $2,400 a year.

For the elderly, drug costs—which are not covered by Medicare—are a significant hardship. A recent survey by AARP estimated that 8 million people skimp on necessities like food and heating fuel to pay for their prescriptions.

Drug coverage was included in the landmark, but short-lived, 1988 Medicare catastrophic insurance law. The law would have paid for prescriptions but favored cheaper generic brands. Pharmaceutical companies, which saw the provision as the first step toward cost controls, fought back with video news releases and professionally orchestrated grass-roots opposition. When a weaker version became law, the industry played a role, along with various seniors' groups, in stirring up the revolt among the elderly that shocked lawmakers—who thought they had done something clearly positive for once—into repealing it the next year.

"It was a very negative, cynical effort that was not appreciated by members of Congress," says one Senate aide. But it worked.

Two years ago the drugmakers suffered a rare, if partial, loss in Congress. But the battle left a bitter residue of racial politics, which had been used to weaken the reform measure. And since the cost-containment bill became law, the industry has struck back to recover its losses.

The chief mover of the bill was once again Pryor, though the White House's Office of Management and Budget made a similar proposal. Their goal: Get drugmakers to cut their prices to Medicaid, the federal-state health program for the very poor. Since Medicaid pays for close to 15 percent of all prescriptions sold—about $5.5 billion in 1991—why not use that market clout to bring down drug prices and save the government money?

The industry made its usual pitch. But this fight took an especially depressing turn when, as some critics saw it, PMA played the race card.

The trade group hired civil rights veteran Vernon E. Jordan, former president of the National Urban League and partner with the law and lobbying firm Akin Gump Hauer & Feld, to help make its case. (Jordan recently served as chairman of the transition team for President Bill Clinton.) Jordan urged minority groups to oppose the proposal; they did, saying its provisions would mean "second-class medicine" for poor blacks. One letter from the National Black Caucus of State Legislators to another group characterized the Medicaid proposals as coming from "mean-spirited bigots [who] want to strike at the black underclass"—Pryor's strong civil rights record notwithstanding.

PMA even persuaded Jesse Jackson and other minority leaders to write participants in the 1990 budget summit and voice their opposition to the Medicaid measures, according to the *National Journal*. The National Black Nurses Association, the League of United Latin American Citizens and others amplified the "second-class medicine" argument with a press conference, maintaining that provisions favoring the use of less expensive medications would limit Medicaid recipients' access to drugs.

But Pryor's aides point out that the bill contained an override allowing doctors to prescribe any drug they deemed "medically necessary." Many third-party payers and hospitals nationwide use rules similar to those the bill would have imposed, they maintain.

Although it was reported that some of the bill's opponents had longstanding financial and other ties to the drug industry, and the bill had many supporters—

AARP, the American Public Welfare Association, the National Governors Association, the National Caucus and Center on the Black Aged, and others—the damage had been done.

As a result, the bill that eventually passed, while still a win for Medicaid, was watered down. It requires manufacturers to charge Medicaid the "best price" they give other bulk purchasers, a formula that should lead to discounts of at least 15 percent by 1993. Stripped from the legislation were measures that could have encouraged use of less expensive drugs.

And, after a year-and-a-half under the law, the industry has recovered part of its loss. Many firms raised their "best prices" to other bulk purchasers, so the scale for establishing the Medicaid price was ratcheted up. Within a year, the Department of Veteran Affairs, for example, was hit with drug price increases averaging 21 percent, but in some cases much more, costing it an estimated extra $90 million in 1991. One 76-year-old disabled veteran, Ralph Beckwith, wrote Rep. Mike Synar (D–Okla.) about price hikes on his eye medicine—which he has to pay for, along with his other medications, out of a $400 monthly income. "Must I go blind now," Beckwith wrote, "so some pharmaceutical company can get rich off of the old people?"

ORPHAN DRUGS

PMA's Mossinghoff says the industry can't afford to pass along the same deep discounts it once gave the veterans to the much larger Medicaid market, so it's natural that all prices would rise. Several bills to address the problem have been proposed, but the PMA's arguments have a familiar ring. For the government to step in again, Mossinghoff testified, "would cause an unwarranted and unprecedented disruption of the U.S. free market system—at a time when free market principles are sweeping the world."

Drug firms, of course, don't operate in a pure free market environment, and one of the more generous government-granted benefits is called orphan drug status. While many feel it's been exploited, fixing it is harder than it seems.

The nine-year-old Orphan Drug Act gives pharmaceutical makers research tax breaks and a seven-year monopoly for new drugs developed to treat patients with rare diseases—small and normally unprofitable markets that drug companies might otherwise ignore. It's worked: more than sixty orphan drugs are on the market, and without the law important breakthroughs might not have occurred.

Two problems, though. One is that some of the drugs are priced beyond the reach of those who need them—"ransom" for a captive market, says Sen. Howard Metzenbaum (D–Ohio). A year's supply of Genzyme's Ceredase, for example, developed to treat Gaucher's disease, can cost more than $300,000.

And while a drug may be developed for one malady, other uses sometimes develop. While its market burgeons, it still retains orphan drug status—and the manufacturer can raise prices substantially. Fujisawa USA's aerosol pentamadine was developed to treat a rare form of pneumonia that affects just a few hundred people in this country. Then it turned out that AIDS victims often get the same sickness. The drug's sales have soared—and so has its cost.

Pending before the Senate now is a bill cosponsored by Metzenbaum and Sen. Nancy Kassebaum (R–Kan.) to trim exclusive marketing rights for orphan drugs to two years; the monopoly can continue for up to nine years if a drug's sales don't top $200 million. Industry lobbying helped convince President Bush to veto more modest changes to the law in 1990.

"What's happened is more and more companies have abused and violated the intent of the act," says Abbey Meyers, executive director of the National Organization for Rare Disorders, which supports the changes. Senate staffers say the industry has at least one lobbyist covering each member of the Senate Labor and Human Resources Committee. One of the best-credentialed: Former committee member Paula Hawkins (R–Fla.). Hawkins, who lost her Senate seat in1986, earns $120,000 annually as a consultant to Genentech and rents a limo when she comes to town, according to lobbying disclosure reports.

Industry has gained the support of the NAACP and others in the minority community. They argue that anything that could discourage drug R&D could hurt minorities because they tend to get sick more often. More important for this fight, the industry has split the rare-diseases groups, which often rely on their money to help finance projects and special events. The Cystic Fibrosis Foundation (CF), in particular, broke with most other rare-diseases groups to enthusiastically line up on industry's side. CF has a close relationship with Genentech, one of the loudest opponents of the bill, in part because the firm is preparing to market a new orphan drug for the disease. CF also has a business alliance with Genzyme, the maker of costly Ceredase: Though Ceredase is not a cystic fibrosis treatment, the foundation's mailorder pharmacy has exclusive East Coast marketing rights to the drug.

The foundation sent out fliers to its pharmacy customers earlier this year with a bold headline—"Urgent! Your Lives are Being Threatened"—asking them to write to Capitol Hill opposing changes in the law. It has hired two lobbying and public relations firms to help put together what it calls the Coalition for Orphan Drug Research. But each time the foundation has sent to Capitol Hill a list of its members, all of whom ostensibly oppose changes in the law, there have been "problems," says a Senate aide. Some listed organizations actually support the amendments or have taken no position, such as the Retinitis Pigmentosa Foundation, which wrote an angry letter demanding that its name be removed.

Jeffrey Kerr, a vice president of CF, denies any overreaching. "There are a couple of groups that have changed their minds" after being listed, he says. Some of CF's opponents charge that the industry is paying for the coalition and the foundation's other lobbying efforts against the bill; Kerr denies it. Still, divisions about CF's outspoken lobbying on the bill have arisen even within its own board of directors.

The drug industry also cares deeply about hanging onto its monopoly rights for larger market drugs. Normally drug patents last seventeen years, but industry argues that the Food and Drug Administration (FDA) is so slow in approving products that few years are left before competitors can enter the scene. With more than thirty of the 100 leading drugs scheduled to lose their patents by 1995, drug companies have begun pushing the House and Senate judiciary committees for valuable patent extensions.

"We definitely see more lobbying on this issue these days," says Dennis Burke, a Senate Judiciary staffer.

Congress last granted a patent extension in 1988, when a reprieve for a Warner-Lambert drug was quietly attached to a big trade bill. But in June, Rep. William Hughes (D–N.J.) and the judiciary subpanel he chairs approved three extensions—including one to American Home Products that had not been the subject of hearings or debate. That company's CEO, joined by veteran drug industry lobbyist J.D. Williams, called on virtually every member of the House and Senate Judiciary committees, Hill staffers say. Hughes denied he was influenced by lobbyists.

The bill, which passed the full committee, paradoxically toughens standards for future extensions while not applying those criteria for the three it approves. An attempt to rush it through on the House floor without debate in early August was slowed when Rep. Pete Stark (D–Calif.) demanded a roll call vote, questioning "whether billions of dollars should be given away to three of the largest, most profitable pharmaceutical manufacturers in this country who already enjoy generous" government support. Even so, it passed.

FRIENDS IN HIGH PLACES

The industry also had good friends in the Bush administration. The drug industry complained about the FDA to then-Vice President Dan Quayle's Council on Competitiveness. And last November, after meetings with the PMA, the Industrial Biotechnology Association, the Association of Biotechnology Companies, and representatives of Eli Lilly (based in Quayle's home state of Indiana), the council announced several recommendations for speeding up the drug approval process, some of which closely resembled a drug industry wish list.

George Bush was a Lilly board member in the late 1970s, and company executives gave generously to Quayle's political campaigns. Lilly Vice President Mitchell Daniels Jr., a former Regan White House official, cohosted a November 1991 Bush–Quayle fundraiser—right around the time the Quayle council announced its recommended FDA reforms. The council played a key role in Bush's 1990 pocket veto of orphan drug reforms and the U.S. decision to bow out of the global biodiversity treaty last year. Daniels later joined the Bush–Quayle campaign.

Proponents of the FDA reforms say they will cut the average time for drug testing and approval from ten years to six. But the changes, which include hiring private research labs to review some new drug applications, have provoked concern on Capitol Hill. Some members warn that outside review, for instance, raises the danger of conflicts of interest.

Critics say what's really needed is to beef up the FDA's budget, decimated during the 1980s, and give it new enforcement powers. They cite examples of drug firms that have withheld safety data from the agency and the FDA bribery scandal involving generic drug firms several years ago.

David Pryor has joked that pharmaceutical industry lobbyists shouldn't schedule their vacations during the first 100 days of the Clinton Administration—not that they're likely to. Pending are his bill attacking their Puerto Rican tax credits, the orphan drug legislation, the patent extension issue and other measures.

Then there is the emerging debate over national health-care reform. In June 1992, PMA joined the Healthcare Equity Action League, a coalition that is fighting comprehensive reform measures. Industry lobbyists are keeping an eye on the dozens of bills on Capitol Hill, many of which call for cost controls on the health-care industry and drug coverage under Medicare or some other comprehensive national health insurance program.

The Clinton presidency is another source of concern. During the campaign, he often mentioned drug costs in his discussions of health-care reforms, and Clinton is close to industry nemesis and fellow Arkansas Democrat Pryor.

Under increasing attack, some drug companies have begun subsidizing heart and AIDS treatments for the poor and elderly, providing rebates on drugs given out by federally financed public health programs, and giving away experimental drugs to patients with life-threatening diseases. Several firms have vowed to limit price hikes, for now, to the inflation rate.

But underestimating the drug lobby is a proven mistake. Nothing is expected to dampen the zeal of the drug firms for fighting every perceived threat to their surprisingly free rein, and industry analysis still expect drug company earnings to climb at double-digit rates.

"If the debate and vote on [the Puerto Rico tax breaks] is any indication of how long it is going to take to reform the health-care system in this country," says Pryor, "it is clear to me that we have a very long way to go. If Congress cannot stand up to the pharmaceutical industry—for which we spend less than 10 percent of our health-care dollars—how in the world are we going to stand up to the other entrenched health-care interests?"

AIDS Drugs & the Pharmaceutical Industry: A Need for Reform*

Mary T. Griffin**

I. INTRODUCTION

The modern pharmaceutical industry has grown up over the past fifty years. Its first twenty-five years were marked by phenomenal successes and growth in an atmosphere relatively free from criticism or stringent regulatory requirements. The country was grateful for advances in health care made by the industry. Relative to hospitalization, the cost of drug therapy was cheap. Beginning in the early 1960s, however, the industry's pricing practices and profit margins came into question. Hearings addressing concerns about the industry revealed huge markups, the lack of price competition in the pharmaceuticals market and the sizable profits enjoyed by the industry.

In spite of extensive investigations into the industry over the past twenty-five years, the industry has done little to alter its practices. During the 1980s, criticism of the industry heightened in the midst of price increases far in excess of the general rate of inflation. A number of cost control devices were implemented, but

* This Article is adapted from a thesis done in partial satisfaction of an L.L.M. from George Washington University Law Center. The author wishes to thank Teresa Schwartz for her support and guidance with this Article.

** Mary T. Griffin, J.D., 1985, Temple University School of Law; L.L.M., 1991, George Washington University Law Center; Food and Drug Law Institute Fellow.

American Journal of Law & Medicine, V. 17, n.4, 1991.

they have not achieved the goal of reducing the overall level of drug prices. The industry continues with its practice, begun in the 1960s, of blaming its high prices on the escalating costs of research and development caused by the costs of the lengthy approval process and regulatory requirements. To assist the industry in dealing with burgeoning research and development costs, Congress provided a number of financial incentives through legislation passed in the 1980s.

Into this atmosphere of increasing prices and mushrooming research and development budgets came the AIDS crisis. By the second half of the decade, a number of pharmaceutical companies had become involved in the search for AIDS drugs. In response to pressure from AIDS activists and in recognition of the need to expedite drug therapy for people with AIDS, the government has instituted a number of regulatory and policy changes in the drug development and approval process. These changes have significantly reduced the time it takes to develop a drug. Nevertheless, the industry has priced these drugs as some of the most expensive drugs ever produced.

To ensure people with AIDS access to these drugs, a method to control the costs of such therapy should be instituted. Cost control systems implemented thus far have proven unsuccessful and present special problems for AIDS drugs, many of which are subject to monopolistic pricing because they are single-source products. The time has come for a system of direct price control, coordinated by the government, to address the prices charged for AIDS drugs.

This Article explores the history and economics of the pharmaceutical industry, and the failed attempts of government to reduce prices. This analysis demonstrates the need for a system of national price regulation to address the problem of AIDS drugs, some of the most needed and yet most expensive drugs the industry has to offer.

II. THE PHARMACEUTICAL INDUSTRIAL REVOLUTION

The extensive research efforts involved in the search for drugs to treat HIV disease and AIDS-related illnesses[1] represent the extent to which society relies upon and believes in drug therapy in providing medical care to its suffering citizens. The view that virtually every ailment can be treated with drug therapy predominates in this country: one expects and desires a drug when illness strikes. This perception probably explains why the United States leads other countries in per capita expen-

1. Drugs are currently used to treat people who are HIV-positive but display no symptoms of the opportunistic infections which signify AIDS, as well as those who are experiencing "full blown" AIDS. Anti-viral drugs, such as AZT and ddI are used by people who are HIV-positive to attack the virus and delay the onset of symptoms. Other drugs, such as Pentamidine, are used to treat the various infections which people with AIDS experience. This Article deals with all drugs which are used in various ways to combat HIV and the diseases that it causes. For the sake of clarity, all such drugs are here referred to as "AIDS drugs." The reader is reminded that many people who are presently asymptomatic but HIV-positive receive these drugs.

ditures on drugs.[2] Another explanation can be gleaned from the way in which drugs and the pharmaceutical industry developed in this country.

In the first part of this century, pharmaceutical companies supplied bulk chemicals to pharmacists who then prepared prescriptions and sold them to consumers.[3] During that time, the United States was involved primarily in manufacturing drugs, relying on Germany for a supply of bulk synthetic drugs distributed to pharmacists.[4]

World War II and the discovery of sulpha drugs transformed the industry into one focused on research and development (R & D). It was not until 1932, with the discovery and patenting of Prontosil, the first sulpha drug, that the pharmaceutical industry made the big leap from manufacturing to R & D.[5] The industry's expansion into R & D proved to be extremely successful, as more sulpha drugs were developed.[6] The United States, along with the United Kingdom, Germany, France and Switzerland, became involved in a race to discover new and extremely profitable drugs.[7] The relatively moderate cost of developing a new drug in relation to its financial success, the patent and trademark protection provided to new discoveries, and the systematic marketing and promotion of brand name products contributed to the industry becoming one of the most profitable of all manufacturing industries. The industry produced new chemical entities (NCEs) at a steady rate during the 1940s and 1950s, and many of these became leading drugs.[8] Through patents on these discoveries, companies secured monopolies in particular therapeutic markets and maintained high prices.[9] The combination of these factors with the low debt level of the industry contributed to profit levels for pharmaceutical companies which averaged in excess of 7% above the average profit levels of all United States manufacturing concerns.[10]

The growth of the drug industry was phenomenal: in 1939 the sales volume

---

2. *Skyrocketing Prescription Drug Prices: Hearings Before the Senate Special Comm. on Aging*, 101st Cong., 1st Sess. 9 (1989) [hereinafter *Hearings on Skyrocketing Prices*] (statement of G. Adrianssens, Belgian Consumers Ass'n).

3. United States Bureau of Consumer Protection, Drug product Selection 15 (1979) [hereinafter Drug Product Selection].

4. *See* H. Redwood, The Pharmaceutical Industry: Trends, Problems and Achievements 37–40 (1987).

5. M. Silverman & P. Lee, Pills Profits & Politics 4 (1974).

6. *Id.*; H. Redwood, *supra* note 4, at 33. The intensified research efforts, and the discovery in 1937 that sulfonamide was the active ingredient in Prontosil, led to the discovery of many more sulpha drugs and to the development of industrial research laboratories to accommodate the research. *Id.* Prior to the development of these laboratories, much research had taken place in small laboratories and pharmacies, and by doctors experimenting with drugs to develop treatments for patients. H. Dowling, Medicines for Man: The Development, Regulation, and Use of Prescription Drugs 24–25 (1970).

7. H. Redwood, *supra* note 4, at 40.

8. *Id.* at 45, 47. The term "leading drug" refers to the level of sales volume obtained on the particular drug and may vary depending upon the source.

9. *Id.* at 46.

10. M. Silverman & P. Lee, *supra* note 5, at 328 table 2 (1974); United States Dep't of Health Educ. & Welfare Task Force on Prescription Drugs, The Drug Makers and Drug Distributors 45–47 (1968) [hereinafter HEW Task Force, The Drug Makers].

for the industry was $149 million and by 1957 it had increased elevenfold to $1,677 million.[11] The industry's high rate of return on its investment in R & D between 11% and 18%, led to its increased commitment to R & D.[12] In 1955, the industry spent approximately $91 million on R & D; by 1965, that figure had tripled to $328 million.[13] The drug industry led all other industries in the percentage of self-financing of R & D.[14]

During the 1940s and 1950s, the investment had proven to be worth the return. While the cost of developing an NCE tripled, the revenue from the drug increased five times.[15] By 1956, brand or trade name drugs had saturated the market: almost 90% of the prescriptions filled were brand name drugs.[16] Prices of prescription drugs increased and per capita expenditures nearly doubled between 1950 and 1960.[17] Congress expressed concerns over the lack of competition in the industry, but it was not until 1959, after the Federal Trade Commission (FTC) for the first time treated the pharmaceutical industry separately from the chemical industry in reporting on industry profits, that the extent of the industry's profits was exposed.[18] This revelation, along with reports of false and deceptive promotion practices, led to the Kefauver hearings.[19] 1960 marked not only further investigative hearings, but also the beginning of the decline in the number of new

11. Lasgna, *1938–1968: The FDA, the Drug Industry, the Medical Profession, and the Public*, in SAFEGUARDING THE PUBLIC: HISTORICAL ASPECTS OF MEDICINAL DRUG CONTROL 171 (J. Blake ed. 1970) [hereinafter SAFEGUARDING THE PUBLIC].

12. D. SCHWARTZMAN, THE EXPECTED RETURN FROM PHARMACEUTICAL RESEARCH 42–46 (1975).

13. PHARMACEUTICAL MFR. ASS'N, PRESCRIPTION DRUG INDUSTRY FACT BOOK 39 (1986) [hereinafter PMA FACT BOOK].

14. *Id.* at 40.

15. M. STATMAN, COMPETITION IN THE PHARMACEUTICAL INDUSTRY: THE DECLINING PROFITABILITY OF DRUG INNOVATIONS 28 (1983).

16. PMA FACT BOOK, *supra* note 13, at 63. Brand or trade name products are typically single-source or patented drugs developed by R & D intensive pharmaceutical companies. Brand name products are often referred to as "pioneer" drugs to distinguish them from generic (copied) drugs. Generic drugs are multi-source products marketed under the generic or abbreviated universal name developed for the drug, and are either copies of previously patented products or drugs which have never been the subject of patents. *See, e.g.*, *Generic Drugs: Still Safe?*, CONSUMER REPORTS, May 1990, at 310–13

Prior to the proliferation of brand and trade name drugs in the 1940s, the majority of prescriptions were written generically and were pharmacy-filled, as opposed to factory-filled products. H. REDWOOD, *supra* note 4, at 11. For a discussion of the generics market in relation to the brand name market, see *infra* text accompanying notes 252–256.

17. M. SILVERMAN & P. LEE, *supra* note 5, at 335 table 8.

18. *Id.* at 110-12.

19. *Id.* at 111–14. Beginning in the late 1950s, the Senate Committee on the Judiciary, Subcommittee on Antitrust and Monopoly, began a series of hearings on administered prices in specific industries. Senator Estes Kefauver, Chair of the Subcommittee, held extensive hearings to examine pricing practices of the pharmaceutical industry in the early 1960s. The hearing culminated in the passage of the Kefauver-Harris amendments to the Federal Food, Drug and Cosmetic Act of 1938. *See infra* text accompanying notes 78–92. *See also* ADMINISTERED PRICES: DRUGS, REPORT OF THE SENATE COMM. ON THE JUDICIARY, BY ITS SUBCOMM. ON ANTITRUST AND MONOPOLY, PURSUANT TO S. RES. 52, S. REP. 448, 87TH CONG., 1st SESS. 155–222 (1961).

drug introductions. The revolution appeared to be coming to an end, or at least changing course.

III. ECONOMICS OF THE PHARMACEUTICAL INDUSTRY

The successes of the pharmaceutical industry and the contributions made by it to health care shielded the industry from closer inspection of its pricing practices and economic structure for some time. The industry successfully integrated the use of patents, trademarks and extensive advertising and promotion campaigns to create a market characterized not by price or quality competition, but by competition based on promotionally achieved product differentiation and the introduction of new, higher priced products. Into this structure the industry implemented a pricing system in which prices were set according to the increase in market share which the sale would yield. This structure enabled drug manufacturers to maintain high price differentials and reap sizable profits from products which were relatively inexpensive to develop by exploiting the public's perception that drugs were effective and inexpensive alternates to hospitalization. It was not until the Kefauver hearings exposed the high profit margins and exploitive pricing practices that the economic structure of the industry was questioned.

Despite years of hearings and investigations, and efforts of outraged members of Congress, the drug industry has not effected many changes in its structure: it continues to charge high prices and accumulate above average profit levels. The AIDS crisis began in the early 1980s in the midst of price increases occurring at rates higher than ever before. The high prices charged for AIDS drugs and the escalating prices in general brought the pricing practices of the industry to the forefront again. Various Congressional committees have made a number of inquiries concerning the escalating prices of drugs. Due to the nature of the disease and the way in which the drugs were developed, however, the AIDS situation presents a particularly compelling reason to reexamine the drug industry's practices and to take action to correct the inequities brought about by the economic structure and practices of the industry.

A. Current Market

The current prescription drug industry is comprised of a number of small firms, which sell mostly generic drugs, and large firms, which sell brand name and, to a lesser extent, generic drugs, and engage in intensive R & D efforts.[20] As R & D costs have steadily increased, and as the industry has allocated more of its revenues to R & D, a consolidation of resources in the form of mergers and acquisitions and joint ventures have taken place, causing a higher degree of concentration in the pharmaceutical industry.[21] The Pharmaceutical Manufactur-

20. United States Dep't of Commerce, Competitive Assessment of the U.S. Pharmaceutical Industry 12 (1984) [hereinafter Competitive Assessment].
21. Standard and Poor's Industry Survey, health Care, H 18–19 [hereinafter Standard and Poor's].

ers Association (PMA), the industry's trade association, has over 100 member companies which discover and develop most of the prescription drugs in the United States, and which account for 95% of the industry's sales.[22] In 1989, PMA member firms devoted 16.7% of their sales, or $7.3 billion, to R & D, up 12.3% from 1988.[23]

The industry continues to command above average profit levels.[24] Over the past thirty years, the overall price increase to consumers for drugs has been three to four times greater than the increase in prices for all other items. Unlike other markets, this has not resulted in decreased sales. Many have made inquiries into the drug industry's practices to determine how these trends continue. The answers, for the most part, lie in the economic structure of the industry.

B. The Economic Structure of the Drug Industry

Certain characteristics of the drug industry set it apart from other industries and help explain the industry's ability to steadily increase prices and profits in the midst of fluctuating market conditions. One major difference in the prescription drug market is the lack of consumer control over the selection of the product. Another relevant characteristic, the lack of price competition among drug companies, stems from a variety of factors. The prevalence of patent protected products and the proliferation of brand name products have enabled drug companies to create and sustain leading market positions in certain therapeutic drug markets. These characteristics operate together in the market to deprive consumers of the opportunity to effectuate control over the market and enable drug manufacturers to continue to raise prices and profits.

1. The Professional Intermediary and Access to Information The more knowledge that a consumer has about the effectiveness and quality of a product, the greater the ability of that consumer to control the selection process and thereby exert influence over the market. Consumers have very little access to information about the safety and effectiveness of prescription drugs.[25] The consumer must rely

---

22. *Industry Will Invest $8.2 Billion to Discover, Develop New Medicines*, in PHARMACEUTICAL MFR. ASS'N, NEW DRUG APPROVALS IN 1989 8 (1990) [hereinafter PMA, 1989 NEW DRUG APPROVALS].
23. *Id.*
24. UNITED STATES DEP'T OF COMMERCE, BUREAU OF THE CENSUS, QUARTERLY FINANCIAL REPORT FOR MANUFACTURING, MINING AND TRADE CORPORATIONS, at XXIV table B & XXVI table D (2d Quarter 1988). The percentages are based on the last two quarters of 1987 and the first two quarters of 1988. PMA, 1989 NEW DRUG APPROVALS, *supra* note 22. Figures based on PMA members' sales. STANDARD AND POOR'S *supra* note 21, at H 17 (based on 1987 figures). Freudenheim, *Price Revolt Spreading on Prescription Drugs*, N.Y. Times, Nov. 14, 1989, at D1, col. 4 (citing United States Department of Labor statistics); Interview with Christopher Jennings, Deputy Staff director of the Senate Select Committee on Aging, Sept. 22, 1990 (citing to Consumer Price Index figures on prescription drugs provided by the Bureau of Labor Statistics, United States Department of Labor for the years 1980–1990) [hereinafter Interview with Christopher Jennings].
25. S. WIGGINS, THE PHARMACEUTICAL INDUSTRY 5–6 (1985).

on the experience and knowledge of the prescribing physician or the dispensing pharmacist; but typically doctors are not well informed about a variety of drugs because information gathering is a costly process.[26] Because the cost of information is high, and the one who exerts control over the selection process generally does not make a selection on the basis of price, drug manufacturers are able to maintain high price differentials.[27]

The drug industry's intensive promotion and advertising campaigns and, in particular, its use of drug company representatives, or "detail men," have encouraged brand name practices by physicians.[28] Despite the revival of generics and pressure to contain costs, physicians typically do not consider price differentials when prescribing.[29] The costly and time consuming nature of the information gathering process leads to physicians' reliance on the *Physicians Desk Reference (PDR)* and detail men for much of their information.[30]

Another source of knowledge upon which doctors rely is experience with certain drugs.[31] If detail men and brand name promotion, along with other practices, such as providing free samples of drugs to doctors, are successful in bringing about brand name loyalty, then the doctors will continue to prescribe according to their experience with patients; that is, they will prescribe brand name drugs. This cyclical process ultimately benefits the drug manufacturers.

2. The Lack of Price Competition: Higher Priced Products and Patent Protection Price competition is an integral part of the free market enterprise system in this country, but not of the pharmaceutical industry.[32] According to one model of perfect competition, prices are set close to manufacturing costs to ensure both sales and profits.[33] Consumers choose among products on the basis of price, quality and value, and thus influence the market. Manufacturers respond to changes in consumer demand by lowering prices or by innovating to lower costs. Theoretically, this model invites innovation because a higher quality or lower priced product will attract consumers. But pharmaceutical manufacturers exert

26. *Id.* at 9.

27. M. STATMAN, *supra* note 15, at 54. Figures used in this Article may be based on those which relate to member firms of the PMA or to the pharmaceutical industry as a whole. Since the PMA members develop more than 95% of drugs, however, figures will be used interchangeably.

28. *See* M. SILVERMAN & P. LEE, *supra* note 5, at 110.

29. *See, e.g.*, DRUG PRODUCT SELECTION, *supra* note 3, at 5–6.

30. *See* W. WIGGINS, *supra* note 25, at 9–12.

31. *Id.* at 10. Based on numbers of prescriptions physicians write each year and the type of drugs prescribed, Wiggins found that doctors who write 500–1,000 new prescriptions each year, those who write 2,000 new prescriptions each year, and those who write 3,500 new prescriptions each year prescribe each drug an average of 10–11 times per year. *Id.* Wiggins concluded that these numbers indicate a lack of experience with particular drugs on the part of the physicians. *Id.* at 11.

32. H. DOWLING, *supra* note 6, at 105.

33. *See, e.g.*, H. REDWOOD, *supra* note 4, at 46. *See generally* HEW TASK FORCE, THE DRUG MAKERS, *supra* note 10, at 37–44 (discussing the role of patents and trademarks on competition in the pharmaceutical industry).

much more control over the market and continue to increase prices to pay for the type of competition in which the industry engages: developing and promoting new products.[34]

When the search for new drugs expanded after the discovery and patenting of the first sulpha drugs in the 1930s, drug manufacturers quickly realized the profitability of wonder drugs. Improved health justified the cost to the patient, and patents assured manufacturers a monopoly for seventeen to twenty years.[35] The prospect of patents motivated manufacturers to develop new, therapeutically different drugs to displace existing therapies at higher prices. The relatively low cost of developing a drug and the high rates of return led to an increased emphasis on R & D in the search for new, patentable drugs. Many attribute at least part of the success of the United States drug industry in the world pharmaceutical market to its ability to obtain extensive patent coverage, including both product and process patents, over new therapies.[36]

Critics charge that pharmaceutical manufacturers develop "me-too" products, that is, drugs differing only slightly from previously developed drugs with arguably little or no added therapeutic value, in order to obtain patents and higher prices for the new products.[37] Trademarks—product designations for the exclusive use of the registrant manufacturer—are used in conjunction with large advertising and promotion campaigns to create and proliferate a market for the product. Manufacturers justify higher prices, create a market for the drug and enjoy a monopoly for the life of the patent (and perhaps longer), even for products containing little or no added therapeutic value. In this way, manufacturers charge higher prices for promotionally achieved product differentiation.

3. Drug Prices and Profits The pricing of drugs involves two mysterious and complex processes: the setting of the price of the drug and the pricing structure of the various markets once a drug is introduced. The factors involved in pricing drugs are not easy to assess since the cost of any given drug includes the cost of developing other products. The drug industry pricing structure involves various policies and practices of differential pricing and discounting, making it extremely difficult to determine the actual price levels of certain drugs. Clearly, however, consumers subsidize the price differentials, ensuring continued high profit levels

34. M. STATMAN, *supra* note 15, at 1.

35. Not everyone agrees as to the extent of improvement in health care realized by the drug revolution. Many risks and health problems, i.e., adverse reactions and side effects, are associated with drug therapy. In addition, while drugs often manage diseases and symptoms, they do not always provide cures. For a discussion of the risks and benefits associated with the widespread introduction of drugs into our society, see M. SILVERMAN & P. LEE, *supra* note 5, at 1–23.

36. H. REDWOOD, *supra* note 4, at 46. The antibiotics market, one of the largest therapeutic markets, experiences the greatest price competition and has the lowest percentage of patient protected products. HEW TASK FORCE, THE DRUG MAKERS, *supra* note 10, at 39.

37. P. BROOKE, RESISTANT PRICES: A STUDY OF COMPETITIVE STRAINS IN THE ANTIBIOTICS MARKET 19 (1975).

for the industry. When called upon to explain the high prices and profit levels, drug manufacturers often refuse to divulge specific information relating to costs asserting trade secret protection, and blame the prices on the high and increases costs of R & D.

a. Setting the Price of a Drug Pricing factors include direct manufacturing costs, research and development costs, overhead, clinical factors, marketing and distribution costs, and profit potential. Because drug manufacturers allocate marketing, R & D and other costs over a number of their products, the actual cost of a drug is far less than the price charged.[38] The price of any successful drug also reflects the costs of research failures.[39]

A drug is priced according to what the market will bear, taking into consideration the therapeutic advantages of the product and the cost of alternative therapies.[40] For example, a major breakthrough in a new therapeutic category where no substitutes exist, as in the case of AIDS drugs, carries a high profit potential and will be priced according to such potential.[41] Where products offer an improvement over existing drugs, the manufacturer will set the price higher than that of existing therapies to maximize the profit potential of the improvement.[42]

Price increases usually occur in the first years of a drug, to capitalize on the period of fastest growth.[43] Decreases typically occur, if at all, after a drug has been on the market for a number of years and after costs have been cut or after the manufacturer recognizes the high profits obtained in the past from the drug.[44] Theoretically, the expiration of the patent and the entry of generics should increase competition and reduce the price of a drug. But manufacturers often increase prices soon after patient expiration to maximize profits while the drug still controls the market share and to offset the expected losses from generic competition in the future.[45]

b. Effective Patent Life A patent provides an inventor with protection from the unauthorized use of the invention for a period of seventeen years.[46] Patents on

38. HEW TASK FORCE, THE DRUG MAKERS, *supra* note 10, at 33.
39. *Id. See* S. WIGGINS, *supra* note 25, at 14.
40. HEW TASK FORCE, THE DRUG MAKERS, *supra* note 10, at 33; P. BROOKE, *supra* note 37, at 17.
41. For a discussion on AIDS drug pricing, see *infra* text accompanying notes 194–202.
42. *See* HEW TASK FORCE, THE DRUG MAKERS, *supra* note 10, at 33–34. Clinical factors include the size and characteristics of the population which will take the drug; whether there will be short or long term use; quantity of drug to be ingested; and frequency of use. *Id.* at 33.
43. *See id.* at 33–35. *See, e.g.*, M. STATMAN, *supra* note 15, at 22–25 (nine year average introduction stage before plateau is reached). The annual rate of growth in sales revenue for NCEs during the period of introduction was determined by the author to be 11.5% for those drugs introduced between 1940 and 1974. *Id.* at 23.
44. HEW TASK FORCE, THE DRUG MAKERS, *supra* note 10, at 35–36.
45. *See, e.g.*, Statman, *The Effect of Patent Expiration on the Market Position of Drugs*, in DRUGS AND HEALTH: ECONOMIC ISSUES AND POLICY OBJECTIVES 145 (R. Helms ed. 1981) (over 50% of drugs under study experienced price increases at time of or after patent expiration).
46. 35 U.S.C. § 154 (1988).

drugs are typically issued prior to FDA approval.[47] The effective patent life (EPL) is thereby reduced by the length of the approval process.[48] In 1984, brand name manufacturers obtained patent term extensions through the Drug Price Competition and Patent Term Restoration Act (PTRA).[49] These manufacturers argued that the reduction in the EPL allowed for generic opportunity before the drug's profit potential could be realized,[50] hindering innovation because of the manufacturers' fear that R & D costs would not be recoupled.[51]

Due to successful promotion, advertising, and brand naming practices, however, the expiration of a patent does not always bring an end to a monopoly. Studies demonstrate that an effective monopoly on a single source patented product continues after the introduction of generic copies. Prices on the brand name products are not automatically reduced upon arrival of generics into the market.[52]

c. Pricing Structure Although the actual prices paid for drugs are difficult to determine due to the industry's multi-pricing structure,[53] the rate of increase, by any index, in drug prices over the past ten years has out-paced the rate of inflation. Price differentials, in conjunction with promotion and advertising efforts, bring drugs to the attention of those who exert the most influence over the market: physicians and institutional purchasers.[54]

Drug manufacturers traditionally charge hospitals and certain government institutions lower prices than those charged to community pharmacies,[55] in some instances more than 90% lower.[56] As the number of Health Maintenance Organizations (HMOs) increases, manufacturers have also begun to reduce prices of

47. *See* Wheaton, *Generic Competition and Pharmaceutical Innovation: The Drug Price Competition and Patent Term Restoration Act of 1984*, 35 CATH. U.L. REV. 433, 451 (1986).

48. *Id.* at 451.

49. Drug Price Competition and Patent Term Restoration Act, Pub. L. No. 98–417, 98 Stat. 1585 (1984) (codified as amended at 21 U.S.C. § 321 (1984)). For an account of the genesis of the PTRA and its predicted effects on competition and pharmaceutical innovation, see generally Wheaton, *supra* note 47.

50. Wheaton, *supra* note 47, at 454–55.

51. *Id.* at 455.

52. *See, e.g.*, Statman, *supra* note 45, at 145, 149.

53. *See, e.g.*, M. SILVERMAN & P. LEE, *supra* note 5, at 171–83.

54. COMPETITIVE PROBLEMS IN THE DRUG INDUSTRY, 1972: A SUMMARY AND ANALYSIS AND DISCUSSION OF ISSUES ON HEARINGS BEFORE THE SENATE SUBCOMM. ON MONOPOLY, SELECT COMM. ON SMALL BUSINESS DURING THE NINETIETH AND NINETY-FIRST CONGRESSES, 92ND CONG., 2D SESS. 17 (Comm. Print 1972) [hereinafter SUMMARY AND ANALYSIS OF HEARINGS].

55. UNITED STATES DEP'T OF HEALTH, EDUC. & WELFARE TASK FORCE ON PRESCRIPTION DRUGS, FINAL REPORT 11 (1969) [hereinafter HEW TASK FORCE, FINAL REPORT]. *See also* M. SILVERMAN & P. LEE, *supra* note 5, at 174.

56. *See, e.g.*, STAFF OF SENATE SPECIAL COMM. ON AGING, PRESCRIPTION DRUG PRICES: ARE WE GETTING OUR MONEY'S WORTH?, 101ST CONG., 2D SESS. 31 app. I (Comm. Print 1989) (examples in table) [hereinafter ARE WE GETTING OUR MONEY'S WORTH?]; SUMMARY AND ANALYSIS OF HEARINGS, supra note 54, at 15 (prices charged retail and institutional markets often vary by as much as several thousand percent); Williams, *More Firms Give Medicaid Breaks on Drugs*, L.A. Times, Sept. 17, 1990, at D1, col. 5 (review of prices of 8 drugs reveals price differentials of 14%–35% between average wholesale price and prices charged to hospitals).

drugs sold to those institutions. This practice has been extremely successful in bringing drugs to the attention of physicians and creating brand loyalty. Brand loyalty is created in two ways: the physician obtains experience and knowledge about a particular drug and the physicians becomes *accustomed* to prescribing the brand name drug, a result referred to as brand name recall, or habitual prescribing.[57] There is no doubt about the effectiveness of this process: the majority of prescriptions written are for brand name, not generic drugs.[58]

Another industry practice, offering discounts on drug purchases, is more pervasive than, yet often hard to distinguish from, price differentials. The average wholesale price (AWP) of a drug published in drug price list books serves as an umbrella under which prices are discounted rather than reflecting actual prices.[59] Manufacturers have elaborate pricing systems using the AWP as a ceiling and discounting according to the benefits to market share expected from the sale.[60] Community pharmacies, usually charged the highest prices, rarely pay more than 10% below the AWP, and often pay much less.[61] AWPs often go unchanged for years because they have so little to do with the actual prices of the drugs.[62]

IV. GOVERNMENT REGULATION OF THE PHARMACEUTICAL INDUSTRY

The drug industry was able to grow rapidly not only because its structure evolved in an atmosphere relatively free from close examination, but also because it developed in a fairly unrestrictive regulatory setting. Laws passed early in the industry's history were directed at adulteration and preventing outlandish and false claims made directly to consumers. Requirements for proof of safety did not come about until the Federal Food, Drug and Cosmetic Act of 1938.[63] The 1962 amendments to the Act added a number of requirements to the drug approval process, including proof of efficacy, thereby transforming the drug approval

57. *See* Leffler, *Persuasion or Information? The Economics of Prescription Drug Advertising* 24 J.L. & Econ. 45, 52–64 (1981) (examination of drug advertising to determine effects on physicians and market, concluding that getting the drug to the doctor through promotion provides information to doctors and promotes "brand name recall' or "habit formation" in prescribing practice and is worth the cost).

58. *See, e.g.*, United States Dep't of Commerce, United States Industrial Outlook—1991 (Drugs) 45-3,4 (1991) (generics accounted for 30% of the value of all prescriptions dispensed in 1989).

59. *See, e.g.*, Medical Econ Co., Drug Topics' Red Book 109–752 (1989) (yearly list of AWPs and retail and direct prices, where provided).

60. *See, e.g.*, HEW Task Force, The Drug Makers, *supra* note 10, at 32–33 (statement of drug industry employee commenting on drug industry's elaborate "selling plans").

61. *See, e.g.*, Are We Getting Our Money's Worth?, *supra* note 56, at 12 (independent retail pharmacists typically receive 13% discounts); Conlan, *AWP Prices for Medicaid Plans Comes Under New Attack*, Drug topics, Dec. 11, 1989, at 48 (citing 15.5% below AWP discount figure).

62. Are We Getting Our Money's Worth?, *supra* note 56, at 12.

63. Federal Food, Drug and Cosmetic Act of 1938, ch. 675, 52 Stat. 1040 (1938) (codified as amended at 21 U.S.C. §§ 301-392 (1988)).

process and giving the FDA much more authority over the process.[64] The drug industry lobbied for changes soon after the 1962 amendments were enacted, asserting that the Act's burdensome requirements caused a decline in the rate of innovation and added unnecessary costs to the drug development process.[65] Although the industry did not succeed in implementing major changes, many of its proposals have been integrated into the drug approval process for AIDS drugs and for other drugs made to treat life threatening conditions.[66] Despite extensive government cut backs in the regulatory process for AIDS drugs, and contrary to drug industry representations that the lengthy drug approval process was the reason behind the escalating prices, the drug industry has failed to respond with lower prices for AIDS drugs.

A. Early Attempts at Policing the Industry

Although Congress had passed legislation aimed at prohibiting the importation of adulterated drugs as early as 1848, it was not until the late nineteenth and early twentieth centuries that Congress took measures to prohibit the sale of adulterated drugs produced in this country.[67] While the Federal Pure Food and Drugs Act of 1906[68] prohibited false and misleading statements in the labeling of drugs, it did little to prevent the sale of impure or unsafe drugs.[69] The 1906 Act was amended in 1912 to prohibit false therapeutic claims, but the Act was still unable to reach issues of safety.[70]

Enforcement of the Act was far from rigorous in the midst of the pro-business political climate of the 1920s. The responsibile agency took the approach of regulating through negotiation and was consequently accused of colluding with

64. Kefauver-Harris Amendments to the Federal Food Drug and Cosmetic Act, Pub. L. No. 87–781, 76 Stat. 780 (1962) (codified as amended at 21 U.S.C. §§ 321, 331, 332, 348, 351–353, 355, 357–360, 372, 374, 376, 381 (1988)).

65. *See, e.g.,* PMA FACT BOOK, supra note 13, at 42 (noting observers' conclusions that decline in innovation was the result of cost of drug amendments).

66. *See infra* test accompanying notes 95–113.

67. Young, *Drugs and the 1906 Law* [hereinafter Young, *Drugs and the Law*], *in* SAFEGUARDING THE PUBLIC, *supra* note 11, at 147–57. Between 1871 and 1905, approximately 200 bills addressing food and drug adulteration were introduced. M. SILVERMAN & P. LEE, *supra* note 5, at 83.

68. Federal Pure Food and Drugs Act of 1906, Pub. L. No. 384, ch. 3915, § 8, 34 Stat. 768, 771 (1906).

69. *See* H. GRABOWSKI, DRUG REGULATION AND INNOVATION: EMPIRICAL EVIDENCE AND POLICY OPTIONS 12–14 (1976). There was no distinction made between prescription and proprietary, or over-the-counter, drugs for purposes of labeling requirements under the 1906 Act. *Id.* at 12 n.2.

70. The Sherley Amendment, ch. 352, 37 Stat. 416 (1912). The Sherley Amendment of 1912 banned false and misleading therapeutic claims made by patent or proprietary brand or trade name medicines directly to the public medicine manufacturers, i.e., manufacturers who sell. The amendment was passed in response to Johnson v. United States, 221 U.S. 488 (1911), in which the Supreme Court agreed with the drug manufacturers that the prohibition in the 1906 Act against false and misleading statements did not apply to therapeutic claims.

the industry.[71] The agency believed that more could be achieved by assisting the industry with its technological quality control problems than through the product seizures provided for in the Act.[72]

B. Regulating a Growing Industry: Concerns about Safety

The Depression brought about heightened public scrutiny of business and an atmosphere of fierce competition characterized by false and deceptive practices by the industry, prompting increased enforcement efforts by the FDA.[73] In response to numerous deaths resulting from the sale of an elixir sulpha drug, Congress passed the Federal Food, Drug and Cosmetic Act in 1938 which enhanced the government's authority over false and misleading claims, and, most importantly, required the FDA to approve drugs on the basis of safety criteria.[74] On opposing this Act, the pharmaceutical industry argued that requiring evidence of safety would cripple research efforts and cause a delay in getting new drugs to market.[75]

Under section 505 of the Act, the manufacturer was required to submit a New Drug Application (NDA) with evidence attesting to the drug's safety.[76] If the application satisfied the regulatory criteria and the FDA took no action within a specified period of time, then the application became ''effective'' and the drug was approved for marketing.[77]

C. Congress is Ready to Regulate

In 1959, the Kefauver hearings into drug pricing and competition in the pharmaceutical industry commenced. Kefauver believed that regulatory legislation was needed to cure many of the ills which were revealed during the hearings: above average profit levels, false and misleading claims made in promoting the drugs, the lack of price competition in the industry, the huge markups on drugs, and the amount of money spent on promotion. Despite these obvious problems, Kefauver lacked the necessary support to enact regulating laws.[78]

In the 1950s, however, a crisis reminded the public and Congress of the benefits of regulating the drug industry: the effectiveness of existing safety guidelines prevented the drug Thalidomide from harming large numbers of people in

---

71. Young, *Social History of American Drug Legislation*, in DRUGS IN OUR SOCIETY 217, at 154–55 (P. Talalay ed. 1964). *See also* J. YOUNG, THE MEDICAL MESSIAHS: A SOCIAL HISTORY OF HEALTH QUACKERY IN TWENTIETH CENTURY AMERICA 98–103 (1967) [hereinafter J. YOUNG, MESSIAHS].
72. Young, *Drugs and the Law, supra* note 67, at 154.
73. *See* J. YOUNG, MESSIAHS, *supra* note 71, at 101–04.
74. Federal Food, Drug and Cosmetic Act, ch. 675, 52 Stat. 1040 (1938) (codified as amended at 21 U.S.C. §§ 301-392 (1988)).
75. M. SILVERMAN & P. LEE, *supra* note 5, at 87.
76. Federal Food, Drug and Cosmetic Act, ch. 675, § 505, 52 Stat. at 1052–53 (1938).
77. *Id.*
78. *See* M. SILVERMAN & P. LEE, *supra* note 5, at 112–14.

the United States.[79] Congress reacted by strengthening existing regulations by enacting the most stringent laws that it had ever passed in the area of drug regulation, the 1962 Kefauver-Harris Amendments.[80]

The major changes made by the amendments include the following: pre-marketing FDA approval;[81] substantial proof of efficacy requirements;[82] and substantial evidence of safety and efficacy from adequate and well-controlled studies over which the FDA was given more authority.[83] Subsequent regulations required that drug promotion be limited to claims the veracity of which had been established before the FDA, and that the promotions include information about side effects and contraindications.[84]

The 1962 amendments increased FDA involvement in the pre-market testing and clinical trial process. The drug manufacturer is now required to submit an Investigational New Drug application (IND) and information about preclinical testing of the drug to the FDA for review.[85] To promote quality control in manufacturing, the provisions for registration and inspection of manufacturing establishments were added.[86] With the added criteria of effectiveness and requirements for more clinical studies, there was no doubt that the 1962 amendments would change the drug development process, increasing the amount of time that it would take to get a drug through the approval process and increasing the safety and efficacy of drugs which ultimately reached the consumer.

The present drug approval process involves pre-clinical R & D, clinical testing and the FDA review of the NDA. After pre-clinical R & D—testing in animals for biological activity and safety—the drug's sponsor files an IND with the FDA to obtain approval for clinical testing in humans.[87] The clinical trial process includes three distinct phases of testing, each building on and dependent upon the results of the previous phase.[88] These trials test for safety and effectiveness and assess the risks, side effects and adverse effects of the drug;[89] they take five to seven years to complete.[90]

Upon completion of the third phase of testing, the drug company or sponsor

---

79. *See* H. Dowling, *supra* note 6, at 200–02.
80. The Kefauver-Harris Amendments, Pub. L. No. 87-781, 76 Stat. 780 (1962) (codified as amended at 21 U.S.C. §§ 321, 331, 332, 351-353, 355, 357-360, 372, 374, 376, 381 (1988)).
81. 21 U.S.C. § 355(a).
82. *Id.* at § 355(d).
83. *Id.* at § 355(e) (l).
84. S. Peltzman, Regulation of Pharmaceutical Innovation: The 1962 Amendments 9 (1974) (discussing effects of 1962 amendments on R & D and on the drug development process).
85. 21 U.S.C. § 355(i).
86. *Id.* at § 360.
87. 21 C.F.R. § 312.23 (1990); Gordon, *The Drug Development and Approval Process*, in Pharmaceutical Mfr. Ass'n, New medicines in Review 5 (1990).
88. 21 C.F.R. § 312.2(a)-(c) (1990); Gordon, *supra* note 87. Ember, *FDA Presses to Speed Life-Saving Drugs to Marketplace,* Chemical & Engineering News, Sept. 25, 1989, at 10.
89. 21 C.F.R. § 312.21(c) (1990); Ember, *supra* note 88. Under 21 C.F.R. § 312.42 (1990), the FDA has the authority to place a clinical hold on the clinical trial process halting the studies until the problems are resolved.
90. 21 C.F.R. § 312.21(a)-(c) (1990); Gordon, *supra* note 87; Ember, *supra* note 88.

files an NDA to obtain FDA approval for marketing.[91] The FDA reviews the information, which takes two to three years, and either issues an approval letter or takes other action, such as a request for further information.[92]

D. Government Regulation in Response to the AIDS Crisis

The entire drug development process takes approximately ten to twelve years.[93] For people with AIDS and other life-threatening diseases for which drug therapy is the only available treatment, ten years is a frighteningly long period of time. In response to the life-threatening nature of the disease and to pressure from AIDS advocates and pharmaceutical manufacturers, the FDA has been streamlining its drug approval process in a variety of ways, allowing for the approval of a number of AIDS drugs in an unusually short time. The FDA continues to develop policies and regulations to address the needs of people with life-threatening illnesses. The process involves balancing the need for access to these drugs with the FDA's duty to assure that only drugs which meet established safety and efficacy criteria reach consumers.

1. Expedited Review Process In 1987, the FDA created the "1-AA" designation process, an expedited approval process to assure that all potential AIDS therapies received the highest priority for review.[94] This classification system, an extension of the existing review system for NDAs significantly shortened the time required to approve a drug. Azidothymidine (AZT), the first drug approved for the treatment of HIV infection, completed the NDA portion of the approval process in a record-setting three and one-half months.[95] The expedited review process may also bring drugs used to treat AIDS-related illnesses to market at a much faster rate than would have occurred in the normal drug approval process.[96]

Another reason for AZT's speedy approval was the early consultation between the FDA and the drug manufacturer, Burroughs-Wellcome, regarding the design of preclinical and clinical trials. Successes in early trials led the FDA to the rare decision to combine Phase II and Phase III trials[97] and provide greater

91. *See generally* 21 C.F.R. Part 314 (1990).

92. *See* 21 C.F.R. § 314.100–314.170 (1990).

93. *See, e.g.*, Jackson, *Unpublished Study Pegs Cost of New Drug at $231 Million,* THE SCIENTIST, June 25, 1990, at 5 (unpublished study conducted by Tufts University Center for the Study of Drug Development concluded that it now takes 12 years to bring a drug to market).

94. OFFICE OF THE SECRETARY OF HEALTH, STATUS OF PRODUCTS FOR THE TREATMENT OF AIDS AND AIDS-RELATED DISEASES 3–08 (draft) (March 5,1990) [hereinafter STATUS OF AIDS DRUGS].

95. *See* Ember, *supra* note 88, at 9–10.

96. *Id.* at 11. Cancer drugs have received highest priority status as well under the "1C" designation. *Id.* Many have gone through the FDA approval process in one year or less. *Id.*

97. Phase III trials involve a sample of 1,000 to 3,000 people afflicted with the specified disease. These trials are designed to obtain further information about the safety and effectiveness of the drug in order to assess the risks and benefits associated with the use of the drug. 21 C.F.R. § 312.21(c); Gordon, *supra* note 87.

access to the drugs.[98] In 1988, the FDA formalized this process, often referred to as the Bush Initiative, through regulations which provide sponsors with the opportunity to consult FDA officials regarding the clinical testing of products intended to treat life-threatening or severely debilitating illnesses early in the development process.[99]

These regulations provide the FDA with more flexibility in the drug approval process. If the studies demonstrate that the benefits of the drug outweigh the risks, the FDA is authorized to cancel Phase III studies and request that the sponsor submit a treatment protocol which allows people outside the clinical trial process to receive the drug for treatment use.[100] While the treatment protocol is in effect, the sponsor assembles and submits data to the FDA for review and eventual marketing approval the drug.[101] If the FDA approves the drug, it may ask the sponsor to conduct "Phase IV" post-approval trials to provide additional information on the risks, benefits, and optimal use of the drug.[102]

2. Treatment IND In addition to the regulations providing for an early consultation process, the AIDS crisis hastened the implementation of the "Treatment IND" mechanism. The Treatment IND, similar to the treatment protocol, allows for the earlier treatment use of the drug in people not involved in clinical trials.[103] This option is only available for drugs under clinical investigation for serious or immediately life-threatening diseases in people "for whom no comparable or satisfactory alternative drug or other therapy is available."[104] Under the Treatment IND, participants receive the drug either free of charge or at cost.[105] They may be monitored through collaborative efforts of their physicians, the government or academic medical centers, and the drug sponsor.

Both the Bush Initiative and the Treatment IND are designed for drugs that treat such illnesses as AIDS or cancer. Most would agree that these illnesses present extreme examples of the risk-benefit relationship and that it is more humane to provide the drugs at an earlier time. The decision to distribute the drug

98. Gordon, *supra* note 87.
99. 21 C.F.R. § 312.82 (1990). The process involving early consultation was referred to as the "Bush Initiative" after the then vice-president who chaired the President's Task Force on Regulatory Reform, which was involved in these regulations. Ember, *supra* note 88, at 11. Prior to the AZT review process and the passage of these regulations, drug manufacturers typically did not meet with FDA reviewing officials until the end of Phase II trials. Phase II trials involve 200 to 300 people afflicted with the specified disease, and are "conducted to evaluate the effectiveness of the drug for a particular indication or indications in people with the disease or condition under study" and to determine side effects and risks associated with ingestion of the drug. 21 C.F.R. § 312.21(b).
100. 21 C.F.R. § 312.83 (1991).
101. *Id.*
102. *Id.* at § 312.85 (1991).
103. *Id.* at § 312.84 (1990).
104. *Id.* at § 312.34 (a) (1991).
105. Ember, *supra* note 88, at 11. The drug manufacturer cannot receive profits from sales to people in the Treatment IND program. *Id.*

outside the clinical testing process or eliminate portions of that process, however, cannot be viewed lightly considering the benefits derived from thorough investigation. In the absence of these clinical trials, Phase III in particular, the drug would be tested on only a few hundred subjects and for only three years. This creates the risk of placing drugs on the market which have unknown adverse side effects or long term negative effects.

In referring to the implementation of the Bush Initiative, one FDA reviewing official commented that "[t]here is no question that the initiative arose directly from the urgency people felt about getting answers about AIDS."[106] Without the efforts of AIDS advocacy groups and others both inside and outside of the FDA bureaucracy, it is unlikely that either the Bush Initiative or the Treatment IND would have been incorporated into the FDA regulations.

3. Parallel Track Proposal The need and demand for earlier access to AIDS drugs has prompted a third proposal, the parallel track approach, which has been suggested as a policy by the Public Health Service in coordination with the FDA.[107] According to the published proposed policy statement, the parallel track mechanism, or expanded access protocol, would provide expanded availability of investigational drugs for people with AIDS and HIV-related diseases.[108] This approach places certain carefully selected drugs on a "fast track," giving people not involved in the clinical trials access to the drugs after safety has been established in Phase I trials.[109] The drugs chosen would be distributed through physicians who would be required to report safety and efficacy data.[110] The information provided by the physicians in the "studies" would not be as extensive as the information collected through the clinical trial process but the policy allows for wider participation in the investigative process. To be eligible for the parallel track program, a person must have an HIV-related illness, be unable to participate in the controlled trials, and be unable to take the standard treatment of approved drugs.[111]

The evidence of safety and effectiveness required before a drug could be approved under the expanded access protocol is less than that required for Treatment IND approval. In addition, before a company could charge for drugs provided through the parallel track program, it first must obtain approval from the

106. *Id.* at 12 (quoting Robert J. Temple, Director of FDA's Office of Drug Evaluation I).
107. Public Health Service, Expanded Availability of INDs through Parallel Track Mechanism for People with AIDS, Proposed Policy Statement, 55 Fed. Reg. 20,856 (1990).
108. *Id.*
109. *See* Ember, *supra* note 88, at 9–13; Status of AIDS Drugs, *supra* note 94, at 3–09. Phase I trials are conducted on a relatively small group of approximately 20–80 people with AIDS or other diseases, or on healthy volunteers. These trials are designed to ascertain the safety of the drug by determining the metabolism and pharmacologic actions of the drug and any side effects associated with increased dosage. 21 C.F.R. § 312.21(a) (1990); Ember, *supra* note 88, at 10.
110. 55 Fed. Reg. 20,858–20,859.
111. *Id.* at 20,858.

FDA,[112] which would monitor the studies and could terminate them if certain criteria are present.[113]

Although, for obvious reasons, AIDS advocacy groups would prefer earlier access to the drugs, the parallel track approach presents problems. Most would agree that drugs should be subject to rigorous and controlled testing, particularly against placebos, and that such studies further important research goals and provide assurances as to the safety and efficacy of the drugs. The parallel track would allow people to receive the drug after fewer than 100 subjects have received the drug in a highly controlled setting. This raises concerns about the effects on those people who receive the drug outside the clinical trial setting and who do not have the benefit of strict review and monitoring given to participants in clinical trials. Side effects and serious adverse effects may go unnoticed or untreated. In addition, earlier and expanded access to the drugs may encourage participants in clinical trials to abandon those studies or alter those studies' results by taking other drugs. This may be detrimental to the validity and effectiveness of the ongoing trials.

The drug approval process has never before experienced the rapid changes brought about in response to the AIDS crisis. The effect of these changes may not be realized for years, but it is clear that in the case of the AIDS drugs approved thus far, the changes have brought drugs to market at a much faster rate than those drugs subject to the normal drug approval process. The risks and benefits to be considered are much more extreme and in some ways easier to examine in the context of AIDS.

As a result of the speedier drug approval process, one would expect lower priced products. As discussed below, this has not been the case with AIDS drugs. The industry, demonstrating its inability to enact rapid changes in its pricing policies, continues to justify its prices and profits on the costs of R & D.

IV. THE INDUSTRY'S JUSTIFICATION FOR PRICES AND PROFITS: RESEARCH AND DEVELOPMENT

Since the time that the pharmaceutical industry discovered the profitability of penicillin and other wonder drugs, it has continuously devoted more and more resources to R & D in the search for newer, more profitable products and has justified its prices and profits on the costs of R & D. While it was true during the first twenty years of the R & D intensive industry that pumping more and more into R & D produced pharmaceutical innovations, the 1960s brought that theory into doubt. Beginning in 1960, the rate of new drug introductions began to decline rapidly and has never returned to the pre-1960 "golden era," despite huge increases in R & D budgets. The industry has blamed this decline on the requirements of the 1962 amendments to the Federal Food, Drug and Cosmetic Act and the "drug lag" produced by them. The industry blames the escalated costs of R

112. *Id.* at 20,859.
113. *Id.* at 20,802 (1990) (to be codified at 21 C.F.R. pt. 312) (proposed May 21, 1990).

& D and, in turn, the prices of drugs on the number and extent of tests required and the lengthy approval process. Others, however, attribute the decline in innovation to the lack of efficiency in the industry and the depletion of scientific knowledge, or the ''scientific plateau,'' brought about by the number of advances made in the 1940s and 1950s, and the industry's unwillingness to reassess the direction of its R & D efforts in light of these factors.[114]

The AIDS crisis has provided a testing ground for the industry's arguments. Manufacturers developed AIDS drugs in record time, at a cost well below the most recent estimate of $231 million to develop one drug.[115] Government agencies have conducted more research on AIDS drugs than in any other area of drug research, with the possible exception of cancer drugs. Government and industry have rarely worked so closely and quickly to develop new drugs. Despite the hurried regulatory setting in which AIDS drugs are developed, they are some of the most expensive drugs that the industry has to offer, and they no doubt provide a large profit to the companies that manufacture them. In justifying these prices, charged to the people most in need of treatment, the industry cannot hide behind the rubric of high costs of R & D and the lengthy approval process.

A. Past Successes of the Industry

The early years of the modern R & D intensive pharmaceutical industry read more like a fairy tale than the development of an American industry. During the 1940s, 192 NCEs were discovered.[116] The 1950s brought continued and greater success with the discovery of thirty-four NCEs.[117]

The industry experienced not only unparalleled success in discoveries, but also in sales and profits. In 1951, for example, thirty-four NCEs were introduced at a cost of $1.5 million per drug[118] in an average time of one year.[119] Twenty years after the introduction of those drugs, the average annual rate of growth in sales revenue was 10.8%.[120]

Although the industry had been regulated by the federal government, it was unique in comparison to other R & D industries in that it did not rely on federal financing for its R & D activities.[121] The industry's reluctance may have been due, in part, to a desire to maintain control over the profits realized from research.[122] As of 1960, only 2% of the industry's R & D budget was obtained through government contracts; the remainder was industry financed.[123]

---

114. *See generally* H. Grabowski, *supra* note 69, at 17–25 (discussing the various courses associated with the decline in innovation).
115. *See* Jackson, *supra* note 93, at 5.
116. PMA Fact Book, *supra* note 13, at 40.
117. M. Statman, *supra* note 15, at 28.
118. *Id.*
119. *Id.* at 29.
120. *Id.* at 71 (for the years 1967–1975, for drugs introduced in 1951).
121. HEW Task Force, The Drug makers, *supra* note 10, at 15.
122. *Id.* at 15. The Task Force pointed out that certain patents developed with the assistance or financing of federal monies revert to the federal government. *Id.*
123. PMA Fact Book, *supra* note 13, at 38 (figures relate to PMA member corporations).

The 1960s brought a decline in the level of innovation. There were eighteen fewer drugs introduced in 1960 than in 1959, signifying a change in the trend established in the prior two decades.[124] By 1962, the number had decreased to twenty-six drugs, with the cost of development increasing by 30% over the costs of developing drugs in the late 1950s.[125] The total number of NCEs introduced in the 1960s was 215, 38% less than in the 1950s, and at eight to ten times the cost.[126] While the industry complained that the high cost of R & D resulted from the changes made by the Kefauver-Harris amendments, the National Academy of Sciences/National Research Council found[127] that over 15% of the drugs approved prior to 1962 were ineffective for all the conditions for which they were intended.[128] According to the *Medical Letter on Drugs and Therapeutics*, only thirty-two significant therapeutic advances were introduced in the 1960s.[129]

Although the industry historically has dominated in the field of drug research and development, the government has expanded its involvement in the area of chemical drug research. The first big leap came in 1955 when the National Cancer Institute initiated a program to find drugs to cure cancer.[130] Since then, a number of drug research programs have been established by the various Institutes of Health and other agencies.[131] The government has provided its most extensive research and development efforts in the area of AIDS and cancer drugs, and has obtained a number of patents on drug discoveries, usually licensing their development and manufacture to private firms.[132]

In the case of AIDS research, collaborative efforts among the industry, academia and government have brought about the development of AIDS drugs through advances made in the areas of immunology and virology. Despite the collaborative nature of these efforts, however, pharmaceutical companies have not been forthcoming in acknowledging the contributions made to AIDS drugs by the government.[133]

B. The Industry's Response to the Law of Diminishing Returns

By 1970, it was fairly clear that the golden era of drug discovery had come to an end and that there needed to be an assessment of the direction that the industry

---

124. M. STATMAN, *supra* note 15, at 28.
125. *Id.*
126. *Id.* The cost of developing a drug in 1960 was $5 million; in 1970, the cost was $48 million. *Id.*
127. P. BROOKE, *supra* note 37, at 22.
128. *Id.*
129. Council on Economic Priorities, *In Whose Hands? Safety, Efficacy, and Research Productivity in the Pharmaceutical Industry*, in 4 ECON. PRIORITIES REP. 48 table 10 (Aug./Nov. 1973).
130. H. DOWLING, *supra* note 6, at 36.
131. *Id.*
132. For a discussion on the development of drugs for the treatment of AIDS, *see infra* text accompanying notes 151–193.
133. *See* Haigler, *Reduced Dosage Cuts Cost of AIDS Drug*, N.Y. Times, Sept. 16, 1989, at A26 (Letters), col. 3; Mitsuya, *Credit Government Scientists With Developing Anti-AIDS Drug*, N.Y. Times, Sept. 28, 1989, at A26 (Letters), col. 3 (responding to Haigler letter, providing a chronology of AZT's development and pointing out the essential role of government scientists in developing the drug).

was taking. Prompted by reports of continued high profit margins and increasing prices, Congress conducted an investigation into the industry in the late 1960s and early 1970s.[134] The years of hearings and voluminous reports revealed the industry's use of patents on drugs offering little or no therapeutic improvements, to gain a competitive edge in the market.[135] The duplicative research efforts of companies, which only served to produce more therapeutically similar products at a cost borne by consumers, was criticized as wasteful.[136] Although firms in the industry continued to increase their R & D budgets, the rate of growth slowed as did the rate of new product introduction.[137] Along with the 1980s came the most dramatic increases in R & D expenditures, quadrupling in the span of ten years from $2 billion in 1980 to $8.2 billion in 1990.[138]

Increased R & D expenditures represent the industry's continued adherence to the theory that more money will automatically result in more innovation. The 1980s have demonstrated the fallacy of that assumption. By one estimate, the top twenty-five drug makers spent $7 billion to bring fifty-four NCEs, with little or no potential of therapeutic gain over existing therapies, to market between 1981–1988.[139] As one author points out, "the development of New Chemical Entities of this kind [offering little or no therapeutic improvement to existing therapies] will be costly as that of drugs with revolutionary impact on hitherto unsolved problems of therapy."[140]

C. Financial Incentives for the Industry

Competition in the pharmaceutical industry has been characterized by the introduction of new, higher priced drugs. According to a study partially funded by the PMA, the cost of developing a new drug has soared to $231 million,[141] almost double the $125 million reported in 1985.[142] Prices have increased phenomenally since 1980; in that period, the consumer price index for prescription drugs has risen 150%.[143] The industry has argued that the regulatory delay in the approval process accounts for the increased costs of R & D and the increased prices.[144]

134. *See generally Competitive Problems in the Drug Industry, Hearings Before the Senate Subcomm. on Monopoly of the Select Comm. on Small Business*, Parts 1–23 (1968–1973).
135. SUMMARY AND ANALYSIS OF HEARINGS, *supra* note 54, at 26.
136. *See id.* at 27–31.
137. *See, e.g.*, PMA 1989 NEW DRUG APPROVALS, *supra* note 22 (R & D investment chart); Grabowski, *An Analysis of US International Competitiveness in Pharmaceuticals*, MANAGERIAL & DECISION ECON. (Special Issue) 27, 28 (1989).
138. PMA, 1989 NEW DRUG APPROVALS, *supra* note 22.
139. ARE WE GETTING OUR MONEY'S WORTH?, *supra* note 56, at 7.
140. H. REDWOOD, *supra* note 4, at 194.
141. Jackson, *supra* note 93, at 5.
142. The $125 million figure has been cited often since it was first reported through a study in 1986 conducted for PMA. *See, e.g.*, Gordon, *supra* note 87.
143. Interview with Christopher Jennings, *supra* note 24.
144. *See, e.g.*, *Health and the Environment—Part 2: Hearings on H.R. 1663 Before the Subcomm. on Health and the Environment, House Comm. on Energy and Commerce*, 97th Cong., 1st Sess. 83–84 (1981) (prepared statement of Lewis Engman, President of PMA, in which he discusses the effects of regulatory burdens on the costs of R & D).

While it is true that drugs are subject to one of the most intensive regulatory processes, they have received a considerable amount of "special treatment" through legislation designed to enhance the incentives for their development. In recent years, Congress has provided the industry with patent term extension legislation,[145] tax credits for R & D activity,[146] and seven year marketing exclusivity privileges under the Orphan Drug Act.[147] Additionally, profits from manufacturing operations in Puerto Rico and other United States territories are exempt from federal taxes,[148] under laws originally enacted over fifty years ago, to provide incentives for economic development in these areas.[149]

Despite these financial incentives, the industry and many of its proponents continue to call for more tax breaks for R & D activity, an accelerated regulatory process, and higher prices.[150] AIDS-related drugs are subject to a number of these R & D cost breaks *and* an accelerated drug approval process. Contrary to theory and the industry's argument, however, providing these financial incentives to manufacturers has not brought down the prices charged for these drugs.

VI. THE DEVELOPMENT OF AIDS DRUGS

Just as the industry began to devote unprecedented amounts to its R & D budgets and geared up to address the increased competition coming from Japan, the AIDS crisis hit. Although the industry was slow to respond with drug development, R & D intensive firms, particularly those involved in anti-viral research, jumped in after the virus was discovered and after the extent of the affected population

145. Drug Price Competition and Patent Term Restoration Act of 1984, Pub. L. No. 98–417, 98 Stat. 1585 (1984) (codified as amended at 15 U.S.C. §§ 68b, 68c, 70b (1988); 21 U.S.C. §§ 301, 360cc (1988); 28 U.S.C. § 2201 (1988); 35 U.S.C. §§ 156, 271, 282 (1988)). Next to Sweden, which has a 28 month drug approval period, the United States has the longest drug approval process, at 23 months. COMPETITIVE ASSESSMENT, *supra* note 20, at 48.

146. 26 U.S.C. § 41 (1988). *See also* ARE WE GETTING OUR MONEY'S WORTH?, *supra* note 56, at 8.

147. The Orphan Drug Act, Pub. L. No. 97–414, 96 Stat 2049 (1983) (codified as amended at 21 U.S.C. §§ 360aa-360ee (1988)).

148. *See, e.g.*, Goozner, *Tax Laws Taking Jobs, Workers Claim,* Chicago Tribune, Sept. 27, 1990, § 2 at 1 (large pharmaceutical plant in Illinois to be closed to shift production to facilities in Puerto Rico built three years ago to take advantage of tax benefits); *see also* Pharmaceutical Mfr. Ass'n, Information Packet Accompanying Slide Presentation 26 (1989) (lists Puerto Rico's political status among the 12 issues pending for the industry).

149. *See, e.g.*, Wolpert, *Pharmaceutical Capital of the World,* GLOBAL TRADE, July 1988, at 38. Lyphomed, for example, the manufacturer of one of the leading AIDS-related drugs, Pentamidine, recently set up manufacturing facilities in the Virgin Islands to take advantage of the tax breaks. LYPHOMED, INC., ANNUAL REPORT 1989 6–7 (1990) [hereinafter LYPHOMED 1989 REPORT] (damage caused by Hurricane Hugo limited 1989 tax benefits attributable to Puerto Rican operations). *See also* sources cited *supra* note 148.

150. *See* Miller, *Productivity and Competition: A Look at the Pharmaceutical Industry,* COLUM. J. WORLD BUS., Fall 1988, at 85–88 (pharmaceutical industry is one of the most competitive in the international market and needs to be given larger tax breaks for funds to promote innovation); Vagelos, *R & D: Good Medicine for the World,* ACROSS THE BOARD, May 1987, at 22, 27 (need for stronger national and international incentives).

became known. Currently sixty-four firms are involved in the development of eighty-eight drugs and vaccines.[151]

Despite intensive government involvement and resources, changes in the regulatory and policy processes of drug approval, and hefty financial incentives, AIDS drugs are expensive. The government has helped the industry achieve success in the area of AIDS drugs; it is now time for the industry to respond by lowering prices. Thus far, changes in prices as well as in regulations and policy have come about primarily through political pressure exerted by AIDS activists and groups. The following discussion explains the development of AIDS drugs and provides insight into why the government and AIDS activists are calling for an end to industry price gouging.

A. The First AIDS Drug is Developed

April 1984 brought the first major breakthrough in AIDS research: the discovery of the human immunodeficiency virus (HIV), a retrovirus referred to as human T-cell lymphotropic virus type III (HTLV-III).[152] Despite the prevailing view that drug development was inherently unfeasible for treating human retroviruses, the National Cancer Institute (NCI), in conjunction with the National Institute of Health (NIH), developed a drug screening system in mid-1984.[153] The NCI asked pharmaceutical companies to make drugs in their stocks available for testing on the virus.[154] Burroughs-Wellcome (B-W) sent azidothymidine (AZT).[155] AZT was first synthesized in 1964 through research funded by the NCI. Although thought at the time to be a possible antitumor agent, AZT proved ineffective for that use.[156]

In February 1985, the NCI conducted experiments with AZT and determined that the drug inhibited the HTLV-III in vitro.[157] After the drug's activity against the virus was determined, B-W and the NCI reached an agreement that B-W would continue to supply the drug for possible future injection into human beings and the NCI would make available to B-W a supply of thymidine, a necessary component of AZT, while B-W searched for a supplier.[158]

After successful initial testing, AZT was given to humans in clinical trials.[159] When, in September 1986 during Phase II testing, the results revealed a significant

151. PHARMACEUTICAL MFR. ASS'N, AIDS MEDICINES IN DEVELOPMENT, 1991 [hereinafter, 1991 AIDS MEDICINES].

152. *See generally* Gallo, Salahuddin & Popovic, *Frequent Detection and Isolation of Cytopathic Retroviruses (HTLV-III) From Patients With AIDS and at Risk for AIDS,* 224 SCIENCE 500 (1984) (discussing AIDS-causing virus).

153. *See* Yarchoan & Broder, *Development of Antiretroviral Therapy of the Acquired Immunodeficiency Syndrome and Related Disorders: A Progress Report,* 316 NEW ENG. J. MED. 557, 558 (1987).

154. *AIDS, Drugs, Need and Greed,* N.Y. Times, Sept. 29, 1989, at A34, col. 1.

155. *Id.*

156. *AIDS Issues (Part I): Cost and Availability of AZT: Hearings Before the House Subcomm. on Health and the Environment, Comm. on Energy and Commerce,* 100th Cong., 1st Sess. 31 (1987) (Statement of R. Windom) [hereinafter *Hearings on AZT*].

157. *Id.* at 33.

158. *Id.* at 31.

159. *Id.* at 7 (statement of T. E. Haigler).

difference in survival rates between patients who received the placebo and those treated with AZT, the trials were halted.[160] A Treatment IND was then approved to allow more patients access to AZT.[161] This highly unusual action of foregoing trials resulted in the approval of AZT in March 1987, only two and a half years after the NCE's initial request for drugs.[162]

Zidovudine, as the drug is now called, was provided to people with AIDS under this Treatment IND, through a system of AIDS Treatment Evaluation Units (ATEUs).[163] Participants in the clinical trials received the drug free of charge; those who received it outside the clinical trial process could be charged for the drug but the manufacturer was not permitted to reap a profit from the sales.[164] Clinical testing on AZT continues through the various protocols.

B. Other AIDS and AIDS-Related Drugs

The government was not only a primary moving force behind the development of AZT, but it has developed and owns two other promising drugs, both of which are analogues of AZT. The drug Dideoxyinosine (ddI), licensed to Bristol-Myers Squibb Company, has received unusual treatment from the FDA.[165] After encouraging results were observed in early trials, the FDA agreed to approve a treatment IND and allowed wider availability of the drug under an open safety protocol in parallel with the Phase II controlled clinical trials.[166] This expanded access program the first of its kind allowed for distribution of the drug to 23,000 patients.[167] In October 1991, the FDA approved ddI although tests have not been completed.[168] As one scientist stated about the controversial decision, "It is a decision based on scientific hunch and a policy decision that we need another drug other than AZT."[169]

The second drug developed by scientists at the NIH was Dideoxycytidine (ddC). It was licensed to Hoffman-LaRoche and was also approved for participation in an expanded access program.[170] In order to be eligible for the program, however, a person must be unable to take AZT or ddI.[171] AIDS activists have criticized this restriction, arguing that any person with AIDS who has not benefitted from AZT, regardless of whether that person has taken ddI, should be allowed the opportunity to try ddC.[172]

---

160. Yarchoan & Broder, *supra* note 153, at 562.
161. *Hearings on AZT, supra* note 156, at 32 (statement of R. E. Windom).
162. *Id.* at 33.
163. *Id.* at 30.
164. *Id.* at 8 (statement of T. Haigler); Ember, *supra* note 88, at 11.
165. Dideoxyinosine (ddI) is manufactured by Bristol-Myers Squibb Co., under the trade name VIDEX. 1991 AIDS MEDICINES, *supra* note 151, at 2.
166. Marx, *New AIDS Drug Passes First Clinical Test,* 245 SCIENCE 353, 353 (1989).
167. Gladwell, *Second AIDS Drug Given Conditional Approval,* Wash. Post, Oct. 10, 1991, at A4, col. 1.
168. *Id.*.
169. *Id.*
170. Hilts, *More Eligible for AIDS Drugs,* N.Y. Times, June 1, 1990, at B5, col. 4.
171. *Id.*
172. *Id.*

Other AIDS drugs are being developed, including genetically engineered products, but AZT, ddI and ddC continue to be the primary therapies for the treatment of HIV and AIDS-related illness. Due to the harmful side effects of these drugs and the gradual resistance to them, people with AIDS now typically take the three drugs either in combination at lower doses or in sequence.[173] Doctors now recommend that patients use drug therapy at earlier stages of the disease, as studies show that earlier use of the drugs maintains the functioning of the immune system for longer periods.[174] Many scientists believe that AIDS will be treated with a combination of drug therapies administered at various stages of the disease and that no one drug will be the answer.[175]

Until the recent approval of ddI, AZT had been the only approved medicine for treatment of HIV disease for five years.[176] For the treatment of illnesses associated with AIDS, most significantly pneumocystis carinii pneumonia (PCP) and Kaposi's sarcoma, twelve drugs have been approved.[177] In response to concern expressed by AIDS activists over the pace of research on drugs for AIDS-related illnesses, the National Institute for Allergic and Infectious Diseases (NIAID) approved more clinical trials on drugs designed to treat AIDS-related diseases.[178] As of October 1991, eighty-eight drugs and vaccines were under development and undergoing clinical testing for the treatment of HIV and AIDS-related diseases.[179] In addition, to assist the clinical trial process, the government established a community-based trial approach—Community Based Clinical Trial (CBCT) Network—in which doctors in the community serve as investigators to supplement the investigations conducted in the traditional large institutional settings.[180] This represents the first time in which community doctors have played such an integral role in the drug research process. As one investigator noted, "[i]f we could develop in this country a research network that could reach even the poor in the trenches, we might get the answers to a lot of questions more quickly."[181]

C. The Orphan Drug Act and AIDS Drugs

In addition to support from the federal government in the form of an accelerated drug approval process and financial and research assistance, developers of AIDS drugs

---

173. Stroud, *Will New Drugs Help Tame the AIDS Virus?,* Investor's Daily, June 27, 1990, at 1; *Experimental AIDS Therapies,* L.A. Times, June 25, 1990, at A21, col. 2.
174. Knox, *Earlier Use of AZT Urged for Those With AIDS Virus,* Boston Globe, June 22, 1990, at 57, col. 1.
175. *See* Stroud, *supra* note 173.
176. 1991 AIDS MEDICINES, *supra* note 151, at 2.
177. *Id.* at 11.
178. *See id.* at 2.
179. *Id.* at 1.
180. Stroud, *AIDS Spurs Novel Approach to Drug Trials,* Investor's Daily, July 31, 1990, Health-Care Business Section, at 1. Currently, 45 cities are involved in the Network across the United States. AMERICAN FOUND. FOR AIDS RESEARCH (AMFAR), AIDS/HIV TREATMENT DIRECTORY 107–08 (Summer 1991).
181. Stroud, *supra* note 180.

have been aided by the Orphan Drug Act (ODA).[182] The ODA was enacted in 1983 to provide financial incentives for the development of orphan drugs, defined under the current Act as drugs for the treatment of diseases or conditions which affect fewer than 200,000 people or for which the sale of the drug would not be profitable enough to cover development costs.[183] By 1990, the FDA had granted 375 orphan designations and had approved forty-one orphan drugs.[184] Congress has amended the ODA three times since 1983,[185] and in 1990, Congressman Henry Waxman moved unsuccessfully to reform the ODA again to address the windfall profits that some manufacturers have realized as a result of orphan drug designation.[186]

The ODA provides two major financial incentives: seven year marketing exclusivity periods, which go into effect after approval of the drug for sale,[187] and tax credits for clinical research conducted on orphan drugs.[188]

AIDS drug developers have taken advantage of the ODA. One half of the drug currently approved for HIV and AIDS-related illnesses have been granted orphan drug status.[189] Of those drugs in development and undergoing clinical testing, over 40% are designated as orphan drugs. This designation delays the onset of competition from other AIDS drugs and enables a manufacturer to charge whatever the market will bear.

Concerned about the abuse of the ODA and the windfall profit levels attained on much needed drugs, AIDS activists have unsuccessfully pressured the FDA's Office of Orphan Products Development to discontinue orphan drug status for certain AIDS drugs,[190] bringing to light some of the problems with the ODA.

---

182. Orphan Drug Act, Pub. L. No. 97-414, 96 Stat. 2049 (1983)(codified as amended at 21 U.S.C. §§ 360aa-360ee (1988)). For a comprehensive review of the Orphan Drug Act, see C. ASHBURY, ORPHAN DRUGS: MEDICAL VERSUS MARKET VALUE (1985).

183. 21 U.S.C.A. § 360bb(a)(2) (West Supp. 1990).

184. *See* HOUSE REPORT ON ORPHAN DRUG AMENDMENTS OF 1990, H.R. REP. NO. 635, 101st Cong., 2d Sess. 3 (1990) [hereinafter HOUSE REPORT ON ORPHAN DRUG AMENDMENTS].

185. The Health Promotion and Disease Prevention Amendments of 1984, Pub. L. No. 98-551, § 4, 98 Stat. 2815, 2817, amended the act to define "rare disease or condition" as one that affects fewer than 200,000 persons. Prior to this amendment, the Act provided no numerical ceiling. This gap created difficulties for the agencies in determining which diseases were "rare." The Orphan Drug Amendments of 1985, Pub. L. No. 99-91, § 2, 99 Stat. 387, 387 removed the provision that only nonpatentable drugs could be granted orphan status. The Orphan Drug Amendments of 1988, Pub. L. No. 100-290, § 2(a), 102 Stat. 90, 90, established the time period for filing a request for orphan designation.

186. *See* HOUSE REPORT ON ORPHAN DRUG AMENDMENTS, *supra* note 184, at 2–3.

187. 21 U.S.C. § 360cc(a). PMA President Gerald Mossinghoff has called the exclusivity provision "by far the most important incentive offered by the Orphan Drug Act." BIOTECHNOLOGY NEWSWATCH, May 7, 1990, at 4.

188. 26 U.S.C. § 28 (1988).

189. *See* OFFICE OF ORPHAN PRODUCTS DEVELOPMENT, ORPHAN DESIGNATIONS THROUGH AUGUST 31, 1991 [hereinafter 1991 ORPHAN DESIGNATION].

190. *See* Letter from Marlene E. Haffner, M.D., Director of the Office of Orphan Products Development, to Jean F. McGuire and Jeffrey Levi, AIDS Action Council (Nov. 30, 1989) (stating in response to a previous letter, that there was no sound basis for discounting the designation of products for AIDS treatment as orphan products), *reprinted in Orphan Drug Act: Hearings Before the Subcomm. on Health and the Environment of the House Comm. on Energy and Commerce*, 101st Cong., 2d Sess. 52–54, (1990)(included in prepared statement by Jean F. McGuire) [hereinafter *Hearings on Orphan Drug Act*].

One such problem is that drugs are designated as orphan drugs at a time when the number of patients is low, but by the time the medicines reach the market, the patient population is large.[191] Another drawback is the exclusivity provision[192] which denies any cost recovery to competitors who are not the first to develop a particular drug. There is no mechanism to allow for shared marketing for drugs developed simultaneously or to revoke the orphan drug status if either the costs of developing the drug have been recovered quickly or if the patient population exceeds the 200,000 mark.[193] In the case of AIDS drugs, such mechanisms are warranted. Companies manufacturing AIDS-related products report substantial profits from constantly increasing sales. The ODA's impact on AIDS drugs is yet another example of assistance provided to drug developers without a corresponding price benefit to people with AIDS.

VII. THE COST OF AIDS DRUGS

The need for AIDS drugs has been the motivating force behind regulatory changes that the drug industry has been advocating for years. The drug development process has been shortened, and the federal government has served as an ally in the research and testing of AIDS drugs. Yet these changes are not reflected in the prices of these drugs, which are some of the highest in the prescription drug market and bring companies ever-mounting revenues and profits.

A. R & D and the Cost of AIDS Drugs

Questioned in Congressional hearings about the $8,000–$10,000 price per patient for AZT, B-W gave as reasons the difficulty in differentiating AZT from other antiviral research, the medical costs associated with caring for the clinical trial participants, the competitor drugs predicted to arrive on the market in the next few years, and the expense of the drug.[194] No dollar figure, however, was given.

The $231 million estimated cost of developing a drug[195] is based on a ten to twelve year development period.[196] That figure includes the costs of preclinical and clinical trials and data collection and monitoring.[197] In the case of AZT, the govern-

191. 21 U.S.C. § 360bb(a)(2) (the determination of whether the drug is an orphan drug is made on the basis of facts and circumstances existing at the time of the request for designation).
192. *Id.* at § 360b(c)(2)(F)(i).
193. *See* House Report on Orphan Drug Amendments, *supra* note 184, at 2–3. The amendment, H.R. 4638, would have required the FDA to make projections three years into the future in determining the number of persons affected for purposes of the orphan drug designation ceiling of 200,000. *Id.* at 4. The amendment also mandates that orphan drug designation be taken away if the affected population exceeds 200,000. *Id.* The amendment further provides for limited competition to thwart the excessive profits reported on some orphan drugs by allowing for the marketing of simultaneously developed orphan drugs. *Id. See also* Gladwell, *Drug Law Splits Biotech Firms,* Wash. Post, Apr. 1, 1990 at H1, col. 1.
194. *Hearings on AZT, supra* note 156, at 13 (statement of David Barry, V.P. of Research, Burroughs-Wellcome).
195. Jackson, *supra* note 93, at 5.
196. *Id.*
197. *Id.*

ment conducted the initial testing on the drug and provided resources throughout the clinical trial process, and it continues to do so. The government also provided an initial supply of thymidine to B-W to produce the drug for testing purposes.[198]

Only two and one-half years had elapsed from the time of the initial tests conducted by B-W to the date of approval for marketing. The usual clinical trial and approval period had been cut by 80%. Considering that intensive research on AZT began in 1985 and that the drug was approved in 1987, it is not difficult to understand why Congressman Waxman was not satisfied with the response from B-W: "the cost, particularly of clinical trials, is not less than the cost of . . . the development of most other drugs. . . ."[199]

Similar explanations about the cost of the development of another drug, pentamidine, have also been far from adequate, given the benefits provided under the ODA and the relatively short time in which it was given market approval.[200] Pentamidine's developer, Lyphomed, like B-W, has not been forthcoming in providing the cost of developing the drug, and its price has gone up 300% since it first appeared on the market in 1984.[201] It strains the imagination to explain why the company quadrupled the price of the product, other than a desire to increase profits.[202]

1. AZT Burroughs-Wellcome submitted an NDA on AZT in late 1986, and the drug was approved in March 1987.[203] The patent, a first in a series, was granted in February 1988, providing BW with exclusive rights to the drug for the treatment of AIDS and HIV disease until 2005.[204] Although AZT was approved for marketing before BW had received its patent, the company had exclusive marketing privileges for a period of seven years under the ODA.[205] BW reported sales of

198. *Hearings on AZT, supra* note 156, at 31 (statement of R. Windom).
199. *Id.* at 13 (statement of David Barry, V.P. of Research, Burroughs-Wellcome).
200. 1991 ORPHAN DESIGNATIONS, *supra* note 189, at 22; Conlan, *AIDS Advocates Move to Import Pentamidine for Lower Price,* DRUG TOPICS, Oct. 16, 1989, at 92.
201. *See infra* text accompanying notes 220–230.
202. Siler, *LyphoMed's Vital Signs are Stabilizing,* BUSINESS WEEK, July 3, 1989, at 46.
203. *Hearings on AZT, supra* note 156, at 8 (statement of T. E. Haigler); Ember, *supra* note 88, at 11.
204. GENETIC TECH. NEWS, Mar. 1988, at 12.
205. AZT was designated as an orphan drug in July 1985. When the drug was approved for marketing in March 1987, exclusive marketing privileges were granted to B-W pursuant to 21 U.S.C. § 360cc(a). During the past year, two suits have been filed in relation to B-W's patents on AZT. The first suit, instituted by potential AZT users (represented by the Public Citizen Litigation Group), alleges that the B-W use patent is invalid because, among other reasons, B-W failed to name certain government scientists as co-inventors. The government was also named a defendant. Due to issues involving standing, the suit may be dismissed. People With AIDS Health Group v. Burroughs Wellcome Co., HEALTH SPAN: THE REPORT OF HEALTH BUSINESS AND LAW, July/Aug. 1991 [hereinafter HEALTH SPAN], at 25 (D.D.C. Mar. 18, 1991).

The second law suit was initiated by B-W in response to a generic firm's entry into the AZT market. Despite B-W's patent, the generic drug manufacturer filed an application for a generic copy of AZT, alleging that B-W's patent is invalid. The generic firm also cited B-W's failure to list government scientists as co-inventors. The NIH issued a press statement supporting the generic firm's allegations and, in a highly visual action, granted a non-exclusive license to the firm to manufacture and market AZT. Burroughs Wellcome Co. v. Barr Laboratories, HEALTH SPAN, *supra,* at 25–26 (E.D.N.C. May 14, 1991).

$25 million for the months that the drug was on the market during 1987.[206] Although the wholesale price of the drug was between $8,000 and $10,000, the cost to people receiving the drug as treatment ranged from $10,000 to $12,000 because of the 5-20% markup charged by pharmacies.[207] In late 1987, under pressure from AIDS activists and government officials, BW reduced the price by 20%.[208]

As the number of people receiving AZT grew, sales increased to $158 million in 1988.[209] In 1986, B-W's after-tax profits rose by approximately 10%, jumped by 60% in 1987, and soared another 30% in 1988.[210] Undoubtedly, investors were pleased with the 50% rise in earnings per share between 1985 and 1988,[211] but people with AIDS, AIDS activists, and government officials were fuming.

Rather than submit to more questions as to the reasons for the prices and be forced to explain why a capsule that costs an estimated 40¢ to produce should cost the person with AIDS or the government $1.50,[212] BW decided to reduce the price of AZT by another 20%.[213] For those with full symptoms of AIDS, the price for a one year supply of AZT is now between $4,000 and $6,000.[214] AZT, however, has not lost its status as one of the most expensive prescription drugs available.

As of early 1990, there were an estimated one million people with HIV or AIDS in the United States, and six to eight million worldwide.[215] In March 1990, the drug was approved for a wider range of indications, expanding the drug's market from 60,000 people to over one million or more in the United States.[216] In addition, the drug has been approved for pediatric AIDS treatment.[217] BW reported sales in excess of $140 million during the first half of 1990, representing

206. WELLCOME PLC, ANNUAL REPORT 1989 13, 39 (1990) [hereinafter B-W ANNUAL REPORT] (calculated on the basis of 16 million pounds sterling at the dollar exchange rate of 1.55 as listed by B-W in the annual report).
207. *See* Weiss, *Charges, Countercharges, and Confusion on AZT Prices,* DRUG TOPICS, Sept. 7, 1987, at 92.
208. Cimons, *Maker of Only AIDS Drug Cuts Price 20%,* L.A. Times, Dec. 15, 1987, at I22, col. 1.
209. B-W ANNUAL REPORT, *supra* note 206, at 13, 39 (calculated on basis of 90 million pounds sterling at the dollar exchange rate of 1.76).
210. *Id.* at 39.
211. *Id.* (7.5 earnings per share in 1985; 15.1 earnings per share in 1988).
212. *See* Freudenheim, *One Hope For AIDS Patients is Hostage to the Market,* N.Y. Times, Sept. 3, 1989, at E5, col. 1 (citing estimate provided by analyst with Shearson, Lehman & Hutton).
213. *See* Taravella, *AIDS Drug Brings Providers Challenge of Distribution,* MODERN HEALTHCARE, Sept. 29, 1989, at 38–39 (referring to price reduction announced in previous week).
214. *Id.* Estimates of prices of the drug vary from $2,800 to $6,500 for a one year supply. *See, e.g.,* Knox, *supra* note 174 ($4,000 per year); Pollack, *Orphan Drug Law Spurs Debate,* N.Y. Times, April 30, 1990, at D1, col. 3 ($6,500 per year).
215. Steinbrook, *AIDS Conference Ends on Note of Confidence,* L.A. Times, June 25, 1990, at A1, col. 2.
216. Oran & Marsh, *Wellcome AIDS Drug Wins US Approval,* Fin. Times, March 3, 1990, at I4 (an estimated 400,000-600,000 people with AIDS or HIV worldwide were using drug at time of expanded approval).
217. Cimons, *AZT Cleared for Children's Use, First Such AIDS Drug,* L.A. Times, May 4, 1990, at A4, col. 1.

an increase of 50% over sales during the same period in the previous year and an increase in profits of 28%.[218] The total sales of AZT are now in excess of $540 million[219] and still the company has disclosed nothing regarding the costs of developing the drug.

2. Pentamidine The pricing practices for the AIDS-related drug pentamidine also have come under sharp criticism. In 1983, the drug had not been approved for marketing in the United States, primarily because PCP was so rare that it was not commercially profitable for drug companies to manufacture the drug.[220] The Centers for Disease Control (CDC) contacted Lyphomed, a small genetics firm which had a special process conducive to manufacturing pentamidine, and asked them to produce the drug as an orphan drug.[221] Although injectable pentamidine was approved for the treatment of PCP in 1984, the approval in June 1989 of Lyphomed's aerosolized version allowed for its wider, prophylactic use.[222]

As preventive medicine, pentamidine has a huge and growing market. When pentamidine was first introduced in 1984, the price of a vial was approximately $25.[223] Despite the increased use of the drug, the wholesale price now hovers around $100 per vial.[224] Although pentamidine is not the only approved treatment for PCP, it is now the drug of choice for treating PCP and can be given to people who demonstrate an intolerance to other drugs.[225] With an increasing patient population of over 200,000, and marketing exclusivity rights on the aerosolized version until 1996, it is likely that Lyphomed will be able to recover the costs involved in developing the drugs while making a sizable profit.

The company states that pentamidine's exorbitant price is due to Lyphomed's status as a small (but growing) genetics firm, not equipped with large R & D reserves. Lyphomed claims that it therefore must recover its R & D costs from the sales of the pentamidine.[226] There may be some truth to this assertion, but a more accurate explanation for the continued high prices may be the company's desire to post large profits to improve its financial status, harmed by losses as a result of the FDA's discovery of quality control problems.[227]

---

218. WELLCOME PLC, INTERIM REPORT (1990) (chairman's statement).
219. B-W ANNUAL REPORT, *supra* note 206, at 13, 39 (using exchange rates listed, this figure was as of mid-1990).
220. *See* R. SHILTS, AND THE BAND PLAYED ON: POLITICS, PEOPLE AND THE AIDS EPIDEMIC 54 (1987).
221. *Hearings on Orphan Drug Act, supra* note 190, at 162–63 (statement of Brian Tambi, Lyphomed).
222. Leary, *F.D.A. Approves Drug that Fights Leading Killer of AIDS Patients,* N.Y. Times, June 16, 1989, at D16, col. 1.
223. Kolata, *Criticized on AIDS Drug, Maker Will Give it to Some,* N.Y. Times, Oct. 12, 1989, at A26, col. 6.
224. *Id.*
225. *See* LYPHOMED, INC., ANNUAL REPORT 1988 15 (1989) [hereinafter LYPHOMED ANNUAL REPORT].
226. Kolata, *supra* note 223, at A26, col. 5–6.
227. Siler, *supra* note 202, at 46.

Between 1984 and 1988, Lyphomed's reported average annual sales growth was 45%.[228] In 1988, sales were down to $130 million, an estimated 30% of which was attributable to pentamidine sales, with a net loss of $21 million.[229] The approval in June 1989 of the aerosolized version sent Lyphomed's stock soaring and helped the company come out of the slump recovering with a $30 million increase in income.[230] Lyphomed should be commended for its efforts in developing pentamidine, but people with AIDS should not be called upon to bear the entire burden of ensuring the company's profitable status.

The usual justifications for high drug prices—escalating R & D costs, extensive clinical trials, and a lengthy and slow approval process held up by the FDA bureaucracy—are not applicable in the case of AIDS drugs. Given the ways in which the government has assisted the development and approval of AIDS drugs, disappointment in the drug companies' response is justified.

B. The Government and the Cost of AIDS Drugs

The development of AIDS drugs represents the most extensive involvement that the government has had in the area of drug development and one of the most effective collaborative efforts among government, industry, and academia. In the case of AZT, government involvement can be traced to the invention of the drug in 1964 by researchers working under a grant from the NCI. In addition, it was government scientists who took the risks and conducted the first in vitro and human testing to establish that AZT acted against HTLV-III.[231]

The drugs ddI and ddC also arose out of government research and represent another successful collaborative effort.[232] Unlike AZT, however, the government applied for patents on ddI and ddC to recover some of their outlays through licensing agreements and royalties and, more importantly, to retain a degree of control over the prices charged for the drugs.[233] The licensing agreement with Bristol-Myers for ddI includes a clause which requires that the company charge a reasonable price.[234] This licensing agreement provides a test to determine whether such a device serves to control prices.

---

228. Lyphomed Annual Report, *supra* note 225, at 16.
229. *Id. See* Siler, *supra* note 202, at 46.
230. Lyphomed 1989 Report, *supra* note 149, at 6–7. Lyphomed reported a net income loss in 1989 of $18 million despite a substantial increase in gross profit and sale. Lyphomed provided a number of reasons for the loss, including the cost involved with a stock acquisition by Fujisawa. However, the company gave credit to Nebupent for enhancing its economic status. *Id.* at 6.
231. Mitsuya, *supra* note 133.
232. Marx, *supra* note 166, at 353; *Yarchoan, In vivo Activity Against HIV and Favorable Toxicity Profile of 2¾-3¾-dideoxyinosine,* 245 Science 412, 412 (1989).
233. Freudenheim, *supra* note 212.
234. The licensing agreement between the NIH and Bristol-Myers Squibb Co. for the manufacture and development of ddI contains a clause requiring that the drug be sold at a "reasonable price." Chase, *Burroughs Wellcome Reaps Profits, Outrage from its AIDS Drug,* Wall St. J., Sept. 15, 1989, at A1, col. 1. The agreement was entered into pursuant to provisions of the Technology Transfer Act, which was enacted in 1986 to serve as an incentive for innovation.

In addition to the extensive amount of resources that the government has allocated to research activities, it is also the primary third-party payor for the drugs. The exact amount of money that the government spends to supply drugs to people with HIV and AIDS is difficult to ascertain, but many receive federal assistance for drugs through Medicaid and Medicare.[235] Federal spending on AIDS care under these programs has greatly increased in recent years.[236] In addition, approximately $200 million in Social Security funds was spent on people with HIV and AIDS in 1990.[237]

Even these expenditures are inadequate, however, as not all Medicaid programs cover the costs of all AIDS drugs,[238] and many private insurers either do not cover the cost of prescription drugs or impose a cap on reimbursement levels.[239] Additionally, many people with HIV and AIDS are simply uninsured.[240]

Since Medicaid covers 40% of people with HIV and AIDS, taking into consideration the expanded uses of AZT and a cost of $4,000-$6,000 per year per person with full blown AIDS, it would not be unreasonable to estimate government spending for AZT to be in the range of $240 million.

These figures do not include the government's cost of pentamidine, which has a target patient population estimated to be in excess of 200,000.[241] Using the conservative estimate of $1,000 annual cost per person for pentamidine, the federal government may spend $80 million for this drug. The figure of $320 million (for only two drugs) represents almost 50% of the total federal Medicaid dollars devoted to AIDS treatment in 1990.[242] Considering that drugs are only a

---

The Act provides for government employees to profit from their inventions and sets up a mechanism for transferring technology to the private sector while ensuring that the government retains ownership rights. *Id.*

235. *See* Spolar, *Footing the Bill: The Politics Behind the Money*, Wash. Post., June 19, 1990, at 29; Boodman, *The Dilemma of AZT: Who Can Afford It?*, Wash. Post, Aug. 8, 1989, at 26.

236. OFFICE OF THE SECRETARY OF HEALTH, AIDS—TOTAL FEDERAL GOVERNMENT SPENDING (Feb. 23, 1990)[hereinafter TOTAL FEDERAL SPENDING REPORT]; HEALTH CARE FINANCING ADMINISTRATION, ESTIMATED FEDERAL MEDICAID AND MEDICARE COSTS OF AIDS (Dec. 8, 1989) (includes impact of AZT).

237. TOTAL FEDERAL SPENDING REPORT, *supra* note 236.

238. *See* NAT'L GAY RIGHTS ADVOCATES, ACCESS TO AIDS-RELATED DRUGS UNDER MEDICAID: A FIFTY STATE ANALYSIS 8-11 (1989) (listing which drugs are covered by various state Medicaid programs); UNITED STATES CONG. RESEARCH SERVICE, MEDICAID SOURCE BOOK 485–94 (1988), *reprinted in* AIDS: CASES AND MATERIALS 578, 578–79 (M. Closen, et al. eds. 1989). *But see* Weaver v. Reagen, 701 F. Supp. 717 (W.D. Mo. 1988) (Missouri Medicaid program's refusal to place AZT on drug list violates federal regulations), *aff'd*, 886 F.2d 194 (8th Cir. 1989).

239. Arno & Green, *The Economics of AIDS*, in THE AIDS KNOWLEDGE BASE 10.1.1-8-9 (P. Cohen, M. Sande & P. Volberding eds. 1990).

240. *Id.* at 10.1.1-5 (study revealing 54% of hospitalization costs for people with AIDS covered by Medicaid while only 17% covered by private insurance); Lambert, *AIDS Insurance Coverage is Increasingly Hard to Get*, N.Y. Times, Aug. 7, 1989, at A1, col. 1 (substantial number of people with AIDS are denied coverage through variety of mechanisms such as insurer's knowledge of HIV screening tests performed on insured).

241. *See supra* text accompanying notes 223–225.

242. *See* Fed. News Serv., Jan. 29, 1990 (Department of Health and Human Services briefing); States News Serv., Sept. 27, 1989.

portion of the treatment cost for a person with HIV or AIDS, approximately $50,000 annually per person,[243] this estimate of 50% means one of two things: the estimate is completely off or there are people with HIV or AIDS not receiving AZT and other drugs.

If Medicaid is not providing for all people in need of drugs, and if there is a portion of the HIV-infected population not covered by insurance or Medicaid, which there is, there are people with HIV or AIDS who do not have access to the drugs due to cost. Lowering the price of the drugs would certainly go a long way towards ensuring that all of those in need receive the drug.

VIII. COST CONTROL SYSTEMS

In 1990, the nation's health care costs exceeded 12% of the gross national product,[244] or $675 billion;[245] the government's share was 41% of that amount.[246] In response, Congress is searching for ways to cut health care costs. The government spent an estimated $3.3 billion on prescription drugs in 1989, accounting for 10% of the industry's domestic sales.[247] Although prescription drug costs are not the largest portion of health care expenditures, they are the fastest rising.[248]

In response to escalating drug prices, federal and state governments, as well as private insurers, hospitals and HMOs have implemented a variety of cost controls. While some of these devices have resulted in cost savings for the particular institutions employing them, they have not achieved the goal of reducing prices. Most of these mechanisms rely on the use of lower priced generic products and/or the practice of purchasing drugs in large volumes rather than on the direct control of prices. Despite the need for a system to control the prices of AIDS drugs, none of those systems in place appear to provide the solution, since AIDS drugs are not yet subject to generic opportunity and no alternatives to drug therapy exist.

Over the years, proposals to reduce prices involving more direct price control devices have been presented but were successfully opposed by the pharmaceutical industry as well as by other interest groups, such as the American Medical Association (AMA).[249] The industry has argued successfully that systems involving more

243. Arno & Green, *supra* note 239, at 10.1.1 ($40,000-$60,000 to treat people with AIDS based on one year median survival period); Perlman, *Scientists Optimistic at AIDS Conference,* San Francisco Chronicle, June 25, 1990, at A8 (citing government study).

244. Kemper & Novack, *The Great American Health-Care Sellout,* Wash. Post, Oct. 13, 1991, at C4, col. 2.

245. United States Dep't of Commerce, U.S. Industrial Outlook 1991 44-1 (1991).

246. *Id.*

247. PMA, 1989 New Drug Approvals, *supra* note 22; Freudenheim, *supra* note 22.

248. Bureau of the Census, Statistical Abstract of the United States 1990 470 table 761 (1990) [hereinafter Bureau of Census Abstract] (between 1980 and 1987, the consumer price index rose for medical care by 55.2 and for drugs by 68.3).

249. M. Silverman & P. Lee, *supra* note 5, at 113–16 (the PMA and the AMA fought against the inclusion of compulsory licensing in the 1962 amendments to the Federal Food, Drug and Cosmetic Act of 1938).

direct control over prices would endanger the incentives for innovation and would result in the loss of the United States industry's status as world leader in the area of drug development.[250] The industry has asserted that the lengthy drug approval process and extensive regulatory requirements force firms to charge such prices.[251] In the area of AIDS drugs, however, these arguments do not provide a satisfactory justification for the high prices. Since most cost control systems have not achieved a reduction in prices and are not effective means to reduce the price of AIDS drugs, it is time to consider direct price controls for AIDS drugs.

A. Cost Control Systems in Place

1. Generics While other countries have opted for the use of direct price control systems,[252] the United States has gone the route of generics[253] to contain rising drug costs and prices.[254] Until the 1940s, generic prescribing was the norm, but the promotion and proliferation of brand name prescription drugs changed prescribing habits, and by the 1950s most prescriptions were written for brand name products.[255] In the 1970s, generics began to reappear in the market. Several factors aided the revival of generic products, including the expiration of many patent covers providing the "opportunity" for generics, the repeal of many anti-substitution laws, and the absence of price control systems.[256] Despite a mush-

---

250. *See id.* at 87 (industry fought against compulsory licensing, arguing threat to industry innovation); Hudson, *State Medicaid Officials Battle Drug Firms in War to Cut Costs,* HOSPITALS, Apr. 5, 1990, at 30 (arguments against proposals to lower prices charged to Medicaid put forward by industry include a decrease in incentive to produce innovative new drugs).
251. *See Health and the Environment—Part 2: Drug Patent Restoration: Hearings Before the Subcomm. on Health and the Environment of the House Comm. on Energy and Commerce,* 97th Cong., 1st Sess. 350–52 (1981)(statement of Lewis Engman)(industry asserted that patent restoration legislation, by restoring patent time lost to lengthy approval process, would exert downward pressure on prices of drugs).
252. H. REDWOOD, *supra* note 4, at 156.
253. Before describing the generics market, it will be useful to explain the nomenclature. Drug products have three names: the brand or trade name; the generic name; and the chemical name. HEW TASK FORCE, THE DRUG MAKERS, *supra* note 10, at 8. The chemical name describes the chemical structure or makeup of the drug. *Id.* The generic name is a shorter, established name, often an abbreviated chemical name, which is universally recognizable. *Id.* The brand name, or trademark name, is the name that the manufacturer assigns to the drug and uses to distinguish it from competitors' products. *Id.* A generic drug is one that can be interchanged with a brand name drug because it has the identical active ingredient. COMPETITIVE ASSESSMENT, *supra* note 20, at 11; INTERNATIONAL RESOURCE DEVELOPMENT INC., GENERIC DRUGS IN THE 1990s 46 (1988) [hereinafter GENERICS IN THE 1990s]. Generic may describe the interchangeable drug or the process of prescribing or dispensing interchangeable drugs. COMPETITIVE ASSESSMENT, *supra* note 20, at 11. Generic prescription drugs include drugs which have never been subject to a patent cover or are copies of products the patents on which have expired. H. REDWOOD, *supra* note 4, at 232. Generic drugs may be "branded," marketed under product or house brand names, or "unbranded," sold only by the generic name of the drug and with little promotion or advertising. COMPETITIVE ASSESSMENT, *supra* note 20, at 12.
254. H. REDWOOD, *supra* note 4, at 231–32. Some European countries do not allow substitution of generics. *Id.* at 233.
255. *See id.* at 230–32.
256. *Id.* at 231–32; GENERICS IN THE 1990s, *supra* note 253, at 13.

rooming generic drug market, however, the move to revive generics has not produced a reduction in drug prices. With regard to AIDS drugs, price competition from generics is a distant prospect because of patents and marketing exclusivity periods.

2. Formularies The growth of the generics has increased the use of formularies as cost control mechanisms. A "formulary" is a list of preferred drugs developed by a professional assessment of comparative safety, efficacy, usefulness in patient care, and/or economy.[257] Including less expensive products (therapeutically equivalent or generic products), the formulary controls costs by promoting volume purchases of less expensive alternative drugs, for which institutions can negotiate discounts.

Despite their increased use, formularies have not been entirely successful in controlling costs. Drug manufacturers have successfully thwarted attempts by state programs to negotiate lower prices. Pharmaceutical manufacturers have fought state legislative efforts that would allow medical assistance programs to negotiate lower prices through the solicitation of bids from manufacturers. They also have refused to negotiate with state programs to offer rebates to secure their drug's place on the formulary and have supported legislation which bans any restrictions on Medicaid prescriptions.[258] A number of studies reveal that the use of formularies result in little or no cost savings.[259]

In the case of AIDS drugs, the formulary system does not provide a solution for the high prices because there are no approved alternatives to the patented drugs now in use.

3. Other Cost Control Systems In addition to the use of generics and formularies, other cost control systems include maximum allowable cost programs,[260] bulk

257. MAJORITY STAFF OF SENATE SPECIAL COMM. ON AGING, 101ST CONG., 2D SESS., SKYROCKETING PRESCRIPTION DRUG PRICES: TURNING A BAD DEAL INTO A FAIR DEAL 28 (Comm. Print 1990)[hereinafter DRUG PRICES]; Perrin, *Formularies and Pharmacy: The Uneasy Bond,* DRUG TOPICS, July 3, 1989, at 32, 34.

258. *See* DRUG PRICES, *supra* note 257, at 11–14; Hudson, *supra* note 250, at 30–34; Shroeder, *Congress Looks to Pharmacists for Clues on Drug Buying,* DRUG TOPICS, Dec. 11, 1989, at 47–48; Freundenheim, *Cutting the Cost of Medicaid Drugs,* N.Y. Times, Jan. 30, 1990, at D2, col. 1.

259. *See, e.g., Hearings Before the Subcomm. on the Health of Families and the Uninsured of the Senate Comm. on Finance,* 102nd Cong., 1st Sess. 6 (1990) [hereinafter *Finance Hearings*] (statement of Gail Wilensky, Administrator of Health Care Financing Administration)(citing study by Systemetrics/McGraw-Hill on California's Medi-Cal program which revealed a 15% increase per year since 1984 despite restrictive formula); Kreling, Knocke & Hammel, *The Effects of an Internal Analgesic Formulary Restriction on Medicaid Drug Expenditures in Wisconsin,* 27 MED. CARE 34, 39–43 (1989).

260. In 1976, the Department of Health and Human Services (DHHS) instituted a Maximum Allowable Cost/Estimated Acquisition Cost (MAC/EAC) system for all its health care programs. Under MAC, payments for high volume multisource drugs are limited to the lowest prices at which they are available. The DHHS Reimbursement Board was created to set the limit for a particular drug at the lowest unit price at which the drug is widely and consistently available. The MAC price becomes the basis upon which the level of reimbursement is determined.

The EAC program is state directed, requiring states to establish EAC limits for *all* drugs

purchasing and bidding practices,[261] chargeback and rebate systems,[262] and mail order prescription plans.[263] Each of these systems may result in cost savings for the particular organization or consumer. Evidence of widespread savings to the consuming public from the increased use of these systems, however, is scant. Over the past decade, per capita expenditures on drugs increased by 60%.[264] The

---

supplied under the Medicaid program. The states estimate the prices that pharmacies pay for drugs and may use various methods to determine these prices, as long as they reflect the actual prices paid. The EAC limit, like the MAC limit, becomes the basis upon which reimbursement amounts are calculated. *Prescription Drug Price Increases: Hearings Before the House Subcomm. on Health and the Environment of the House Comm. on Energy and Commerce,* 99th Cong., 1st Sess. 330–37 (1986) [hereinafter *Hearings on Price Increases*](statement of Robert Helms, Acting Assisting Secretary for Planning and Evaluation, HHS). The MAC program saved the federal government $10 million in 1985, *id.* at 334, but the program later was abandoned due to a number of drawbacks in the administration of the program and to the time-consuming nature of the notice and comment rulemaking procedure which was required to set or change MAC limits. *See id.* at 341–43.

A number of options to the MAC system were proposed, but in 1987 the DHHS decided to leave reimbursement decisions in the hands of the states. *See* Robinson, *New Medicaid Drug Rules: Reform or Retreat?,* DRUG TOPICS, Sept. 7, 1987, at 54–55. The Health Care Financing Association issued general guidelines, however, for determining the "aggregate limits" on drug costs which were based on 150% of the lowest average wholesale prices. *Id.* at 54.

261. Bulk purchasing simply refers to the practice of buying in large quantities to obtain discounts on particular high volume drugs. Typically, large institutional purchasers, either individually or with other institutions, will negotiate for discounts on the basis of the amount purchased. Some community pharmacies also have joined together to purchase in bulk in an attempt to control costs. In addition, large institutions, particularly governments, will make calls for bids on particular drug products. This practice inspires competition and lower prices but brand name manufacturers drop prices only when they perceive that a gain in market share will result. Many manufacturers have refused to participate in price bidding; have argued that states have no authority to negotiate prices; and have lobbied for legislation which would prohibit states from negotiating prices. *See* DRUG PRICES, *supra* note 257, at 11–12; Freudenheim, *supra* note 258; Shroeder, *supra* 258.

262. Chargeback and rebate programs involve institutions contracting with drug manufacturers for drugs at discount rates. The institutional purchasers reimburse the pharmacies at the undiscounted rates which the pharmacies paid for the drugs dispensed to the beneficiaries of the institution or program, and the purchasers then recover the difference through a chargeback or rebate from the manufacturer. *See* Shroeder, *supra* note 258, at 47.

263. Purchasing prescriptions through the mail is one of the fastest growing methods of containing costs. The mail order prescription business now boasts sales in excess of $1.6 billion. *See Should You Buy Drugs by Mail?,* CONSUMER REPORTS: HEALTH LETTER, May 1990, at 33. Drugs by mail plans are offered through a variety of groups including mail service firms, chain drugstores, hospitals and a growing number of employers whose prescription drug costs are increasing faster than are other components in their health benefits packages. Handel, *Employers Can Control Prescription Drug Costs Through Innovative Plans,* PENSION WORLD, Apr. 1989, at 14–17. Cost benefits of mail order plans are achieved through increased generic dispensing, lower ingredient costs, lower dispensing fees and lower administrative costs. Barbieri, Sydlaske & Wilson *A Case-Specific Experience Study of the Cost Effectiveness of Mail Service Drug Option Plans,* BENEFITS QUARTERLY 80–82 (1988). Studies of individual plans reveal costs savings of 15–30%. *Id.* The extent of cost savings, however, is difficult to assess because only certain drugs are sent through the mail and there is evidence of waste due to the large quantities which typically are dispensed, i.e., 90-day supplies which often are not needed or used. *See* Vibbert, *How to Restrain Ballooning Drug Benefit Costs,* BUSINESS AND HEALTH, Apr. 1989, at 44.

264. BUREAU OF CENSUS ABSTRACT, *supra* note 248, at 94 table 137 (based on 1980–1987 figures; per capita expenditures on drugs rose from 73 in 1980 to 120 in 1987; per capita expenditures for all health care rose 50% from 577 to 1,115).

skyrocketing prices of drugs during that same time period served to offset any savings that might have been realized by the consumers and other purchasers.

B. Proposed Cost Control Devices

1. Compulsory Licensing Compulsory licensing, that is, requiring that a patent holder license the use of the patent to another after a specified period of time, has been proposed as a method to reduce prices.[265]

In the late 1960s, government and political bodies exposed the practice of price differentials and the high net profits reaped by the industry,[266] and revealed the wasteful nature of the R & D activity on which the industry justified its profit levels.[267] At the heart of the industry's monopolistic pricing practices was the use of drug patents to create and control markets on particular drug therapies.[268]

Compulsory licensing was one of several suggestions resulting from hearings and reports by Congress. The suggested scheme for compulsory licensing involved requiring the patent holder to license "any other manufacturer who desired to produce and market the drug on a royalty basis" after a specified period of time.[269] This would enable a drug manufacturer to recoup R & D costs plus a reasonable profit while promoting price competition among rivals by allowing other firms to enter the product market.[270]

The Public Health Price Protection Act, proposed in 1972,[271] would have required that a drug patent be made available for licensing when the Federal Trade Commission (FTC) determined that certain conditions were met.[272] Under the proposal, the FTC would be given authority to determine a reasonable royalty rate for the drug.[273] Despite precedent in other areas of the law and the need for regulation, the bill, introduced on several occasions, never became law.

Compulsory licensing represents a rational approach to the current monopolistic nature of the drug industry. In the long run, the public interest is served by widening the availability of drugs through reduced prices while ensuring profits to maintain incentives for innovation. In the case of AIDS drugs, compulsory licensing would benefit the public interest by providing access to the only form of therapy available to people with HIV or AIDS. In the short run, however,

---

265. M. Silverman & P. Lee, *supra* note 5, at 113–14.
266. *See generally Competitive Problems in the Drug Industry: Hearings Before the Senate Subcomm. on Monopoly of the Select Comm. on Small Business,* 93d Cong., 1st Sess. 9733-35 (1973)(statement of J. S. Turner).
267. HEW Task Force, Final Report, *supra* note 55, at 7–8, 13–14.
268. *Id.* at 12–13.
269. HEW Task Force, The Drug Makers, *supra* note 10, at 43. The period of time recommended was three years, in recognition of the fact that the greatest portion of sales on a new drug occurs in the first few years after the drug is approved for marketing. *Id.*
270. *Id.*
271. 118 Cong. Rec. 32,931 (1972)(introduced as Amendment No. 1659 to the National Drug Testing and Evaluation Center Bill).
272. *Id.* at 32,932.
273. *Id.*

compulsory licensing will not serve the needs of people with HIV or AIDS. With a disease such as AIDS where time is of the essence, three years—the time period before licensing would be required—is too long a time to wait. In addition, there is the risk that drug manufacturers, knowing that licensing will be required, would charge even higher prices to recoup as much as possible during the initial exclusivity period. Since people with HIV or AIDS have no alternatives, the drug manufacturers could extract such prices.

A more serious problem with compulsory licensing is the probable difficulty of passing such legislation. The industry would likely fight fiercely against it. Furthermore, the lengthy legislative process would have to overcome such obstacles as the force of existing patent laws and the Orphan Drug Act's marketing exclusivity provisions.

2. Use of Patented Products by the Government One of the proposals that has resurfaced in response to the AIDS drugs crisis is a little known but powerful provision of the United States Code.[274] Under this provision, a patented invention can be appropriated for manufacture by or for the government. An inventor's only recourse is to recover reasonable compensation from the government; traditional damages for patent infringement are not available.[275]

Most of the case law dealing with the provision addresses the issue of compensation. A patent holder's claim under the section is treated as an "eminent domain taking of a patent license."[276] Drawing on precedents from eminent domain or "takings" cases, courts have repeatedly stated that the appropriate measure of damages is to be based on what the owner has lost and not on what the taker has gained.[277] Damages are the "reasonable royalty" for the license given prevailing market conditions and royalty fees.[278] Determining the appropriate market and licensing fees, however, has proven to be a difficult and laborious process for courts.[279]

The government could manufacture AIDS drugs or could license the manufacture of AIDS drugs to other companies. The major obstacle is determining the cost savings that the government could reap from such an activity. The level of compensation allowed is "reasonable and entire" but it is not clear if that would include some level of profits for the manufacturer. Although there are guidelines

274. 28 U.S.C. § 1498 (1988).
275. *Id.* at § 1498(b).
276. *E.g.*, Leesona Corp. v. United States, 599 F.2d 958, 966 (Ct. Cl.), *cert. denied,* 444 U.S. 991 (1979).
277. *See id.* at 969; ITT Corp. v. United States, 17 Cl. Ct. 199 (1989).
278. *Leesona,* 599 F.2d at 968. Although the "reasonable royalty" method is the one most often employed, courts use various methods of valuation to determine compensation for government infringement. In Decca, Ltd. v. United States, 640 F.2d 1156 (Ct. Cl. 1980), *cert. denied,* 454 U.S. 819 (1981), the court listed three possible valuation methods: determination of reasonable royalty for the license (the preferred method); awarding percentage of cost savings to the government as a result of the infringement; and awarding lost profits. *Id.* at 1167.
279. *See, e.g., ITT,* 17 Cl. Ct. at 205–10.

provided by the cases, it would still be a difficult task to predict whether the government could actually save money by licensing the drugs. In addition, the government moves slowly as a bureaucracy and is reluctant to involve itself in the production of drugs for widespread distribution. The government has not used this provision extensively in the area of drugs and shows little willingness to do so with AIDS drugs.

3. Direct Price Control: The Situation in Europe One of the complaints consistently lodged against the pharmaceutical industry by members of Congress and others has been that manufacturers charge lower prices for drugs in the export market.[280] Consumers in the United States pay more—often substantially more—for their prescription drugs than do consumers in foreign markets.[281] Many foreign markets employ direct price control systems.[282] In order to remain competitive in those markets, manufacturers charge lower prices which are, in turn, subsidized by United States consumers. Even in those countries that do not employ price control systems, however, the prices are generally lower than those charged in the United States.[283]

The pharmaceutical industry would strongly oppose any move toward direct price control in this country. The industry argues that control over prices would result in less innovation because less funding would be available for research and development. Such a system, however, may force the drug industry to streamline their R & D activities and to focus on developing truly innovative products rather than "me-too" products currently flooding the market.

Australia, New Zealand, Japan, and most European countries employ direct price control systems.[284] Under some of these systems, the manufacturers of new products negotiate with a government agency to determine the price to be charged prior to the introduction of the drugs and periodically thereafter.[285] Other systems also control profit margins of manufacturers and/or wholesalers and retailers.[286] Although the systems vary in how they are structured and administered, prices in controlled markets generally decreased relative to the consumer price index during the 1980s.[287] In Germany, which had employed a free market system but converted to direct price controls this year in response to increasing drug prices,[288] prices had increased at approximately the same rate as inflation.[289]

Comparing prices paid in Europe with prices paid in the United States pres-

280. *See, e.g., Hearings on Price Increases, supra* note 260, at 145–47 (concern expressed that United States consumers were disproportionately financing research).
281. *See Hearings on Skyrocketing Prices, supra* note 2, at 7 table 3.
282. H. Redwood, *supra* note 4, at 156.
283. *See id.*
284. *Id.* at 156.
285. *Id.*
286. *See id.* at 157–58.
287. *See id.* at 160–61.
288. *German Drug Companies Fight Price Cuts,* Pharmaceutical Business News, Sept. 28, 1990, Finance/Business Section at 1.
289. *See* H. Redwood, *supra* note 4, at 158–59.

ents problems: fluctuating exchange rates and the relative strengths of the various currencies; the role of national health care systems in drug pricing; and the myriad of reimbursement systems used in conjunction with direct price controls.[290] However, a study published in 1989 provides invaluable information about drug prices in Europe. The study surveyed drug prices, laws relating to drug prices, and reimbursement systems in European Economic Community (EEC) countries.[291] The price index on selected products surveyed was 86% more in the United States than in those countries with strict price control systems,[292] and average prices in the United States were 54% more than those in the EEC countries.[293]

In addition, the existence of national health care systems in these countries results in lower out-of-pocket drug costs.[294] In the United States, next to physicians' services, prescription drugs account for consumers' highest out-of-pocket expenses.[295] Exacerbating these differences in the United States per capita drug consumption rate, which is higher than in any of the other countries despite the high prices.[296]

One possible conclusion is that a system of strict price controls in the United States would reduce prices and consumption. In light of all the variables involved, however, this conclusion is too simple. While the consumers in Europe have enjoyed decreasing prices relative to inflation over the past ten years, there is evidence that such prices have effected the innovation rates and the health of the industries in those countries.[297] The United States has enjoyed its status as the international leader in both drug innovation and new product introduction; the industry, as well as many economists, would be very concerned about the introduction of strict price controls. Although it is speculative to conclude that direct price control systems are the reason for the decreased rate of innovation in Europe, the industry could make a feasible argument to support such a conclusion. Contrary to this argument, Japan is quickly closing in on the United States' position as leader in new product introductions worldwide, despite its price control systems.[298] Yet, some observers argue that Japan's innovation is duplicative in nature and that many of their new products do not become leading drugs.[299]

---

290. *Id.* at 158–59.
291. Association Belge des Consommateurs, Drug Prices and Drug Legislation in Europe: An Analysis of the Situation in the Twelve Member States of the European Communities (1989).
292. *Hearings on Skyrocketing Prices, supra* note 2, at 7 table 3.
293. *Id.* at 2.
294. *Id.* at 8 table 4.
295. Bureau of the Census, Abstract, *supra* note 248, at 470 table 761.
296. *Hearings on Skyrocketing Prices, supra* note 2, at 9 table 5 (per capita in United States was indexed at 152; 100 represented the EEC average).
297. *See* H. Redwood, *supra* note 4, at 186–91.
298. *See id.* at 189 (between 1961 and 1977, Japan introduced 10% of all NCEs introduced globally; during 1981–1985, that figure rose to 22%).
299. *See, id.* at 189–90 (number of leading NCEs was only eight despite the increased number of NCEs introduced during the early 1980s; the United States had more than 30 leading NCEs, although it led Japan in number of introductions by only 3%).

The United States pharmaceutical industry has led the world in the rate of introduction of new products for some time.[300] Although there are many contributing variables, the industry likely has prospered because our system is founded upon free market principles and the ability to charge what the market will bear. If the profit incentive and the patent and trademark system are taken away, one of our most competitive industries risk losing its status as world leader.

In light of the pervasive attitude which supports free market enterprise and the continued support of the industry by many in Congress and in the academic and business worlds, it is highly unlikely that a system of direct price control will be enacted any time soon. Because of the way in which AIDS drugs were developed and the extensive involvement of the government in the process, however, a proposal for direct price control of such drugs may garner the necessary support.

C. Direct Price Control of AIDS Drugs—A Proposal

The AIDS epidemic has not come to an end; the number of persons afflicted continues to grow while a cure has yet to be discovered. Currently, AIDS drugs are the only hope people with AIDS have of a medical cure. An increasing number of these people are those least able to pay for this treatment. The price of AIDS drugs has increased along with the spread of the disease and the size of the population recommended to receive drug therapy, forcing the government to shoulder an increasing financial burden. Efforts to control the spread of the disease through education and medical research will take time. While these efforts continue, the government can act to reduce the cost of AIDS therapy through the direct price control of AIDS drugs.

Developing a price control system for AIDS drugs can be accomplished through the mechanism of an AIDS Drug Price Control Board. This board could be organized through one of the agencies involved in the AIDS drug development process, such as the NIH, the NIAID, or the NCI. This board will be involved early on in the drug development process to ensure familiarity with and understanding of the extent of the research and development involved, the key players in the process, the structure and cost of the clinical trials, the extent of the patient population to receive the drug, and the predicted success of the drug. The board's task will not be static due to the numerous and varied factors that may come into play in the drug development process, but the areas of inquiry for the board should provide a framework for drug pricing.

The composition of the board will determine whether it is viewed as an objective and capable entity and should be reflective of the various interests affected by the drug development and drug pricing processes. With this in mind, members should be drawn from academia, industry, government, and the community of people with HIV or AIDS. Selection criteria should emphasize a degree of knowledge and familiarity with the AIDS drug development process, the phar-

300. *See, id.* at 147–49, 186–91.

maceutical industry, the structure of the market, and the character of the population affected. At least one member of the board should be an economist familiar with the industry and capable of assessing the effects of the various legislative and market factors on the costs of R & D, predicted rates of return, financial status and needs of the company or companies developing the drug, and other factors relevant to the commercial value of the product. The use of alternate members should be incorporated into the governing document of the board to provide for conflicts of interest.

Before the board can make decisions on the pricing of particular drugs, its members should first agree on a decision-making structure. The structure should allow for a great deal of flexibility to accommodate for the many variables involved, but at the same time must include criteria upon which the board can agree.

Factors to be considered in determining the price of the drug should include the following: 1) the R & D costs directly and indirectly attributable to the development of the drug; 2) the costs of preclinical and clinical studies of the drug; 3) the degree of government involvement and financial assistance; 4) the number of manufacturers of the drug; 5) the patentability of the drug; 6) whether the drug will be developed as an orphan drug; 7) the characteristics and size of population to receive the drug; 8) the financial status of the manufacturer(s) developing the drug; 9) the size and characteristics of R & D activity of the manufacturer(s); 10) the raw material and manufacturing costs; 11) the nature and degree of competition expected from other products; 12) the degree to which other drugs will be used in combination with the product at issue; 13) the rates of inflation; 14) the level of profit requested by the manufacturer(s) and their justifications; and 15) the expected growth of the market. Obviously, this information may not be available until later in development and many drugs will not reach approval. Maintaining supervision throughout drug development, however, will result in a more knowledgeable board and will expedite information gathering.

The drug pricing process will be an ongoing procedure to allow for as much flexibility and negotiation as possible. As the drug nears the marketing approval stage, the board will meet with the manufacturer to discuss a specific price. The manufacturer will be encouraged to support its request and, after the drug has been on the market, could return to the board to request price changes. The early success or failure of the drug and the FDA's desire to expand or restrict use of the drug will be very important factors in determining price changes. Prices need not be set at exact levels, but may be indexed to the rate of inflation. Prices should also reflect the mark-up charged by pharmacies and others in the retail market.

This proposal will be effective only if all involved agree to participate fully. Judging by the drug industry's reaction to other proposals, opposition to this proposal can be expected. The AIDS drug development process, due to the extent and nature of the government's involvement and the nature of the disease, presents a unique set of circumstances. The regulatory changes made to speed the drug development process and the financial incentives provided to manufacturers of AIDS drugs justify the proposal and drug manufacturers must be forced to explain opposition to such a proposal beyond the fear of loss of profit. This program is not a panacea for the high cost of AIDS drugs. Rather, it represents a rational attempt to bring a degree of fairness and equity to the AIDS drug pricing process, or at least initiate discussion about the options available.

IX. CONCLUSION

The pharmaceutical industry has enjoyed above average profit levels for most of its history. When asked to justify such profits, the industry points to the high cost of research and development and the lengthy drug approval process. While the contributions to health care made by pharmaceuticals should not go unnoticed, increasing prices are making them less accessible to the people most in need. Despite the assistance provided by the government in the form of financial incentives and research efforts, AIDS drugs, for many, are simply inaccessible due to their price. Although the need for funds for R & D should not be underestimated, in the case of AIDS, there must be a more equitable approach to drug pricing to ensure access to these much needed drugs. A system of direct price control is a step in the right direction.